Immunotherapy for Solid Malignancies

Editor

ALFRED E. CHANG

SURGICAL ONCOLOGY CLINICS OF NORTH AMERICA

www.surgonc.theclinics.com

Consulting Editor
TIMOTHY M. PAWLIK

July 2019 • Volume 28 • Number 3

ELSEVIER

1600 John F. Kennedy Boulevard • Suite 1800 • Philadelphia, Pennsylvania, 19103-2899

http://www.theclinics.com

SURGICAL ONCOLOGY CLINICS OF NORTH AMERICA Volume 28, Number 3
July 2019 ISSN 1055-3207, ISBN-13: 978-0-323-67825-4

Editor: John Vassallo (j.vassallo@elsevier.com)
Developmental Editor: Laura Kavanaugh

Surgical Oncology Clinics of North America (ISSN 1055-3207) is published quarterly by Elsevier Inc., 360 Park Avenue South, New York, NY 10010-1710. Months of publication are January, April, July, and October. Business and Editorial Offices: 1600 John F. Kennedy Blvd., Ste. 1800, Philadelphia, PA 19103-2899. Customer Service Office: 3251 Riverport Lane, Maryland Heights, MO 63043. Periodicals postage paid at New York, NY and additional mailing offices. Subscription prices are $306.00 per year (US individuals), $533.00 (US institutions) $100.00 (US student/resident), $352.00 (Canadian individuals), $674.00 (Canadian institutions), $205.00 (Canadian student/resident), $422.00 (foreign individuals), $674.00 (foreign institutions), and $205.00 (foreign student/resident). Foreign air speed delivery is included in all *Clinics* subscription prices. All prices are subject to change without notice. **POSTMASTER**: Send address changes to *Surgical Oncology Clinics of North America*, Elsevier Health Science Division, Subscription Customer Service, 3251 Riverport Lane, Maryland Heights, MO 63043. **Customer Service: 1-800-654-2452 (US and Canada). 314-447-8871 (outside US and Canada). Fax: 314-447-8029. E-mail: journalscustomerservice-usa@elsevier.com (for print support); journalsonline support-usa@elsevier.com (for online support).**

Reprints. For copies of 100 or more, of articles in this publication, please contact the Commercial Reprints Department, Elsevier Inc., 360 Park Avenue South, New York, New York 10010-1710. Tel. 212-633-3874; Fax: 212-633-3820; E-mail: reprints@elsevier.com.

Surgical Oncology Clinics of North America is covered in *MEDLINE/PubMed (Index Medicus)* and *EMBASE/ Excerpta Medica, Current Contents/Clinical Medicine, and ISI/BIOMED.*

Contributors

CONSULTING EDITOR

TIMOTHY M. PAWLIK, MD, MPH, PhD, FACS, FRACS (Hon.)
Professor and Chair, Department of Surgery, The Urban Meyer III and Shelley Meyer
Chair for Cancer Research, Professor of Surgery, Oncology, Health Services Management
and Policy, The Ohio State University, Wexner Medical Center, Columbus, Ohio,
USA

EDITOR

ALFRED E. CHANG, MD
Hugh Cabot Professor of Surgery and Professor of Surgery, Division of Surgical Oncology,
University of Michigan Rogel Cancer Center, Ann Arbor, Michigan, USA

AUTHORS

MICHAEL E. AFENTOULIS, MS
Research Associate, Laboratory of Molecular and Tumor Immunology, Robert W. Franz
Cancer Center, Earle A. Chiles Research Institute, Providence Cancer Institute,
Providence Portland Medical Center, Portland, Oregon, USA

CARMEN BALLESTEROS-MERINO, PhD
Research Scientist, Laboratory of Molecular and Tumor Immunology, Robert W. Franz
Cancer Center, Earle A. Chiles Research Institute, Providence Cancer Institute,
Providence Portland Medical Center, Portland, Oregon, USA

GENEVIEVE BOLAND, MD, PhD
Division of Surgical Oncology, Massachusetts General Hospital, Boston, Massachusetts,
USA

PRAVEEN K. BOMMAREDDY, MS, PhD
School of Graduate Studies, Graduate School of Biomedical Sciences, Rutgers University,
New Brunswick, New Jersey, USA

ERIN E. BURKE, MD, MS
Complex General Surgical Oncology Fellow, H. Lee Moffitt Cancer Center, Tampa,
Florida, USA

ALFRED E. CHANG, MD
Hugh Cabot Professor of Surgery and Professor of Surgery, Division of Surgical Oncology,
University of Michigan Rogel Cancer Center, Ann Arbor, Michigan, USA

BRIAN J. CZERNIECKI, MD, PhD
Chair, Department of Breast Oncology, H. Lee Moffitt Cancer Center, Tampa, Florida,
USA

BERNARD A. FOX, PhD
Harder Family Chair for Cancer Research, Laboratory of Molecular and Tumor Immunology, Robert W. Franz Cancer Center, Earle A. Chiles Research Institute, Providence Cancer Institute, Providence Portland Medical Center, Adjunct Graduate Faculty, Department of Molecular Microbiology and Immunology, Member and Co-Leader of the Tumor Immunology Focus Panel, Knight Cancer Institute, Oregon Health & Science University, Cofounder and CEO, UbiVac, Inc., Portland, Oregon, USA

MORGAN L. HENNESSY, MD, PhD
Division of Surgical Oncology, Massachusetts General Hospital, Boston, Massachusetts, USA

TYLER W. HULETT, PhD
Postdoctoral Fellow, Laboratory of Molecular and Tumor Immunology, Robert W. Franz Cancer Center, Earle A. Chiles Research Institute, Providence Cancer Institute, Providence Portland Medical Center, Portland, Oregon, USA

FUMITO ITO, MD, PhD
Center for Immunotherapy, Department of Surgical Oncology, Roswell Park Comprehensive Cancer Center, Department of Surgery, Jacobs School of Medicine and Biomedical Sciences, University at Buffalo, The State University of New York, Buffalo, New York, USA

MOHAMMAD S. JAFFERJI, MD
Immunotherapy and Surgical Oncology Fellow, Surgery Branch, National Cancer Institute, National Institutes of Health, Bethesda, Maryland, USA

SHAWN M. JENSEN, PhD
Senior Research Scientist, Laboratory of Molecular and Tumor Immunology, Robert W. Franz Cancer Center, Earle A. Chiles Research Institute, Providence Cancer Institute, Providence Portland Medical Center, Portland, Oregon, USA

HOWARD L. KAUFMAN, MD
Division of Surgical Oncology, Massachusetts General Hospital, Boston, Massachusetts, USA; Replimune, Inc., Woburn, Massachusetts, USA

EMILY Z. KEUNG, MD
Fellow, Department of Surgical Oncology, The University of Texas MD Anderson Cancer Center, Houston, Texas, USA

NIKHIL I. KHUSHALANI, MD
Vice Chair, Department of Cutaneous Oncology, Moffitt Cancer Center, Associate Professor of Medicine, Department of Oncologic Sciences, University of South Florida Morsani College of Medicine, Tampa, Florida, USA

NICHOLAS D. KLEMEN, MD
Department of Surgery, Yale School of Medicine, New Haven, Connecticut, USA

KRITHIKA KODUMUDI, PhD
Research Scientist III, Clinical Science Lab Department, H. Lee Moffitt Cancer Center, Tampa, Florida, USA

MINYOUNG KWAK, MD, MPH
Division of Surgical Oncology, Department of Surgery, Carter Immunology Center, University of Virginia, Charlottesville, Virginia, USA; Department of Surgery, SUNY Downstate, Brooklyn, New York, USA

KATIE M. LEICK, MD, MS
Division of Surgical Oncology, Department of Surgery, University of Virginia, Carter
Immunology Center, University of Virginia, Charlottesville, Virginia, USA; Department of
Surgery, University of Iowa, Iowa City, Iowa, USA

QIAO LI, PhD
Research Associate Professor, Division of Surgical Oncology, University of Michigan
Rogel Cancer Center, Ann Arbor, Michigan, USA

JANICE REBECCA LIU, MD
Associate Professor, Department of Obstetrics and Gynecology, University of Michigan
Medical School, Ann Arbor, Michigan, USA

SEBASTIAN MARWITZ, PhD
Postdoctoral Scholar, Laboratory of Molecular and Tumor Immunology, Robert W. Franz
Cancer Center, Earle A. Chiles Research Institute, Providence Cancer Institute,
Providence Portland Medical Center, Portland, Oregon, USA

MARIT M. MELSSEN, MS
Division of Surgical Oncology, Departments of Surgery, and Microbiology, Immunology,
and Cancer Biology, University of Virginia, Charlottesville, Virginia, USA; Department of
Immunohematology and Blood Transfusion, Leiden University Medical Center, Leiden,
The Netherlands

DAVID J. MESSENHEIMER, PhD
Senior Scientist, Cancer Immunology and Immune Modulation, Boehringer Ingelheim
Pharaceuticals, Inc., Ridgefield, Connecticut, USA

TARSEM MOUDGIL, MS
Associate Research Scientist, Laboratory of Molecular and Tumor Immunology, Robert
W. Franz Cancer Center, Earle A. Chiles Research Institute, Providence Cancer Institute,
Providence Portland Medical Center, Portland, Oregon, USA

DAVID B. PAGE, MD
Assistant Member, Breast Immunotherapy, Earle A. Chiles Research Institute, Portland,
Oregon, USA

SUNNY J. PATEL, BS
Center for Immunotherapy, Roswell Park Comprehensive Cancer Center, Buffalo,
New York, USA; Medical College of Georgia, Augusta University, Augusta, Georgia,
USA

GANESAN RAMAMOORTHI, PhD
Postdoctoral Research Fellow, Clinical Science Lab Department, H. Lee Moffitt Cancer
Center, Tampa, Florida, USA

LUKE D. ROTHERMEL, MD, MPH
Complex General Surgical Oncology Fellow, Moffitt Cancer Center, Tampa, Florida, USA

KATHERINE SANCHEZ, MD
Immuno-oncology Fellow, Earle A. Chiles Research Institute, Portland, Oregon, USA

AMOD A. SARNAIK, MD
Associate Member, Department of Cutaneous Oncology, Moffitt Cancer Center,
Associate Professor of Surgery, Department of Oncologic Sciences, University of South
Florida Morsani College of Medicine, Tampa, Florida, USA

RICHARD M. SHERRY, MD
Surgery Branch, National Cancer Institute, National Institutes of Health, Bethesda, Maryland, USA

MACKENZIE L. SHINDORF, MD
Surgery Branch, National Cancer Institute, National Institutes of Health, Bethesda, Maryland, USA

CRAIG L. SLINGLUFF Jr, MD
Division of Surgical Oncology, Department of Surgery, University of Virginia, Carter Immunology Center, University of Virginia, Charlottesville, Virginia, USA

VERNON K. SONDAK, MD
Chair, Department of Cutaneous Oncology, Moffitt Cancer Center, Professor of Surgery, Departments of Oncologic Sciences and Surgery, University of South Florida Morsani College of Medicine, Tampa, Florida, USA

WALTER URBA, MD, PhD
Member, Director, and Endowed Chair of Cancer Research, Earle A. Chiles Research Institute, Portland, Oregon, USA

WEIMIN WANG, PhD
Research Lab Specialist, Department of Surgery, University of Michigan Medical School, Ann Arbor, Michigan, USA

JENNIFER A. WARGO, MD, MMSc
Associate Professor, Department of Surgical Oncology, The University of Texas MD Anderson Cancer Center, Houston, Texas, USA

KEITH W. WEGMAN, PhD
Research Scientist, Laboratory of Molecular and Tumor Immunology, Robert W. Franz Cancer Center, Earle A. Chiles Research Institute, Providence Cancer Institute, Providence Portland Medical Center, Portland, Oregon, USA

TAKAYOSHI YAMAUCHI, PhD
Center for Immunotherapy, Roswell Park Comprehensive Cancer Center, Buffalo, New York, USA; Department of Molecular Enzymology, Center for Metabolic Regulation of Healthy Aging, Faculty of Life Sciences, Kumamoto University, Kumamoto, Japan

JAMES C. YANG, MD
Principal Investigator, Staff Clinician, Surgery Branch, National Cancer Institute, National Institutes of Health, Bethesda, Maryland, USA

JING ZHANG, MD
Research Fellow, Division of Surgical Oncology, University of Michigan Rogel Cancer Center, Ann Arbor, Michigan, USA; Department of the 2nd Thoracic Medical Oncology, Hubei Cancer Hospital, Tongji Medical College, Huazhong University of Science and Technology, Wuhan, Hubei, China

WEIPING ZOU, MD, PhD
Charles B. de Nancrede Professor, Professor of Surgery, Pathology, Immunology, and Biology, Co-Director, Cancer Hematopoiesis and Immunology Program, Co-Director, Immunologic Monitoring Core, Director, University of Michigan Surgical Oncology Research Training Program, Director, Center of Excellence for Cancer Immunology and Immunotherapy, University of Michigan Rogel Cancer Center Department of Surgery, University of Michigan Medical School, Ann Arbor, Michigan, USA

Contents

The incidence of melanoma continues to increase even as advances in immunotherapy have led to survival benefits in advanced stages. Vaccines are capable of inducing strong, antitumor immune responses with limited toxicity. Some vaccines have demonstrated clinical benefit in clinical trials alone; however, others have not despite inducing strong immune responses. Recent advancements have improved vaccine design, and combining vaccines with other immunotherapies offers promise. This review highlights the underlying principles of vaccine development, common components of vaccines, and the remaining challenges and future directions of vaccine therapy in melanoma.

Vaccines can be a cost effective preventive measure for both primary prevention of disease and prevention of disease recurrence. Several vaccines targeting breast cancer oncodrivers are currently being tested in clinical trials. Whereas clinical response rates to breast cancer vaccines have been modest despite the induction of strong antitumor T cell responses, it is through these approaches that valuable insight and knowledge have been gained about tumor immunology. With the emergence of new immunotherapies, there is renewed excitement for effective breast cancer vaccine development.

Immunotherapy has led to unprecedented improvement in the treatment and prognosis of high-risk resectable and metastatic disease across cancer types. Nowhere is this better highlighted than in the management of advanced and metastatic melanoma with the introduction of molecularly targeted therapies and immune checkpoint inhibitors. Following their success in melanoma, immunotherapies have also been evaluated and their use approved in the management across a variety of other solid malignancies in the neoadjuvant, adjuvant, and advanced/metastatic setting. This review provides an overview of the current landscape of immune checkpoint inhibition for solid malignancies.

Immune checkpoint inhibitors (ICIs) are therapeutic antibodies that target regulatory molecules on T cells and represent the most widely used FDA-approved class of immunotherapy. ICIs are associated with unique immune-mediated toxicities called immune-related adverse events. These toxicities may affect any organ system, and their precise mechanisms of action remain under investigation. Current evidence suggests that activation of T cells is involved, although other components of the immune response have been implicated. This article summarizes toxicities, potential mechanisms of action, management strategies, and other clinical considerations. Unique mechanisms of action and immune-related toxicities of other FDA-approved classes of immunotherapy are reviewed.

Immunotherapy has revolutionized the treatment of melanoma, with implications for the surgical management of this disease. Surgeons must be aware of the impact of various immunotherapies on patients with resectable and unresectable disease, and how surgical decision-making should progress as a result. We expect that current and developing immunotherapies will increase surgeon involvement for resection of metastatic melanoma, whether for tumor harvests to generate autologous lymphocytes or for consolidating control of disease beyond what immunotherapies alone can achieve. Despite remarkable advancements in the field, significant work is needed to optimize the immuno-modulation that targets cancers while minimizing toxicity for patients.

Oncolytic viruses are naturally occurring, or genetically engineered viruses that can be administered via intralesional injections or intravenously to induce cell death in tumor cells and activate antitumor immune responses. This review summarizes several oncolytic viruses in preclinical and clinical trials, describes challenges in clinical implementation, and important areas of future investigation.

Cancer stem cells (CSCs) are crucial for tumor recurrence and distant metastasis. Immunologically targeting CSCs represents a promising strategy to improve efficacy of multimodal cancer therapy. Modulating the innate immune response involving Toll-like receptors, macrophages, natural killer cells, and $\gamma\delta$T cells has therapeutic effects on CSCs. Antigens expressed by CSCs provide specific targets for immunotherapy. CSC-primed dendritic cell–based vaccines have induced significant antitumor immunity as an adjuvant therapy in experimental models of established tumors. Targeting the tumor microenvironment CSC niche with cytokines or checkpoint blockade provides additional strategies to eliminate CSCs.

The phenotype and functionalities of the major immune cell subsets including myeloid cells, macrophages, dendritic cells, and T cells are altered in the ovarian cancer microenvironment. Immunosuppressive networks including inhibitory B7 family members and regulatory T cell–associated adenosine pathway have been defined in human ovarian cancer. In this review, the authors integrate emerging information on immunosuppressive mechanisms and T cell phenotype and discuss strategies of immunotherapeutic and vaccine regimens. Finally, crucial points regarding design of immuno-oncology clinical trials are reviewed.

The use of immunotherapies for solid and hematologic malignancies has demonstrated durable antitumor effects. Use of checkpoint inhibitors allows for immunologic reactivation of the adaptive immune system against tumor-specific neoantigens and effective rejection. Recent developments in adoptive transfer of T cells has shown effective immune rejection of solid malignancies and durable regression. Adoptive cell transfer involves extraction of in vivo T lymphocytes, selection for or introduction of tumor reactive cells, in vitro expansion, and delivery of the T-cell product back to the patient. This article discusses the different approaches, challenges, and further directions of adoptive T-cell transfer in solid malignancies.

Improvements in systemic immunotherapy are changing the treatment of patients with advanced melanoma and many other tumors. Surgeons may be increasingly called on to manage isolated sites of immunorefractory disease or to provide palliative surgery as a bridge to systemic therapy. Here, the authors describe the biologic rationale for using surgery in patients with immunorefractory disease, provide background on the evolving role of metastasectomy for advanced melanoma, and summarize data on the use of neoadjuvant immunotherapy. Finally, the authors discuss the direction of clinical research in this rapidly evolving field.

Adoptive T cell therapy for solid malignancies is limited because obtaining sufficient numbers of less-differentiated tumor-specific T cells is difficult. This roadblock can be theoretically overcome by the use of induced pluripotent stem cells (iPSCs), which self-renew and provide unlimited numbers of autologous less-differentiated T cells. iPSCs can generate less-differentiated antigen-specific T cells that harbor long telomeres and

SURGICAL ONCOLOGY
CLINICS OF NORTH AMERICA

SERIES OF RELATED INTEREST

Surgical Clinics of North America
http://www.surgical.theclinics.com
Thoracic Surgery Clinics
http://www.thoracic.theclinics.com
Advances in Surgery
http://www.advancessurgery.com

THE CLINICS ARE AVAILABLE ONLINE!
Access your subscription at:
www.theclinics.com

Foreword

Immunotherapy for Solid Malignancies

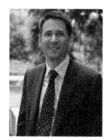

Timothy M. Pawlik, MD, MPH, PhD, FACS, FRACS (Hon.)
Consulting Editor

This issue of the *Surgical Oncology Clinics of North America* is devoted to focusing on the role of immunotherapy for solid malignancies. The guest editor is Dr Alfred Chang. Dr Chang is the Hugh Cabot Professor of Surgery at the University of Michigan. Dr Chang has expertise in the areas of breast cancer, melanoma, sarcomas, liver tumors, and colorectal cancer. He has held leadership roles at the University of Michigan Rogel Cancer Center. Dr Chang runs a laboratory program that has been externally funded for more than 25 years. His research focuses on tumor immunology and immunotherapy. He has been on editorial boards of numerous surgery and oncology journals. He has been a member of the Experimental Therapeutics 2, the Subcommittee D-Clinical Trials, and Clinical Oncology NIH study sections. As such, Dr Chang is ideally suited to be the guest editor of this important issue of the *Surgical Oncology Clinics of North America*.

The issue covers the important topic of immunotherapy for solid cancers. The goal of using the immune system to target tumors and treat solid malignancies has long been an elusive goal. Over the last decade, immunotherapy has evolved significantly to become not only a relevant but also a critical tool in the treatment of patients with solid tumors. While surgery remains the cornerstone of curative-intent therapy for most solid malignancies, immunotherapy has emerged as an important part of the multimodality care. As such, it is critical for surgeons to comprehend the principles of immunotherapy as well as understand the role of employing immunotherapy strategies to treat solid tumors. In this issue of *Surgical Oncology Clinics of North America*, the editors have amassed a wide range of experts across an array of solid tumor types to provide a comprehensive review on the role of immunotherapy. Dr Chang enlisted an incredible group of leaders in their field to cover various aspects of immunotherapy, such as vaccine therapy, oncolytic immunotherapy, and adoptive T-cell therapy. As you will note in reading this issue, Dr Chang and his colleagues have demonstrated the importance

Surg Oncol Clin N Am 28 (2019) xiii–xiv
https://doi.org/10.1016/j.soc.2019.04.001
1055-3207/19/© 2019 Published by Elsevier Inc.

and progress that has been made in the area of immunotherapy for solid tumors. I would like to thank Dr Chang and his colleagues in taking on such an important topic for an excellent issue of the *Surgical Oncology Clinics of North America*.

Timothy M. Pawlik, MD, MPH, PhD, FACS, FRACS (Hon.)
The Ohio State University
Wexner Medical Center
395 West 12th Avenue, Suite 670
Columbus, OH 43210, USA

E-mail address:
tim.pawlik@osumc.edu

Preface

The Dawn of a New Age in Cancer Immunotherapy

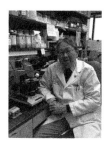

Alfred E. Chang, MD
Editor

It was over one hundred years ago that immunotherapy for cancer was first explored by Dr William Coley with the intratumoral injection of bacterial extracts that resulted in tumor regression in select cases. The emergence of surgical procedures, radiation therapy, and chemotherapy eventually became the mainstay of cancer therapies and relegated immune treatments as an unfulfilled pipedream. Nevertheless, it has been apparent that the immune system can play a role in tumor biology as evident by cases of spontaneous tumor regression and increased cancer incidence among immunosuppressed patients. We have come a long way in understanding the complexities of the immune system, which is highly regulated as it should be to avoid the onset of pathologic autoimmune reactions. Also, we have a greater understanding of the nature of tumor antigens, which act as targets to the immune system and can be highly specific for individual tumors or shared by groups of cancers.

In the past, there have been several approaches to deliver immunotherapy either to enhance the activation of the immune system or to provide agents with tumoricidal activity, such as the use of vaccines, cytokines, monoclonal antibodies, and adoptive cell transfer. These have had encouraging results with limited activity. More recently, approaches to block the regulatory mechanisms that downregulate antitumor immunity (also known as checkpoint inhibition) have had dramatic results in clinical trials involving a variety of solid malignancies. This underscores the notion that antitumor immunity within the host is already present but suppressed in its function. The use of these checkpoint inhibitors allows for the antitumor response to be expressed or maintained. A major focus of current research is to evaluate the combination of these checkpoint inhibitors with other modalities of treatment, such as surgery, radiation, chemotherapy, or other immunotherapies. Another area of success in the application of immunotherapy has been the genetic engineering of T cells with chimeric T-cell receptors (also known as CAR T cells) that are specific for tumor antigens. This has been

Surg Oncol Clin N Am 28 (2019) xv–xvi
https://doi.org/10.1016/j.soc.2019.04.002
1055-3207/19/© 2019 Published by Elsevier Inc.

effective in the treatment of certain B-cell malignancies, where B-cell antigens are well defined. This approach is being explored in solid malignancies, where known tumor-specific antigens are being used to engineer CAR T cells for adoptive cell transfer.

Immunotherapy has become a major modality in oncology, on par with surgery, radiation oncology, and chemotherapy. The Food and Drug Administration has approved many immune agents over the last few years based on efficacy data. One example of this efficacy is demonstrated by the change in the natural history of advanced melanoma. Patients with stage IV melanoma are living longer with some having long-term survival. This issue of *Surgical Oncology Clinics of North America* reviews the recent progress that is occurring with various immune therapies in a variety of solid tumors. It also provides insights as to future directions that cancer immunotherapy is taking. I want to thank all the authors who contributed to this issue, especially the senior authors, who are leaders in the field. I am certain that this is a new dawn, and that many more major advances will take place that will benefit patients with cancer.

Alfred E. Chang, MD
Hugh Cabot Professor of Surgery
Division of Surgical Oncology
Rogel Cancer Center
Michigan Medicine
1500 East Medical Center Drive
Ann Arbor, MI 48109-5392, USA

E-mail address:
aechang@umich.edu

Vaccine Strategy in Melanoma

Minyoung Kwak, MD, MPH[a,b,c,1], Katie M. Leick, MD, MS[a,c,d,1],
Marit M. Melssen, MS[a,e,f], Craig L. Slingluff Jr, MD[a,c],*

KEYWORDS

- Melanoma • Vaccine • Tumor-associated antigen • Neoantigen • Vaccine adjuvant
- T cell

KEY POINTS

- Cancer vaccines are formulated with tumor-associated antigens and vaccine adjuvants to elicit a targeted immune response for tumor control.
- The elicited T cell response to tumor-associated antigens may be discordant with tumor control; current strategies of vaccine antigens and adjuvants are under investigation to improve clinical response rates.
- Many clinical trials are currently underway to determine the optimal combinations for the different types of tumor-associated antigens, vaccine adjuvants, and other immunotherapies such as checkpoint blockade therapy.

Disclosure Statement: Dr C.L. Slingluff Jr has received research funding from Celldex, Merck, and GlaxoSmithKline; provision of drug or equipment for clinical trials: Merck, Celldex, 3M, Theraclion; Consulting fee: Polynoma, Immatics, CureVac (pending), Celldex. These all provide funds to the University of Virginia, not to Dr C.L. Slingluff Jr directly. Dr C.L. Slingluff Jr also is an inventor on patents for peptides used in vaccine trials and receives funds through the University of Virginia Licensing and Ventures Group for this licensed intellectual property. Dr M. Kwak has been supported by three fellowship grants: NIH/NCI T32CA009109, Rebecca Clary Harris memorial fellowship and a grant from the University of Virginia Cancer Center. Dr K Leick has been supported on NIH/NCI T32CA163177, and Dr C.L. Slingluff Jr has been supported by NIH/NCI R01CA178846. The project has also been supported in part by a Clinical Laboratory Integration Project (CLIP) award from Cancer Research Institute, and the UVA Cancer Center Training Grant (P30CA044579).

[a] Division of Surgical Oncology, Department of Surgery, University of Virginia, PO Box 800709, Charlottesville, VA 22908-0709, USA; [b] Department of Surgery, SUNY Downstate, Brooklyn, NY, USA; [c] Carter Immunology Center, University of Virginia, Charlottesville, VA, USA; [d] Department of Surgery, University of Iowa, Iowa City, IA, USA; [e] Department of Microbiology, Immunology, and Cancer Biology, University of Virginia, Charlottesville, VA, USA; [f] Department of Immunohematology and Blood Transfusion, Leiden University Medical Center, Leiden, the Netherlands

[1] M. Kwak and K.M. Leick contributed equally to this article and are considered co-first authors.
* Corresponding author. Division of Surgical Oncology, Department of Surgery, University of Virginia, PO Box 800709, Charlottesville, VA 22908-0709.
E-mail address: cls8h@virginia.edu

INTRODUCTION

The development of vaccines against cancer has driven significant advancements in tumor immunology, leading to a better understanding of the immune response against cancer. There is new expertise on the nature of tumor-associated antigens, making it possible to even genetically engineer immunogenic antigens for melanoma vaccines. This has been achieved through advances in sequencing and manipulating genomes, development of algorithms to define putative T cell antigens, identification of different immune cell types, and unraveling the complexities of the tumor microenvironment.

The promise of cancer vaccines is that vaccines induce targeted, tumor-specific immune responses with long-term memory in cases of recurrence or metastasis, with low risk of toxicity overall. There has been renewed focus on the potential of immunotherapy as a result of the recent success of checkpoint blockade therapy in advanced melanoma. If patients lack a pre-existing immune response to their cancer, they are unlikely to respond to checkpoint blockade; so there is renewed interest in vaccines to induce antitumor immune responses that did not arise spontaneously. There is potential value in combining vaccine therapy with other immunotherapies to improve tumor control. Clinical trials implementing these combination therapies are currently underway. This review summarizes the current antigen and vaccine adjuvant strategies under investigation and highlights the progress made with recent melanoma vaccine therapies in clinical trials.

Background on Tumor Antigenicity and Immune Activation

Cancer vaccines contain tumor-associated antigens and vaccine adjuvants to elicit activation of dendritic cells (DCs) and antigen-specific T cells. Initiation of the immune response against tumor cells occurs through recognition of tumor-associated antigens that must be processed and presented on MHC complexes by antigen-presenting cells (APCs) (**Fig. 1**). Specific T cells recognize these MHC-antigen complexes, leading to their activation and proliferation. Antigen presentation on MHC class I generally activates cytotoxic CD8 T cells (T_{CD8}), whereas presentation on MHC class II activates CD4 helper T cells (T_{CD4}). Elements of both CD8 and CD4 T cells are likely needed to mount an optimal response for tumor control and long-term memory.

Cancer vaccine formulations also incorporate "vaccine adjuvants" to increase T cell stimulation by activating APCs, thereby enhancing antigen presentation and costimulation. Many vaccine adjuvants stimulate pattern-recognition receptors (PRRs) on APCs. These PRRs recognize PAMPs (pathogen-associated molecular patterns) or DAMPs (damage-associated molecular patterns), heat shock proteins, or reactive oxygen intermediates.[1] PAMPs include Toll-like receptor (TLR) agonists, such as CpG sequences. Introducing a tumor-associated antigen with vaccine adjuvants allows for an improved antigen-specific immune response to enhance tumor control.

VACCINE STRATEGIES: ANTIGEN

Antigens used in melanoma vaccines may be shared across patients or may be neoantigens that are uniquely expressed. Different types of antigens have been identified in melanoma (**Fig. 2**), and are summarized in the following. The type of antigen that is selected can determine the tumor specificity, type, and strength of the ensuing immune response.

Shared Melanoma Antigens

Melanocytic differentiation antigens
Melanocytic differentiation antigens are expressed by most melanoma tumors and induce T cell responses.[2,3] The shared aspect of these antigens enables broad

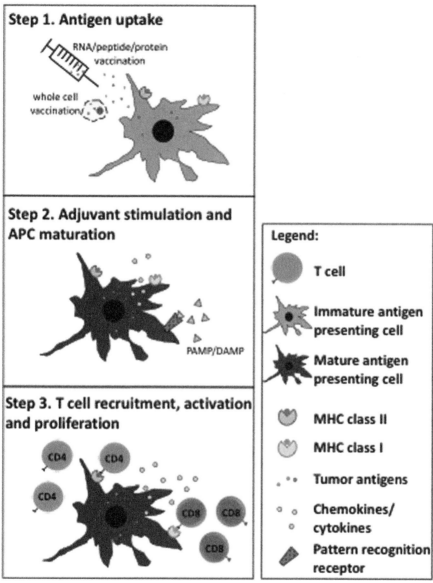

Fig. 1. Mechanism of immune response induction after vaccination. Step 1. Vaccination allows tumor antigen to be taken up by antigen-presenting cells (APCs). Step 2. Adjuvant stimulation supports activation and maturation of APCs. Step 3. APCs present antigen to CD8 T cells by way of MHC class I and to CD4 T cells through MHC class II, resulting in their activation and proliferation and thereby launching an antitumor immune response.

application and generalization of shared antigen-targeting vaccines across multiple patients. Tyrosinase, TRP-2, Melan-A/MART-1, and gp-100 are common source proteins that are also expressed on normal melanocytes and on a few other pigmented cells. Thus, successful immune targeting of melanocytic antigens has the potential to induce autoimmunity to melanocytes. In addition, because these antigens are

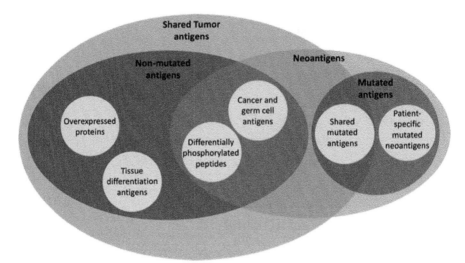

Fig. 2. Different types of tumor-associated antigens in melanoma.

present in some normal tissues, responses to them may be limited by pre-existing central tolerance.[4] Regardless, some vaccine and adoptive therapies targeting these antigens have been successful.[5,6]

Shared mutated antigens

Mutated antigens arise from acquired somatic mutations or single-nucleotide polymorphisms in melanoma cells and are often unique to a given patient tumor, although some are present in a fraction of patients. Because mutated antigens arise through tumorigenesis, they are absent in normal cells. BRAF, KIT, and NRAS mutations are common mutated antigens in melanoma. Antigenic BRAF peptides encompassing the V600E driver mutation of melanoma have been reported,[7–10] inducing BRAF-specific immune responses in humans[9,10] and tumor control in mice.[7,8] These data support further clinical investigation of these mutated antigens in vaccines.

Cancer germ line antigens

Cancer germ line antigens are expressed in the placenta or testis as immune privileged sites[11] and are also uniquely expressed in some malignant tumors. The immunogenicity and unique expression of these antigens in cancers, rather than in normal cells, provides an opportunity to elicit an antitumor immune response using vaccines. Their restricted expression justifies considering them a form of neoantigen. MAGE-A1, MAGE-A3, BAGE, GAGE, and NY-ESO-1 are a few examples of cancer germ line antigens that have been identified. Adoptive T cell therapy using T cells expressing a T cell receptor (TCR) transduced with NY-ESO-1 induced objective clinical responses in 55% of patients with advanced melanoma.[12] Thus, cancer germ line antigens can be effective tumor regression antigens. On the other hand, a MAGE-A3 vaccine failed to enhance survival in a phase 3 trial[13]; so the use of cancer germ line antigens in vaccines remains to be optimized. Although some cancer germ line antigens are solely expressed on tumor cells, a few studies using adoptive T cell therapies have shown cross-reactivity with normal tissues when high-affinity TCRs are used.[14] Some cancer germ line antigens may be sequestered and thus not subject to pre-existing tolerance, whereas others may not be sequestered.[15] Understanding this phenomenon may improve selection of cancer germ line antigens for cancer vaccines.

Phosphopeptides

Phosphorylation of oncogenic proteins supports malignant transformation; thus, targeting them is a promising strategy. Phosphorylated peptides derived from those proteins can be presented by both MHC class I and II molecules, which induces an immune response to the phosphorylated peptide sequence specifically.[16–19] Identification of tumor-specific phosphopeptide antigens may provide opportunities for personalized immune vaccine therapies.[20] A first-in-humans clinical trial has recently been completed (NCT01846143).

Mutated neoantigens

The term neoantigen refers to newly expressed or acquired antigens, as in genomic mutations found within tumors but not in normal somatic cells. Because of its unique genetic sequence, the transcribed DNA, RNA, or translated peptide fragments can be used as a unique source of tumor-associated antigens. The advantage of these mutated neoantigens in vaccines is that it may avoid pre-existing central tolerance that is expected with shared antigens[4] and should reduce risks of on-target autoimmune reactivity. Data also suggest that therapeutic T cells may respond more strongly to mutated neoantigens than to shared antigens.[21,22] Newer approaches have developed algorithms to predict and select advantageous immunogenic features of the mutanome. These mutated epitopes can be engineered into vaccines using a personalized approach.[23] A disadvantage of this personalized technique is the time required for the synthesis of personalized vaccines. Methods to predict immunogenic neoantigens were applied to patients and successfully showed immunogenicity of predicted neoantigens with promising clinical outcomes in a small number of patients.[23–25] However, much research still needs to be done to expand these preliminary results and to optimize immune responses to neoantigens.

Antigen Type and Adjuvants

Selection of an appropriate antigen type can influence the immune response following treatment. Vaccines may use antigen as whole tumor cells, RNA or DNA, single or multiple peptides, or APCs displaying the target antigen. Both efficacy and toxicity can be related to intrinsic immunologic potency, cross-reactivity of vaccine targets to antigen on normal cells, and associated adjuvants.

Peptide vaccines

Peptide vaccines can be synthesized as short or long with single-peptide or multi-peptide mixtures. Peptides are weakly immunogenic when naked peptide is used[26,27]; however, their use in combination with vaccine adjuvants or immune therapies induces potent, and frequently durable, T cell responses.[28–33]

Short peptide vaccines

Short peptide vaccines representing minimal CD8 epitopes (usually 9 amino acids long) thus elicit a cytotoxic T_{CD8} response by binding MHC class I. Their effects on T_{CD8} are advantageous because they activate effector cells directly, thus negating the need for further antigen processing by APCs. Immune response rates may approach 100% in humans, of which 1% to 5% of the T_{CD8} population is peptide-specific effector T_{CD8}.[28,29,31] Minimal epitope vaccines can induce strong T_{CD8} responses alone.[29] One study designed minimal epitope vaccines based on individual patient-mutated neoantigens and generated neoantigen-specific T cell responses in all 3 patients, affecting 23% to 89% of the T_{CD8} population; memory T cells were present for up to 4 months.[24,34,35] Short peptide vaccines may be limited by proteolytic degradation,[36] tolerance due to suboptimal antigen presentation, and less sustained immune responses.[37]

Extensive work has been done with a modified gp100 peptide (gp100$_{209-217}$;209-2M) that is a modified form of peptide naturally presented by HLA-A2 to T_{CD8}. Vaccination with gp100 209-2M alone increased peptide-specific T cells in 97% of patients.[31] Addition of gp100 to IL-2 in a clinical trial involving patients with advanced melanoma significantly increased clinical response rates and improved progression-free survival.[38,39] However, combination of gp100 peptide with checkpoint blockade therapies such as ipilimumab showed no therapeutic benefit compared with ipilimumab alone.[40] Mechanisms underlying this limitation have been explored in mice and suggest the addition of gp100 peptide vaccine in an antigen-depot vaccine with ipilimumab may lead to sequestration and destruction of non–gp100-specific effector T cells, particularly those effector T cells that are induced by ipilimumab.[41] This finding needs to be studied further in patients.

Helper peptide vaccines

Helper T_{CD4} are activated by recognition of peptide presented on class II MHC molecules and induce a multifaceted immune response by supporting APC, T_{CD8} effector function, and T cell memory formation. Thus, immune therapies targeting helper T_{CD4} offer promise for tumor control.[32] A peptide vaccine composed of a mixture of 6 melanoma helper peptides (6MHP) that are recognized by T_{CD4} has been used in clinical trials and induces a Th1 T_{CD4} response without increasing the proportion of T_{regs} (regulatory T cells). T_{CD8} responses also occurred by way of epitope spreading.[27] Sixty-five percent of 6MHP-treated patients with stage IV melanoma developed an immune response, and treatment with vaccine significantly improved overall survival compared with matched controls.[27] Patient survival was associated with antibody response rates and the formation of memory T_{CD4} immune responses.[26]

Long peptide vaccines

Long peptide vaccines refer to lengths of 20 to 30 amino acids and carry the potential benefit of activating both T_{CD8} and T_{CD4} responses. Murine work showed more efficient internalization and processing of long peptides by APCs compared with protein, resulting in more sustained T_{CD8} activation.[42] A phase 1 clinical trial of NY-ESO-1-derived long peptide (30 amino acids) combined with adjuvant induced antigen-specific T cells only when peptide was used in combination with adjuvant, but not with peptide alone.[32] Vaccination with long peptide targeting up to 20 predicted personal neoantigens successfully induced neoantigen-specific T_{CD4} responses to 60% of antigens, whereas T_{CD8} responses were limited to only 16% of unique neoantigens, suggesting preferential activation of T_{CD4} by long peptides.[25] In addition, 4 of 6 patients had no recurrence 25 months after vaccination, suggesting the potential for clinical benefits and long-lasting effects of long peptide vaccines.[25]

RNA, DNA, and protein vaccines

RNA or DNA encoding genes for tumor antigens or immune enhancers can be introduced into APCs or myocytes through bacterial or viral vectors to synthesize peptides and mediate a vaccine effect. Some RNA vaccines involve electroporation of APCs to enable incorporation of mRNA encoding melanoma-associated antigens or immunostimulatory ligands to facilitate antigen-specific T cell responses. In such studies, T_{CD8} responses were detected in 57% to 80% of patients, but no objective clinical responses were observed.[43,44] Some recent RNA vaccines are designed and personalized based on mutations expressed and identified by RNA sequencing and selected for predicted high-affinity binding to MHC class I and II. These are engineered into synthetic RNA and delivered using a vaccine vehicle. Most of the responses induced were T_{CD4} responses,[23] comparable with personalized neoepitope vaccines based on mutated peptides.[25] Neoepitope vaccination also resulted in a broadened repertoire of T cells.[23]

A phase 1 clinical trial of DNA vaccine-encoding genes for immunogenic epitopes for gp100 and TRP2 demonstrated an immune response rate of 84%, comparable with other peptide vaccines using gp100.[38,45] Despite induction of an immune response, DNA vaccines evoke limited objective clinical responses.[45]

Whole cell vaccines

Whole cancer cells can be integrated into vaccines and serve as a source of antigen for APC presentation. They contain numerous mutated neoantigens that are inherent to the tumor, which does not mandate that they be identified before designing and manufacturing the vaccine. Whole cells can be modified to express particular tumor antigens or immune enhancers to further potentiate immune responses. This type of vaccine is typically more proficient at inducing expansion of T_{CD4} than T_{CD8}, resulting in an attenuated antitumor immune response. Despite whole cell vaccines showing initial promise to prolong survival with high clinical response rates, a large randomized phase 3 clinical trial showed no significant clinical benefit.[46] There is currently a phase 3 clinical trial underway (NCT01546571) using a cell-based vaccine derived from cell line supernatants containing antigens shed by tumor cells, which significantly improved disease-free survival in vaccine-treated patients in a previous phase 2 trial.[47]

VACCINE STRATEGIES: VACCINE ADJUVANTS

Vaccine adjuvants are aimed at producing more robust immune responses by increasing antigen uptake and presentation, recruiting other immune cells, or forming a depot effect for sustained release of antigen.[48,49]

Incomplete Freund Adjuvant

A common adjuvant used in peptide vaccines for melanoma is Montanide ISA 51 (Seppic, Inc), a form of incomplete Freund adjuvant (IFA). This is an oil-based agent with droplets of aqueous peptide contained within a surrounding oil phase. This facilitates a depot effect at the vaccine site, allowing for continued antigen exposure in a stabilized oil emulsion.[48] In humans, immune responses to peptides in IFA were greater than peptides pulsed on APCs.[50,51] In mice, the depot effect of IFA may also lead to vaccine-site sequestration of activated T cells against antigen[52] that may prevent T cell homing to tumor. There are data suggesting the added immunologic benefit of other adjuvants such as CD40 stimulating antibody and TLR agonists instead of IFA to avoid these concerns. Human studies have not yet been done to determine whether CD40 antibody plus TLR agonists can induce a much stronger T cell response than IFA alone; however, our studies continue to support the addition of IFA to TLR agonists in melanoma vaccines with short peptides.[53]

Dendritic Cell Vaccines

DC vaccines use autologous DCs to present antigen and to stimulate immune cells by releasing proinflammatory cytokines. In preparation for vaccine synthesis, DCs are isolated from peripheral blood. The vaccine can then be packaged using various adjuvants to induce DC activation, or autologous DCs can be pulsed with antigen ex vivo and administered in the same patient. The vaccination route may determine the tissue site to which the DCs will migrate.[54] A randomized phase 2 trial using autologous DC vaccines with GM-CSF in patients with advanced melanoma showed longer survival compared with a tumor cell vaccine, with 70% reduction in risk of death.[55] However, this trial had low patient numbers and unequal prognostic factors. Other trials demonstrated lower T cell responses with DC vaccines compared with peptide vaccines with adjuvant.[50,51]

Another potential method of further stimulating DCs in murine models is an in vivo method using viral vectors and CD40 stimulating antibodies. CD40 is a costimulatory receptor on DCs that adds to DC maturation and T_{CD8} activation.[56,57] The addition of CD40 antibody to a combination of TLR3 agonists and a neoantigen vaccine against colon adenocarcinoma in mice showed improved survival compared with either agonist alone, with expansion of neoantigen-specific T cells in both the periphery and the tumor microenvironment.[58] These preclinical results show promise in the strength of CD40 for DC activation but still need to be evaluated in humans.

Toll-like receptor agonists

TLR agonists stimulate PRRs on DCs to promote antigen processing and presentation to T cells. A common TLR agonist used in melanoma vaccine adjuvants is the TLR3 agonist poly-ICLC (polyinosine-polycytidylic acid). This agonist matures DCs to generate T_{CD8} and natural killer cells with higher cytotoxic capacity.[59,60] The combination of IFA and poly-ICLC with long NY-ESO-1 peptides showed that both adjuvants had different but beneficial effects on antigen-specific activation of T_{CD4}; emulsification of the antigen in IFA increased antigen-specific T_{CD4}, whereas poly-ICLC induced a Th1 phenotype, leading to increased cell-mediated immunity and inflammatory response.[61]

CpG is an oligodeoxynucleotide fragment rich in cytosine and guanine, similar to bacterial DNA, that is an agonist for TLR9 and induces DC maturation.[62,63] With DC maturation, CpG has also been shown to increase costimulatory surface marker expression with increases in proinflammatory cytokines needed for cytotoxic T_{CD8} costimulation,[62,63] and possibly B cell stimulation.[64] Addition of CpG to IFA has dramatically enhanced T cell responses to a short peptide vaccine.[62] Despite its effectiveness in T_{CD8} promotion, a mouse model suggests it may require decreased levels of immunosuppressive T_{regs} and multiple booster vaccinations to maximize its effect.[65] On the other hand, resiquimod (R848) is an agonist for TLR7 and TLR8 that has been found to decrease the immunosuppressive function of T_{regs}[66] and myeloid-derived suppressor cells (MDSC),[67] supporting increased T cell proliferation.

Systemic Cytokines

Other types of vaccine adjuvants involve the use of immune cell cytokines. GM-CSF (granulocyte-macrophage colony-stimulating factor) is used to attract and activate DCs to further promote peptide antigen–specific responses.[68,69] GM-CSF enhanced immunogenicity of a cell-based vaccine in mice,[68] and combined with a peptide vaccine, increased T cell responses compared with DCs pulsed with the same peptide antigen.[51] However, in a large randomized clinical trial, the addition of GM-CSF to a peptide vaccine significantly decreased responses in both T_{CD8} and T_{CD4} compared with peptide vaccine alone.[70] Also, another large randomized clinical trial revealed that adding GM-CSF to a melanoma cell vaccine resulted in worse survival and early melanoma-related death.[71] The use of GM-CSF as a vaccine adjuvant is cautionary and requires further investigation.

Systemic IL-2 infusions have also been used as a vaccine adjuvant in melanoma due to its overall stimulatory effect on T cells, and its clinical activity as high-dose monotherapy. When IL-2 was combined with the peptide vaccine gp100, clinical responses were significantly higher than with IL-2 alone, with associated longer progression-free survival.[38] Peptide-specific immunogenicity occurred in 19% of patients who received both gp100 and IL-2, but this antigen specificity did not correlate with clinical response. Other studies have failed to show immunologic or clinical benefit of IL-2, GM-CSF, or interferon-alpha in combination with melanoma vaccines.[72,73]

CURRENT MELANOMA VACCINE TRIALS

There are many ongoing clinical trials studying the impacts of various antigen formats and adjuvants on immune responses and clinical outcomes (**Fig. 3**A). Among these, DC and peptide vaccines predominate. Peptide vaccines use a variety of adjuvants, the most common of which is IFA (**Fig. 3**B). DC vaccines, as an adjuvant on their own, do not frequently use additional adjuvants (**Fig. 3**C). Combination therapy with vaccines provides an opportunity to target the immune system through another mechanism to augment antitumor effects and potentiate clinical benefits. The most common combination therapy for peptide vaccines is checkpoint blockade. IL-2 is most common among combination therapies used with DC vaccines, although DC vaccines use more combination therapies overall (see **Fig. 3**B, C).

NOVEL APPROACHES
Prophylactic Melanoma Vaccine

With the success of the generation of a prophylactic vaccine for virus-induced cervical cancer, the idea of prophylactic vaccines against melanoma regains interest. Preclinical in vivo studies have shown the potential of this approach, regardless of whether a DC-based, RNA-based, whole cell–based, or peptide-based antigen vehicle was used.[74–77]

Stem Cell–Based Vaccines

Induced pluripotent stem cells (iPSCs) are immunogenic pluripotent stemlike cells that can be generated from a patient's cells. Their gene expression is similar to embryonic

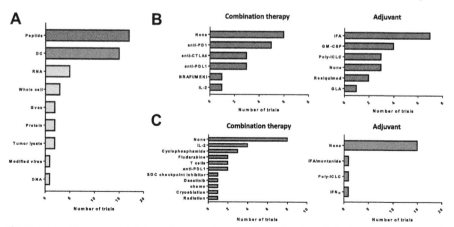

Fig. 3. Current vaccine trials in melanoma. The number of active clinical trials for each melanoma vaccine vehicle as of July 2018 on ClinicalTrials.gov are shown in (*A*). The number of active trials using combination therapies and adjuvants are quantified for peptide vaccines in (*B*) and dendritic cell (DC) vaccines in (*C*).

stem cells and includes expression of many tumor antigens. In preclinical models of melanoma and other solid tumors, immunization and therapeutic vaccination of iPSCs induced robust T_{CD4} and T_{CD8} responses, as well as a reduction in tumor burden.[78] Although these studies are still in the preclinical phase, they show potential for generating effective, personalized vaccines.

SUMMARY

Melanoma vaccine research has shown the potential for vaccines to elicit antigen-specific T cells as well as provide some tumor control. Understanding the importance of specific immunologic effects of antigen vehicle and adjuvant is vital to the progression of a vaccine strategy. As our knowledge base expands through preclinical studies and results from recent clinical trials are finalized, it will be possible to better optimize the approach for sustained tumor control.

Current therapies that involve vaccines alone have limitations due to discordance between antigen-specific T cell expansion and tumor control. Despite cancer vaccines showing lasting immune response rates up to 100%,[28,31] vaccines alone have led to clinical response rates of less than 10% in most studies.[79] This low clinical response may be due to insufficient T cell priming, poor homing to tumor, dysfunction of T cells in the tumor microenvironment, or progressive loss of function. Some of these may be due to defects in antigen presentation or immunosuppressive changes in the tumor microenvironment that could lead to anergic T cells or interference with T cell homing to tumor.[80] The advancement of neoantigen technology, along with newer adjuvant strategies, are all promising additions to increase clinical response. There are other preclinical methods of inhibiting immunosuppressive effects currently under investigation. Therefore, the combination of vaccines with other immunotherapies has clear theoretic advantages as the results of ongoing clinical trials are awaited.

REFERENCES

1. Pradeu T, Cooper EL. The danger theory: 20 years later. Front Immunol 2012;3: 287.
2. Bakker AB, Schreurs MW, de Boer AJ, et al. Melanocyte lineage-specific antigen gp100 is recognized by melanoma-derived tumor-infiltrating lymphocytes. J Exp Med 1994;179(3):1005–9.
3. Reynolds SR, Celis E, Sette A, et al. HLA-independent heterogeneity of CD8+ T cell responses to MAGE-3, Melan-A/MART-1, gp100, Tyrosinase, MC1R, and TRP-2 in vaccine-treated melanoma patients. J Immunol 1998; 161(12):6970–6.
4. Colella TA, Bullock TNJ, Russell LB, et al. Self-tolerance to the murine homologue of a tyrosinase-derived melanoma antigen: implications for tumor immunotherapy. J Exp Med 2000;191(7):1221–32.
5. Rosenberg SA, Yang JC, Schwartzentruber DJ, et al. Recombinant fowlpox viruses encoding the anchor-modified gp100 melanoma antigen can generate antitumor immune responses in patients with metastatic melanoma. Clin Cancer Res 2003;9(8):2973–80.
6. Overwijk WW, Tsung A, Irvine KR, et al. gp100/pmel 17 is a murine tumor rejection antigen: induction of "self"-reactive, tumoricidal T cells using high-affinity, altered peptide ligand. J Exp Med 1998;188(2):277–86.
7. Liu Q, Zhu H, Liu Y, et al. BRAF peptide vaccine facilitates therapy of murine BRAF-mutant melanoma. Cancer Immunol Immunother 2018;67(2):299–310.

8. Cintolo JA, Datta J, Xu S, et al. Type I-polarized BRAF-pulsed dendritic cells induce antigen-specific CD8+ T cells that impact BRAF-mutant murine melanoma. Melanoma Res 2016;26(1):1–11.

9. Somasundaram R, Swoboda R, Caputo L, et al. Human leukocyte antigen-A2-restricted CTL responses to mutated BRAF peptides in melanoma patients. Cancer Res 2006;66(6):3287–93.

10. Sharkey MS, Lizée G, Gonzales MI, et al. CD4(+) T-cell recognition of mutated B-RAF in melanoma patients harboring the V599E mutation. Cancer Res 2004; 64(5):1595–9.

11. Fijak M, Bhushan S, Meinhardt A. Immunoprivileged sites: the testis. Methods Mol Biol 2011;677:459–70.

12. Robbins PF, Kassim SH, Tran TLN, et al. A pilot trial using lymphocytes genetically engineered with an NY-ESO-1-reactive T-cell receptor: long-term follow-up and correlates with response. Clin Cancer Res 2015;21(5):1019–27.

13. Dreno B, Thompson JF, Smithers BM, et al. MAGE-A3 immunotherapeutic as adjuvant therapy for patients with resected, MAGE-A3-positive, stage III melanoma (DERMA): a double-blind, randomised, placebo-controlled, phase 3 trial. Lancet Oncol 2018;19(7):916–29.

14. Johnson LA, Morgan RA, Dudley ME, et al. Gene therapy with human and mouse T-cell receptors mediates cancer regression and targets normal tissues expressing cognate antigen. Blood 2009;114(3):535–46.

15. Tung KSK, Harakal J, Qiao H, et al. Egress of sperm autoantigen from seminiferous tubules maintains systemic tolerance. J Clin Invest 2017;127(3):1046–60.

16. Petersen J, Wurzbacher SJ, Williamson NA, et al. Phosphorylated self-peptides alter human leukocyte antigen class I-restricted antigen presentation and generate tumor-specific epitopes. Proc Natl Acad Sci U S A 2009;106(8): 2776–81.

17. Mohammed F, Cobbold M, Zarling AL, et al. Phosphorylation-dependent interaction between antigenic peptides and MHC class I: a molecular basis for the presentation of transformed self. Nat Immunol 2008;9(11):1236–43.

18. Depontieu FR, Qian J, Zarling AL, et al. Identification of tumor-associated, MHC class II-restricted phosphopeptides as targets for immunotherapy. Proc Natl Acad Sci U S A 2009;106(29):12073–8.

19. Mohammed F, Stones DH, Zarling AL, et al. The antigenic identity of human class I MHC phosphopeptides is critically dependent upon phosphorylation status. Oncotarget 2017;8(33):54160–72.

20. Zarling AL, Obeng RC, Desch AN, et al. MHC-restricted phosphopeptides from insulin receptor substrate-2 and CDC25b offer broad-based immunotherapeutic agents for cancer. Cancer Res 2014;74(23):6784–95.

21. Robbins PF, Lu Y-C, El-Gamil M, et al. Mining exomic sequencing data to identify mutated antigens recognized by adoptively transferred tumor-reactive T cells. Nat Med 2013;19(6):747–52.

22. Lu Y-C, Yao X, Crystal JS, et al. Efficient identification of mutated cancer antigens recognized by T cells associated with durable tumor regressions. Clin Cancer Res 2014;20(13):3401–10.

23. Sahin U, Derhovanessian E, Miller M, et al. Personalized RNA mutanome vaccines mobilize poly-specific therapeutic immunity against cancer. Nature 2017; 547(7662):222–6.

24. Carreno BM, Magrini V, Becker-Hapak M, et al. A dendritic cell vaccine increases the breadth and diversity of melanoma neoantigen-specific T cells. Science 2015; 348(6236):803–8.

25. Ott PA, Hu Z, Keskin DB, et al. An immunogenic personal neoantigen vaccine for patients with melanoma. Nature 2017;547(7662):217–21.

26. Reed CM, Cresce ND, Mauldin IS, et al. Vaccination with melanoma helper peptides induces antibody responses associated with improved overall survival. Clin Cancer Res 2015;21(17):3879–87.

27. Hu Y, Kim H, Blackwell CM, et al. Long-term outcomes of helper peptide vaccination for metastatic melanoma. Ann Surg 2015;262(3):456–64 [discussion: 462–4].

28. Slingluff CL, Petroni GR, Chianese-Bullock KA, et al. Immunologic and clinical outcomes of a randomized phase II trial of two multipeptide vaccines for melanoma in the adjuvant setting. Clin Cancer Res 2007;13(21):6386–95.

29. Slingluff CL, Petroni GR, Olson WC, et al. Effect of granulocyte/macrophage colony-stimulating factor on circulating CD8+ and CD4+ T-cell responses to a multipeptide melanoma vaccine: outcome of a multicenter randomized trial. Clin Cancer Res 2009;15(22):7036–44.

30. Slingluff CL, Petroni GR, Chianese-Bullock KA, et al. Randomized multicenter trial of the effects of melanoma-associated helper peptides and cyclophosphamide on the immunogenicity of a multipeptide melanoma vaccine. J Clin Oncol 2011; 29(21):2924–32.

31. Rosenberg SA, Sherry RM, Morton KE, et al. Tumor progression can occur despite the induction of very high levels of self/tumor antigen-specific CD8+ T cells in patients with melanoma. J Immunol 2005;175(9):6169–76.

32. Sabbatini P, Tsuji T, Ferran L, et al. Phase I trial of overlapping long peptides from a tumor self-antigen and poly-ICLC shows rapid induction of integrated immune response in ovarian cancer patients. Clin Cancer Res 2012;18(23):6497–508.

33. Slingluff CL, Chianese-Bullock KA, Bullock TNJ, et al. Immunity to melanoma antigens: from self-tolerance to immunotherapy. Adv Immunol 2006;90:243–95.

34. Nitschke NJ, Bjoern J, Iversen TZ, et al. Indoleamine 2,3-dioxygenase and survivin peptide vaccine combined with temozolomide in metastatic melanoma. Stem Cell Investig 2017;4. https://doi.org/10.21037/sci.2017.08.06.

35. Zeng G, Li Y, El-Gamil M, et al. Generation of NY-ESO-1-specific CD4+ and CD8+ T cells by a single peptide with dual MHC class I and class II specificities: a new strategy for vaccine design. Cancer Res 2002;62(13):3630–5.

36. Brinckerhoff LH, Kalashnikov VV, Thompson LW, et al. Terminal modifications inhibit proteolytic degradation of an immunogenic MART-1(27-35) peptide: implications for peptide vaccines. Int J Cancer 1999;83(3):326–34.

37. Knutson KL, Schiffman K, Cheever MA, et al. Immunization of cancer patients with a HER-2/neu, HLA-A2 peptide, p369-377, results in short-lived peptide-specific immunity. Clin Cancer Res 2002;8(5):1014–8.

38. Schwartzentruber DJ, Lawson DH, Richards JM, et al. gp100 peptide vaccine and interleukin-2 in patients with advanced melanoma. N Engl J Med 2011; 364(22):2119–27.

39. Kawakami Y, Eliyahu S, Jennings C, et al. Recognition of multiple epitopes in the human melanoma antigen gp100 by tumor-infiltrating T lymphocytes associated with in vivo tumor regression. J Immunol 1995;154(8):3961–8.

40. Hodi FS, O'Day SJ, McDermott DF, et al. Improved survival with ipilimumab in patients with metastatic melanoma. N Engl J Med 2010;363(8):711–23.

41. Hailemichael Y, Woods A, Fu T, et al. Cancer vaccine formulation dictates synergy with CTLA-4 and PD-L1 checkpoint blockade therapy. J Clin Invest 2018;128(4): 1338–54.

42. Bijker MS, van den Eeden SJF, Franken KL, et al. CD8+ CTL priming by exact peptide epitopes in incomplete Freund's adjuvant induces a vanishing CTL response, whereas long peptides induce sustained CTL reactivity. J Immunol 2007;179(8):5033–40.

43. Wilgenhof S, Van Nuffel AMT, Corthals J, et al. Therapeutic vaccination with an autologous mRNA electroporated dendritic cell vaccine in patients with advanced melanoma. J Immunother 2011;34(5):448–56.

44. Wilgenhof S, Van Nuffel AMT, Benteyn D, et al. A phase IB study on intravenous synthetic mRNA electroporated dendritic cell immunotherapy in pretreated advanced melanoma patients. Ann Oncol 2013;24(10):2686–93.

45. Patel PM, Ottensmeier CH, Mulatero C, et al. Targeting gp100 and TRP-2 with a DNA vaccine: Incorporating T cell epitopes with a human IgG1 antibody induces potent T cell responses that are associated with favourable clinical outcome in a phase I/II trial. Oncoimmunology 2018;7(6):e1433516.

46. Faries MB, Mozzillo N, Kashani-Sabet M, et al. Long-term survival after complete surgical resection and adjuvant immunotherapy for distant melanoma metastases. Ann Surg Oncol 2017;24(13):3991–4000.

47. Bystryn JC, Zeleniuch-Jacquotte A, Oratz R, et al. Double-blind trial of a polyvalent, shed-antigen, melanoma vaccine. Clin Cancer Res 2001;7(7):1882–7.

48. Awate S, Babiuk LA, Mutwiri G. Mechanisms of action of adjuvants. Front Immunol 2013;4. https://doi.org/10.3389/fimmu.2013.00114.

49. Temizoz B, Kuroda E, Ishii KJ. Vaccine adjuvants as potential cancer immunotherapeutics. Int Immunol 2016;28(7):329–38.

50. O'Neill DW, Adams S, Goldberg JD, et al. Comparison of the immunogenicity of Montanide ISA 51 adjuvant and cytokine-matured dendritic cells in a randomized controlled clinical trial of melanoma vaccines. J Clin Oncol 2009;27(15S):3002.

51. Slingluff CL, Petroni GR, Yamshchikov GV, et al. Clinical and immunologic results of a randomized phase II trial of vaccination using four melanoma peptides either administered in granulocyte-macrophage colony-stimulating factor in adjuvant or pulsed on dendritic cells. J Clin Oncol 2003;21(21):4016–26.

52. Hailemichael Y, Dai Z, Jaffarzad N, et al. Persistent antigen at vaccination sites induces tumor-specific CD8$^+$ T cell sequestration, dysfunction and deletion. Nat Med 2013;19(4):465–72.

53. Melssen M, Petroni G, Grosh WW, et al. A multipeptide vaccine plus toll-like receptor (TLR) agonists LPS or polyICLC in combination with incomplete Freund's adjuvant (IFA) in melanoma patients. 31st Annual Meeting and Associated Programs of the Society for Immunotherapy of Cancer (SITC 2016). National Harbor (MD), November 10–12, 2016.

54. Mullins DW, Sheasley SL, Ream RM, et al. Route of immunization with peptide-pulsed dendritic cells controls the distribution of memory and effector T cells in lymphoid tissues and determines the pattern of regional tumor control. J Exp Med 2003;198(7):1023–34.

55. Dillman RO, Cornforth AN, Nistor GI, et al. Randomized phase II trial of autologous dendritic cell vaccines versus autologous tumor cell vaccines in metastatic melanoma: 5-year follow up and additional analyses. J Immunother Cancer 2018; 6(1):19.

56. Tacken PJ, de Vries IJM, Torensma R, et al. Dendritic-cell immunotherapy: from ex vivo loading to in vivo targeting. Nat Rev Immunol 2007;7(10):790–802.

57. Hangalapura BN, Timares L, Oosterhoff D, et al. CD40-targeted adenoviral cancer vaccines: the long and winding road to the clinic. J Gene Med 2012;14(6): 416–27.

58. Hoki T, Yamauchi T, Odunsi K, et al. Synergistic anti-tumor efficacy of combined TLR3 and CD40 neoantigen vaccine requires Batf3-dependent dendritic cells. J Immunol 2018;200(1 Suppl):181.7.

59. Alexopoulou L, Holt AC, Medzhitov R, et al. Recognition of double-stranded RNA and activation of NF-kappaB by Toll-like receptor 3. Nature 2001;413(6857): 732–8.

60. Perrot I, Deauvieau F, Massacrier C, et al. TLR3 and Rig-like receptor on myeloid dendritic cells and Rig-like receptor on human NK cells are both mandatory for production of IFN-gamma in response to double-stranded RNA. J Immunol 2010;185(4):2080–8.

61. Tsuji T, Sabbatini P, Jungbluth AA, et al. Effect of Montanide and poly-ICLC adjuvant on human self/tumor antigen-specific CD4+ T cells in phase I overlapping long peptide vaccine trial. Cancer Immunol Res 2013;1(5):340–50.

62. Speiser DE, Liénard D, Rufer N, et al. Rapid and strong human CD8+ T cell responses to vaccination with peptide, IFA, and CpG oligodeoxynucleotide 7909. J Clin Invest 2005;115(3):739–46.

63. Haining WN, Davies J, Kanzler H, et al. CpG oligodeoxynucleotides alter lymphocyte and dendritic cell trafficking in humans. Clin Cancer Res 2008;14(17): 5626–34.

64. Krieg AM. CpG motifs in bacterial DNA and their immune effects. Annu Rev Immunol 2002;20:709–60.

65. Nava-Parada P, Forni G, Knutson KL, et al. Peptide vaccine given with a Toll-like receptor agonist is effective for the treatment and prevention of spontaneous breast tumors. Cancer Res 2007;67(3):1326–34.

66. Peng G, Guo Z, Kiniwa Y, et al. Toll-like receptor 8-mediated reversal of CD4+ regulatory T cell function. Science 2005;309(5739):1380–4.

67. Lee M, Park C-S, Lee Y-R, et al. Resiquimod, a TLR7/8 agonist, promotes differentiation of myeloid-derived suppressor cells into macrophages and dendritic cells. Arch Pharm Res 2014;37(9):1234–40.

68. Dranoff G, Jaffee E, Lazenby A, et al. Vaccination with irradiated tumor cells engineered to secrete murine granulocyte-macrophage colony-stimulating factor stimulates potent, specific, and long-lasting anti-tumor immunity. Proc Natl Acad Sci U S A 1993;90(8):3539–43.

69. Ahlers JD, Dunlop N, Alling DW, et al. Cytokine-in-adjuvant steering of the immune response phenotype to HIV-1 vaccine constructs: granulocyte-macrophage colony-stimulating factor and TNF-alpha synergize with IL-12 to enhance induction of cytotoxic T lymphocytes. J Immunol 1997;158(8):3947–58.

70. Slingluff CL, Petroni GR, Smolkin ME, et al. Immunogenicity for CD8+ and CD4+ T cells of two formulations of an incomplete Freund's adjuvant for multipeptide melanoma vaccines. J Immunother 2010;33(6):630–8.

71. Faries MB, Hsueh EC, Ye X, et al. Effect of granulocyte/macrophage colony-stimulating factor on vaccination with an allogeneic whole-cell melanoma vaccine. Clin Cancer Res 2009;15(22):7029–35.

72. Kirkwood JM, Lee S, Land S, et al. E1696: final analysis of the clinical and immunological results of a multicenter ECOG phase II trial of multi-epitope peptide vaccination for stage IV melanoma with MART-1 (27–35), gp100 (209–217, 210M), and tyrosinase (368–376, 370D) (MGT) +/- IFNα2b and GM-CSF. J Clin Oncol 2004;22(14_suppl):7502.

73. Slingluff CL, Petroni GR, Yamshchikov GV, et al. Immunologic and clinical outcomes of vaccination with a multiepitope melanoma peptide vaccine plus low-

dose interleukin-2 administered either concurrently or on a delayed schedule. J Clin Oncol 2004;22(22):4474–85.

74. Riemann H, Takao J, Shellman YG, et al. Generation of a prophylactic melanoma vaccine using whole recombinant yeast expressing MART-1. Exp Dermatol 2007; 16(10):814–22.

75. Markov OV, Mironova NL, Sennikov SV, et al. Prophylactic dendritic cell-based vaccines efficiently inhibit metastases in murine metastatic melanoma. PLoS One 2015;10(9):e0136911.

76. Phua KKL, Staats HF, Leong KW, et al. Intranasal mRNA nanoparticle vaccination induces prophylactic and therapeutic anti-tumor immunity. Sci Rep 2014;4:5128.

77. van Elsas A, Sutmuller RPM, Hurwitz AA, et al. Elucidating the autoimmune and antitumor effector mechanisms of a treatment based on cytotoxic T lymphocyte antigen-4 blockade in combination with a B16 melanoma vaccine: comparison of prophylaxis and therapy. J Exp Med 2001;194(4):481–90.

78. Kooreman NG, Kim Y, de Almeida PE, et al. Autologous iPSC-based vaccines elicit anti-tumor responses in vivo. Cell Stem Cell 2018;22(4):501–13.e7.

79. Rosenberg SA, Yang JC, Restifo NP. Cancer immunotherapy: moving beyond current vaccines. Nat Med 2004;10(9):909–15.

80. Boon T, Coulie PG, Van den Eynde BJ, et al. Human T cell responses against melanoma. Annu Rev Immunol 2006;24:175–208.

Vaccine Therapies for Breast Cancer

Erin E. Burke, MD, MS[a], Krithika Kodumudi, PhD[b], Ganesan Ramamoorthi, PhD[b], Brian J. Czerniecki, MD, PhD[c],*

KEYWORDS

- Breast cancer • Vaccine therapy • Oncodrivers • Breast cancer immunity

KEY POINTS

- Breast cancer vaccines could provide an effective therapy for both primary prevention of disease and prevention of disease recurrence.
- HER2 and related oncodrivers play a significant role in tumorigenesis and may be ideal targets.
- Several vaccines targeting breast cancer oncodrivers are currently being tested in clinical trials.
- The emergence of new immunotherapies that may be combined with vaccines to increase effectiveness has resulted in renewed efforts in breast cancer vaccine development.

INTRODUCTION

Breast cancer remains the most commonly diagnosed cancer and accounts for the second leading cause of cancer-related deaths in women in the United States.[1] Given that 1 in 8 women will be diagnosed with breast cancer in their lifetime, this disease is a significant public health concern. Since the 1980s, the 5-year survival for patients with breast cancer has improved dramatically.[2] However, for those patients that present with or develop stage IV disease, 5-year survival remains poor at an estimated 27%.[2]

Breast cancer is a heterogeneous disease that has been classified based on histologic characteristics and receptor expression. The most common type of breast cancer is infiltrating ductal carcinoma, representing about 75% of all breast cancers. Infiltrating lobular carcinoma is the second most common subtype of breast cancer accounting for another 5% to 10% of breast cancer diagnoses. Breast cancer is

Disclosures: E.E. Burke, K. Kodumudi and G. Ramamoorthi have no disclosures. B.J. Czerniecki is supported by the CDRMP W81XWH-16-1-0385, the Henle Foundation and Pennies in Action.
[a] H. Lee Moffitt Cancer Center, 12902 Magnolia Drive, Tampa, FL 33612, USA; [b] Clinical Science Lab Department, H. Lee Moffitt Cancer Center, 12902 Magnolia Drive, Tampa, FL 33612, USA; [c] Department of Breast Oncology, H. Lee Moffitt Cancer Center, 12902 Magnolia Drive, Tampa, FL 33612, USA
* Corresponding author.
E-mail address: brian.czerniecki@moffitt.org

then further classified based on the presence or absence of 3 key receptors: estrogen receptor (ER), progesterone receptor (PR), and human epidermal growth factor receptor 2 (HER2).[3] Breast cancers can express 1, 2, all, or none of these 3 receptors, and their pattern of expression can influence both the treatment given as well as the prognosis. The current standard treatment of breast cancer most often requires a multimodality approach with surgery, radiation therapy, and chemotherapy, including cytotoxic chemotherapy, as well as targeted therapies and hormonal therapies. Although this treatment has proved to be effective, it is known to have several side effects. Furthermore, in most cases, with the exception of hormonal therapy, these treatments do little to prevent the disease in the first place. There has been significant interest in the development of therapies that can prevent breast cancer from developing in the first place, as well as therapies that can prevent breast cancer recurrence.

Vaccines are a well-known, cost-effective tool used for disease prevention. Their ability to prevent cancer has recently been shown for cancers caused by infectious agents, such as in the case of human papilloma virus (HPV).[4] But whether a vaccine can be used to prevent a primary cancer not believed to be caused by infection remains unknown. This article aims to review the current data on vaccines for potential primary prevention of breast cancer, prevention of breast cancer recurrence, as well as the potential use of vaccines with other therapies.

ONCODRIVERS IN BREAST CANCER

The aggressive features of breast cancer are mainly driven by the overexpression of important high-affinity transmembrane receptors such as HER2, HER3, EGFR, c-MET, and transmembrane protein epithelial mucin-1 (MUC-1).[5] The HER2 and HER3 receptors belong to the family of human epidermal growth factor receptors and are critically involved in cell growth, proliferation, survival, and differentiation.[6] The overexpression and aberrant activation of HER2 and HER3 constitutively activate downstream signaling cascades that lead to breast cancer cell proliferation, resistance to apoptosis, angiogenesis, invasiveness, and metastatic spread.[7] HER2 overexpression is present in approximately 20% of patients with early-stage breast cancer. The monoclonal antibodies trastuzumab and pertuzumab are currently available therapies for the treatment of patients with HER2 overexpressing breast cancer. Lapatinib (a tyrosine kinase inhibitor) is another treatment alternative that has been approved to treat advanced HER2-positive breast cancer.[8]

MUC-1, a transmembrane protein, has been found to be highly expressed in approximately 90% of patients with breast cancer. An emerging body of research has suggested that MUC-1 is involved in tumor growth, increased cancer cell proliferation, and metastasis in breast cancer.[9] MUC-1 exhibits a novel role in ER-positive breast cancer through enhancing ER-dependent transcriptional activation, which then mediates ER-positive cancer cell growth and survival.[10,11] In addition, MUC1 has been shown to protect against oxidative stress–mediated degradation of EGFR, which further aids the growth of EGFR-positive breast cancer cells.[12]

CELLULAR AND HUMORAL IMMUNE RESPONSE IN BREAST CANCER

In the tumorigenic environment, the uncontrolled growing tumor cells secrete various chemokines, angiogenic factors, and growth factors that promote angiogenesis and tumor invasion.[13] During breast cancer development, tumor-associated macrophages infiltrate the tumor microenvironment and enhance the secretion of VEGF and matrix metalloproteinases, which then aid angiogenesis and tumor invasion. Granulocyte-macrophage colony-stimulating factor (GM-CSF) efficiently controls the activity of macrophages. GM-CSF present in the tumor microenvironment milieu acts on mono-cytes to secrete soluble VEGFR-1 to block and deactivate VEGF-mediated angiogen-esis in breast cancer. In addition, GM-CSF can enhance macrophage-mediated tumor antigen presentation, which induces strong tumor-associated antigen (TAA)–specific immunity.[14,15]

Dendritic cells recognize TAAs in the tumor microenvironment and then migrate to lymph nodes to present TAAs to CD8+ cytotoxic T cells and CD4+ helper T cells, which then create a strong tumor antigen–specific immunity.[16] Strong cytotoxic T lymphocyte and CD4+ T cell–mediated immunity has been identified for various key breast cancer oncodrivers, such as HER2, EGFR, MUC1, hTERT, and CEA, which highlights the crucial role of immune cells in tumor burden clearance.[5,17] Importantly, the HER2-specific and HER3-specific CD4+ Th1 cells immune response are critically essential to reduce tumor growth, eliminate residual disease recurrence, and improve the disease-free survival rate in HER2-expressing breast cancer and HER3-expressing breast cancer.[18,19] Unfortunately, this tumor antigen–associated immunity can easily break down by the action of immunosuppressive cells such as myeloid-derived suppressor cells and CD4+ Foxp3+ CD25+ Treg cells.

Interferon gamma (IFN-γ), a master immune modulating cytokine, also plays a key role in mediating immunity against different cancers. Various types of immune cells, including Th1 CD4+ T cells, CD8+ T cells, and natural killer cells, predominantly pro-duce IFN-γ to mediate specific antitumor immunity.[20] IFN-γ greatly inhibits breast cancer cell growth and proliferation and induces senescence and apoptotic-mediated cancer cell death.[21] IFN-γ has the potential to enhance the expression of major histocompatibility complex (MHC) I and MHC II molecules on antigen-presenting cells as well as tumor cells, which leads to reorganization of TAAs and strong activation of CD4+ T cell and CD8+ T cell antitumor immune response.[22]

Interleukin 21 (IL-21), is another cytokine that plays a diverse role in the immune sys-tem regulation, including the ability to induce differentiation and programming of T cells.[23] IL-21 also efficiently mediates differentiation/maintenance of CD8+ T cells against TAAs. IL-21 has been considered as a potent immunotherapeutic agent for the treatment of HER2 overexpressing breast cancer because of its crucial role in con-trolling the immune response.[24]

VACCINE-BASED THERAPY

Activation and amplification of TAA-specific immunity with prolonged memory T cell immune response can be a great strategy to protect patients from breast cancer recurrence. Vaccine-based therapies have received great attention and have shown some promising outcomes in preclinical studies and clinical trials. Vaccines work by priming the immune system to recognize and respond to antigens that signal either the presence of infection or, in the case of cancer vaccines, an antigen that signals the presence of a tumor cell. Cancer vaccines work by presenting an exogenous source of TAA proteins, peptides, and antigenic epitopes to CD4+ T cells and CD8+ T cells by way of MHC I and MHC II. This further enhances cytotoxic T lympho-cyte and helper T cell–mediated immune response against TAAs (**Fig. 1**).[25]

Therapeutic Vaccines

Peptide-based vaccines
Peptide-based vaccines can be either monovalent or polyvalent. Monovalent vaccines induce an immune response to a single antigen, whereas polyvalent vaccines induce an immune response to multiple antigens. Ideal antigens for monovalent vaccines

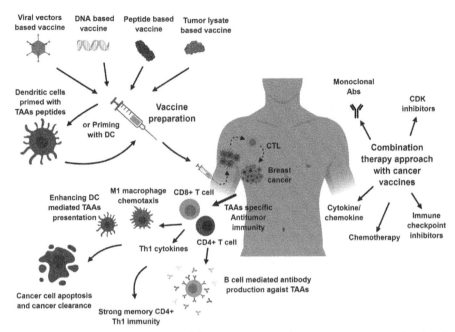

Fig. 1. Overview of the vaccine-based therapies to potentiate strong tumor-associated antigen (TAA)–specific immunity for breast cancer. Breast cancer vaccines can include viral vector–based, DNA-based, peptide-based, tumor lysate–based, or dendritic cell–based vaccines. Breast cancer vaccines promote the presentation of TAAs to CD8+ T cells and CD4+ T cells, which creates an antitumor immune response. The TAA-specific Th1 immunity can further induce chemotaxis of macrophages to the tumor microenvironment, which prevents angiogenesis and breast cancer invasion. In addition, the Th1 cytokines produced by cytotoxic T lymphocytes, CD4+ Th1 cells, and natural killer T cells act on cancer cells to inhibit tumor growth and eradicate their aggressiveness. Some vaccines can activate B cell–mediated antibody production against TAAs and generate long-term memory CD4+ Th1 immune response to avert tumor recurrence in patients with breast cancer.

include antigens that are expressed by most of the tumor cells and are overexpressed in tumor cells. Several monovalent and polyvalent peptide-based vaccines for breast cancer have been proposed.

The E75 peptide vaccine, also known as nelipepimut-S, is a monovalent peptide vaccine that is made up of the E75 peptide, which is derived from the extracellular component of the HER2 protein. It is a vaccine that has been found to stimulate cytotoxic CD8+ T cell response.[26] This vaccine has been studied in combination with use of GM-CSF. Combining the results from 3 early phase trials, a total of 108 women with node-positive or high-risk node-negative disease were treated with E75 vaccine plus GM-CSF and another 79 women were observed (**Table 1**). After follow-up of 60 months, the disease-free survival (DFS) for women who received the E75 vaccine was 89.7% versus 80.2% for the women who were observed ($P = .08$).[27–29] In patients who got the optimal dosing of E75 and GM-CSF, the 5-year DFS was 94.6% for those women who received the vaccine compared with 80.2% in the control group ($P = .05$).[30] Of particular interest was the subgroup analysis from these studies, which showed that patients with tumors that had low levels of HER2 expression had a higher maximum immune response than patients with tumors that had high HER2

Table 1
Summary of completed and ongoing clinical trials looking at vaccine therapy for DCIS and breast cancer

Trial Registration #	Patient Population	Drug	Primary End Point	Secondary End Point	Results
NCT00854789	Breast cancer, negative nodes	E75 + GM-CSF vaccine	Safety, optimal dosing, immune response	Time to disease recurrence	Optimal dosing determined, safety demonstrated, DFS improved in those who got optimal dosing
NCT00841399	Breast cancer, positive nodes	E75 + GM-CSF vaccine	Safety, optimal dosing, immune response	Time to disease recurrence	Optimal dosing determined, safety demonstrated, DFS improved in those who got optimal dosing
NCT01479244	Node-positive breast cancer, low HER2 expression	NeuVax vaccine (E75)	3-y disease-free survival (DFS)	5 and 10-y DFS, overall survival, safety profile	Enrollment complete, study halted for futility
NCT00524277	Breast cancer, node-positive or high-risk node-negative	GP2 peptide + GM-CSF vaccine	DFS	Safety, immune response	No difference in DFS between study arm and control arm
	Node-negative HER2-positive breast cancer	AE37 vaccine	Safety, optimal dosing	Immune response	Safe, optimal dosing determined, able to illicit immune response
	Metastatic breast cancer	Chemotherapy + STn-KLH vaccine (Theratope)	Time to disease progression, overall survival	Safety, quality of life, immune response	No difference in time to disease progression, survival advantage for vaccine plus endocrine therapy

(continued on next page)

Table 1
(continued)

Trial Registration #	Patient Population	Drug	Primary End Point	Secondary End Point	Results
	Stage II breast cancer	Oxidized mannan-MUC-1 vaccine	Recurrence rate	n/a	Significant decrease in recurrence rate in those who received vaccine (12.5% versus 60%)
NCT00179309	Metastatic breast cancer	PANVAC + docetaxel	Progression-free survival	Rate of adverse events	Trend toward improved progression-free survival in vaccine arm
NCT00971737	Metastatic breast cancer, HER2 negative	GVAX and cyclophosphamide plus or minus trastuzumab	Toxicity, progression-free survival, immune responses, pharmacodynamics	Immmune priming, enumeration of CD8+ T cells, characterization of T cell memory pool	Awaiting results
	Breast cancer with depressed immunity	MCF-7 vaccine + GM-CSF and IL-2	10-y disease-specific survival	TAA-specific immunity loss	Significant improvement in DSS in vaccinated patients with immunity loss
Dnr151:785/2001	Metastatic breast cancer, HER2 positive	HER2- plasmid DNA vaccine + GM-CSF and IL-2	Safety and tolerability	Immune response	No toxic effects, immune response identified
	Metastatic breast cancer	hTERT peptide vaccine	Immune response	Overall survival	Immune response demonstrated
	DCIS, HER2 positive	HER2 dendritic cell vaccine	Safety and feasibility	Immune response	Safety demonstrated, 18.5% had no residual DCIS after treatment
NCT02061332	DCIS or breast cancer <5 mm in size, HER2 positive	HER2 dendritic cell vaccine	Safety and tolerability, immune response	Clinical response	Safety and immune response demonstrated, 24% had no residual disease after treatment

expression.[31] In addition, there was a trend toward increased 24-month overall survival for those patients who were vaccinated versus controls in the subgroup of patients who had low HER2 expression (6.8% versus 0%, $P = .8$).[31] A phase 3 trial (PRESENT trial, NCT01479244) aimed to answer the question of the efficacy of the E75 vaccine in patients with node-positive breast cancer and low to intermediate expression of HER2, and this study completed enrollment; however, it was halted by the data safety and monitoring board due to futility (see **Table 1**).[32]

The GP2 HER2 peptide vaccine is another monovalent vaccine that uses a transmembrane portion of the HER2 protein to stimulate the immune system by way of activation of CD8+ cytotoxic T cells. A phase 2 trial investigating this vaccine was completed in which node-positive or high-risk node-negative women were randomized to receive GP2 vaccine with GM-CSF or GM-CSF alone. In a study of 190 patients, no significant difference in DFS was seen at median follow-up of 34 months in the overall study population (see **Table 1**). On subgroup analysis, a trend toward increased DFS was seen in patients with tumors who had overexpression of HER2 and received treatment with the GP2 vaccine and GM-CSF versus patients who received GM-CSF alone; however, this did not reach statistical significance.[33]

Another monovalent HER2 vaccine in development is the AE37 vaccine, and it functions to stimulate the immune system by way of response from both CD4+ helper T cells and CD8+ cytotoxic T cells.[26] This vaccine has been evaluated in a pilot phase 1b study in which a total of 15 patients with node-negative HER-2–expressing breast cancer were treated with the AE37 vaccine and GM-CSF. This study showed significant increase in prevaccination versus postvaccination delayed-type hypersensitivity with no grade 3 or 4 adverse events.[34]

A second target of interest in the development of breast cancer vaccines is MUC-1. The sialyl TN (STn) epitope of MUC-1 has been used as the basis of a vaccine also known as Theratope. This monovalent vaccine was compared with immune adjuvant therapy with keyhole limpet hemocyanin in a phase 3 randomized trial that enrolled patients with metastatic breast cancer previously treated with chemotherapy with responsive or stable disease. In this study, the vaccine did not meet the primary end point of improved disease-free progression.[35] However, in post hoc analysis of this trial, a survival advantage was observed in patients with metastatic breast cancer receiving endocrine therapy plus the sialyl Tn-KLH vaccine. These data suggest the potential for improved clinical outcome by adding the sialyl Tn-KLH vaccine to endocrine therapy in patients with metastatic breast cancer.[36]

More promising results were found in a study of another vaccine that also used the TAA MUC-1. The oxidized mannan-MUC-1 vaccine was evaluated in a pilot phase 3 study in which 31 patients with stage II breast cancer were randomized to injection of the vaccine versus placebo after undergoing standard treatment (see **Table 1**). At 15 years of follow-up, the recurrence rate in those who received placebo was 60% compared with 12.5% in those who received the vaccine ($P = .002$).[37]

Pancreatic vaccine (PANVAC) is a vaccine that encodes for several TAAs seen in breast cancer, such as MUC-1 and CEA, as well as costimulatory molecules. This vaccine was evaluated in a phase 2 trial in which patients were randomized to receive docetaxel with or without PANVAC (see **Table 1**). The primary end point was improved progression-free survival, and there was a trend toward improved progression-free survival in those patients who got both docetaxel and PANVAC versus docetaxel alone (7.9 months versus 3.9 months, $P = .09$).[38]

In a phase 1 clinical trial, the DPX-0907 vaccine, another polyvalent vaccine, composed of 7 MHC I peptides and T helper cell peptide epitope was investigated in patients with breast cancer, ovarian cancer, and prostate cancer. Seventy-three percent of patients showed antigen-specific immune responses to all of the peptides (NCT01095848).[39]

Whole-cell lysate vaccines

Cell-based vaccines induce an immune response by exposing the immune system to an exogenous source of whole cellular or modified cellular components from either tumor or immune cells that can be derived from the patient or a donor. Compared with monovalent vaccines, they should allow for broader activation of the immune system and decreased resistance of tumor cells.[40] One of the early cell-based vaccines comprised autologous breast cancer cells that were infected with Newcastle disease virus to increase expression of interferon-β.[40] In those patients with previously treated metastatic breast cancer, there was a trend toward improved DFS in those who received the high-quality vaccine compared with those who received the low-quality vaccine.[41]

GVAX is an allogeneic cellular vaccine that is derived from irradiated human tumor cancer cells that are transduced to express GM-CSF. This vaccine has previously been studied in other cancers. It is now under investigation for breast cancer in a phase 2 trial in which this vaccine is combined with the use of cyclophosphamide and trastuzumab in patients with metastatic breast cancer (NCT00971737).[42]

The therapeutic potential of a vaccine composed of autologous and allogenic whole tumor cells (MCF-7) in combination with other tumorigenic antigens, such as CA 15-3, CA-125, and CEA was tested in 37 immune-suppressed patients with breast cancer. Adjuvant therapy with 2 biological agents, GM-CSF and IL-2, were provided as standard of care after the completion of vaccination. This study found significantly improved 10-year disease-specific survival (DSS) of 89% after standard care therapy with GM-CSF and IL-2 biological adjuvants in vaccinated patients compared with unvaccinated immune-suppressed historical control patients (DSS 59%).[43]

Viral or DNA-based vaccines

Recombinant DNA or viral vector–based vaccines can potentially be used to provide TAAs to generate TAA-specific cellular and humoral immune response. Previously, a pilot clinical trial in patients with HER2 overexpressing metastatic breast cancer showed the safety and efficiency of DNA plasmid–encoded HER2 vaccine in combination with GM-CSF and IL-2 followed by trastuzumab treatment (see **Table 1**). Strong HER2-specific MHC-II–restricted T cell immune response was observed after long-term follow-up. In addition, an increased level of anti-HER2 antibodies was detected after long-term follow-up in patients who received combination treatment with vaccine, GM-CSF, IL-2, and trastuzumab.[44]

Human telomerase reverse transcriptase (hTERT) has been shown to be highly expressed in various malignancies, including breast cancer.[45] One clinical trial investigated the effect of hTERT peptide–based vaccine in patients with metastatic breast cancer. The hTERT peptide–based vaccine showed 4% to 13% of postvaccine CD8+ cytotoxic tumor-infiltrating lymphocytes (TILs) to be specific against immunized hTERT peptide; these TILs were not present before vaccination. This study also showed increased production of IFN-γ after vaccination. Furthermore, in those who had an immune response to hTERT, median overall survival was improved.[46]

Dendritic cell vaccines

The cell-based vaccines of perhaps greatest interest in breast cancer are those vaccines that use dendritic cells (DCs). Dendritic cells have several characteristics that make them appealing for vaccine development. Dendritic cells are considered the most effective of all antigen-presenting cells, because they are significantly more potent at inducing T cell proliferation and activation than other antigen-presenting cells. DCs are also able to cross prime, which is necessary for the development of antigen-specific cytotoxic T cells.[47] The HER2 DC vaccine, one such DC vaccine, has been investigated in patients with ductal carcinoma in situ (DCIS), an early noninvasive breast lesion that left untreated can progress to infiltrating ductal carcinoma. In a study by Sharma and colleagues,[48] the HER2 vaccine was administered intranodally before surgical resection in 27 patients with HER2 overexpressing DCIS. In 18.5% of patients, there was no evidence of DCIS on final pathology after surgical resection (ie, complete pathologic response). In patients with remaining DCIS, 50% had HER2 expression (a known driver in the progression of breast cancer) that was completely eradicated. In another study looking at HER2 DC vaccine, HER2-positive patients with DCIS or early-stage breast cancer were randomized to receive intralesional, intranodal, or both intralesion and intranodal administration of the HER2 DC vaccine before surgical treatment. In this study, 13 patients (24%) had a complete pathologic response; this rate was higher in those patients with DCIS (28.6%) versus those patients with early-stage breast cancer (8.3%) (see **Table 1**).[49] These results show promise in the development of DC vaccines and are some of the first to show potential for possible primary prevention of breast cancer.

Preventive Vaccines

The preventive or prophylactic vaccine strategy for breast cancer has been proposed for the possible prevention of breast cancer development from its early premalignant lesions. However, the main difficulty in developing preventive vaccines is the development of autoimmune-mediated complications. In contrast, encouraging preclinical results have shown that preventive vaccines are safe and highly effective against animal models for breast cancer.

α-Lactalbumin is a breast-specific differentiation protein that is only expressed during lactation but not in normal breast tissue. Studies have found that α-lactalbumin is highly expressed in about 55% to 60% of breast cancers. Approximately 75% of triple-negative breast cancers (TNBC) express α-lactalbumin.[50] One recent study has shown that α-lactalbumin vaccination prevented the development of breast cancer in mouse mammary tumor virus (MMTV)-neu mice, which develop breast cancer spontaneously. Importantly, α-lactalbumin vaccination greatly enhanced the infiltration of IFN-γ–producing CD4+ Th1 cells and CD8+ cytotoxic T cells and provided strong immunity against tumor development.[51] Another recent preclinical study reported that immunization of experimental mice with α-lactalbumin vaccination prevented tumor growth in BALB/cJ mice bearing 4T1 cell tumors. In addition, a enhanced antitumor response with increased CD4+ T cells and CD8+ T cells was observed when BALB/cJ mice bearing 4T1 cell tumors were treated in combination with α-lactalbumin and tamoxifen.[50] Furthermore, α-lactalbumin vaccine was able to prevent tumor development in BALB/c mice injected with 4T1 TNBC.[52] Collectively, these findings suggest that α-lactalbumin vaccine exhibits promising preventive benefits.

DCs transfected with $_{RGD}$AdVneu have also been investigated in the preclinical setting, and this work has shown that these cells mediate a powerful HER2 tumor antigen–specific CD8+ cytotoxic T cell immune response and humoral immunity in a FVB/NJ transgenic mice model. The $_{RGD}$AdVneu transfected DC vaccine was able to prevent tumor growth in wild-type FVB/NJ mice that had been challenged with HER2-expressing Tg1-1 tumor cells.[53]

Another study has investigated the therapeutic potential of a peptide-based vaccine using 3 different conformational peptide contract sequences, 266 to 296, 298 to 333, and 315 to 333, that mimic regions of the dimerization loop of the HER2 protein. Treatment with each 1 of these peptide vaccines resulted in high-affinity peptide antibodies that inhibited HER2-expressing breast cancer cell proliferation and HER2 cytoplasmic receptor domain phosphorylation resulting in an antitumor effect on tumor growth in vivo. The 266 to 296 peptide vaccine had significantly reduced tumor development in FVB/n and BALB/c transplantable breast cancer models and BALB-neuT and VEGF$^{+/-}$Neu2-5$^{+/-}$ transgenic mice tumor models. These findings suggest that the 266 to 296 epitope peptide should be considered as a promising vaccine for the prevention of HER2-expressing breast cancer.[54]

Finally, a study by Gil and colleagues[55] provided molecular evidence that an HER2-specific MHC class II peptide-based vaccine markedly decreased the development of spontaneous breast cancer in a MMTV-PyMT transgenic mice model through the inhibition HER2. The HER2-specific MHC class II peptide-based vaccine decreased the population of cancer stem cells in MMTV-PyMT transgenic mice.

COMBINATION THERAPY TO IMPROVE VACCINE EFFECTIVENESS

Several possible vaccine and drug combinations are currently being explored to improve outcomes, some of which have already been described. Most of the combination strategies are focused on how to increase the infiltration of T cells at the tumor site. TILs in breast cancer have been associated with improved clinical outcome. The rationale for the multidrug approach to improve vaccine efficacy is discussed in the following sections.

Cytokines/Chemokines

The effect of TERT DNA-based vaccine primed with CCL21 chemokine was tested in a TS/A mouse breast cancer model as a preventive and therapeutic regimen. This study showed that, in TS/A mice, CCL21 treatment followed by addition of TERT DNA vaccine significantly enhanced TERT-specific cell-mediated immune response compared with TERT DNA vaccine alone in preventive as well as therapeutic models. This suggests that the combination therapy of chemokine CCL21 with TERT DNA-based vaccine can prevent breast cancer progression by way of augmented anti-TERT tumor antigen–specific cell-mediated immunity.[56]

Another study has demonstrated that a plasmid DNA (pDNA)–based vaccine that coexpresses HER2 and CCL21 reduced tumor development by mediating a strong Th1 polarized immunity in D2F2/E2 cell syngeneic HER2 BALB/c mice models. The pDNA-based vaccine expressing HER2, CCL21, and GM-CSF protected 70% of experimental mice from tumor growth in D2F2/E2 cell syngeneic HER2 BALB/c mice models. This evidence strongly suggests that pDNA-based vaccines expressing HER2 in combination with biological adjuvants CCL21 and GM-CSF can eradicate residual HER2 breast cancer and ought to be investigated in clinical trials.[57]

Checkpoint Inhibitors

Tumor cells escape the immune response by upregulating immunosuppressive ligands that bind to inhibitory coreceptors on the surface of activated T cells and turn off antitumor immune responses. This has led to limited success in immunotherapy trials including cancer vaccines to activate and expand tumor-specific T cells. Although these immune checkpoint receptors maintain T cell homeostasis, when expressed by tumor-specific T cells, they represent a significant barrier for the induction of maximum antitumor immune responses. Breast tumor cells also express several molecules involved in immune checkpoint regulation. Programmed death ligand-1 (PD-L1) is expressed within breast tumors by malignant mammary epithelial cells, particularly in tumors with high-risk features.[58] Blockade of these receptors has been shown to improve tumor-specific T cell responses. Checkpoint inhibitors PD-/PD-L1 have been investigated in various clinical trials in metastatic breast cancer and TNBCs. For example, the PANACEA trial suggested that the combination of trastuzumab and anti-PD1 resulted in a 15% overall response rate in stage IV HER2-positive patients progressing on HER2 targeted therapies.[59] Those with PDL1 expression or greater than 5% tumor lymphocytes had a response rate of almost 40%.[59] Furthermore, stromal TILs were identified as a potential predictive marker. It is findings such as this that suggest that combining therapies that increase the immune response to breast cancer might also increase the effectiveness of vaccines for breast cancer.

Cyclin-Dependent Kinase Inhibitors

Cell-cycle deregulation in breast cancer is a major hallmark of uncontrolled growth, invasion, and metastasis. Cyclin-dependent kinases (CDKs) and cyclin complex play a critical role in progression and regulation of the cell cycle. The aberrant activation or loss of action of CDKs favors unrestricted cancer cell growth, which suggests that targeting or inhibiting the action of CDKs can be an ideal.[60,61] In particular, the G1/S cell-cycle transition phase has been the focus to investigate the therapeutic potential of various targeted small-molecule inhibitors. Today, the most specific inhibitors, such as palbociclib, ribociclib, and abemaciclib, are available to target CDK4 and CDK6, and their efficiency has been tested in various cancers.[62] Currently, various clinical trials have been evaluating the therapeutic efficacy of these CDK4 and CDK6 inhibitors in combination with intracellular signaling cascade inhibitors or hormone therapy in breast cancer. The results of these studies suggest that, moving forward, they may also be combined with vaccines for improved effect.

SUMMARY

Although clinical response rates to vaccines have been modest despite the induction of strong antitumor T cell responses, it is through these approaches that valuable insight and knowledge about tumor immunology have been gained. The lack of clinical effectiveness of several vaccines thus far should not mean that these vaccine approaches should be abandoned. Rather it should emphasize the need for changes in the application of these approaches for the primary prevention of breast cancer as well as secondary prevention of breast cancer recurrence. Strategies to enhance the potency of vaccines are currently being explored. Some exciting immunotherapeutic strategies, including restoring anti-oncodriver Th1 immune responses, blockade of coinhibitory immune checkpoints as well as combination therapies are in development. Future success is likely to lie in using vaccines in the preventive setting and for prevention of recurrence. Therapeutic vaccines are likely to augment existing treatment modalities and will require approaches to increase their effectiveness.

REFERENCES

1. Cancer.org. Cancer facts & figures. 2018. Available at: https://www.cancer.org/content/dam/cancer-org/research/cancer-facts-and-statistics/annual-cancer-facts-and-figures/2018/cancer-facts-and-figures-2018.pdf. Accessed July 1, 2018.
2. SEER cancer stat facts: female breast cancer. Available at: https://seer.cancer.gov/stsfacts/html/breast.html. Accessed July 1, 2018.

3. Hammond ME, Hayes DF, Dowsett M, et al. American Society of Clinical Oncology/College of American Pathologists guideline recommendations for immunohistochemical testing of estrogen and progesterone receptors in breast cancer. J Clin Oncol 2010;28(16):2784–95.
4. St Laurent J, Luckett R, Feldman S. HPV vaccination and the effects on rates of HPV-related cancers. Curr Probl Cancer 2018;42(5):493–506.
5. Korkaya H, Wicha MS. HER2 and breast cancer stem cells: more than meets the eye. Cancer Res 2013;73(12):3489–93.
6. Nocera NF, Lee MC, De La Cruz LM, et al. Restoring lost anti-HER-2 Th1 immunity in breast cancer: a crucial role for Th1 cytokines in therapy and prevention. Front Pharmacol 2016;7:356.
7. Arteaga CL, Sliwkowski MX, Osborne CK, et al. Treatment of HER2-positive breast cancer: current status and future perspectives. Nat Rev Clin Oncol 2011;9(1):16–32.
8. Larionov AA. Current therapies for human epidermal growth factor receptor 2-positive metastatic breast cancer patients. Front Oncol 2018;8:89.
9. Kufe DW. MUC1-C oncoprotein as a target in breast cancer: activation of signaling pathways and therapeutic approaches. Oncogene 2013;32(9): 1073–81.
10. Rivalland G, Loveland B, Mitchell P. Update on Mucin-1 immunotherapy in cancer: a clinical perspective. Expert Opin Biol Ther 2015;15(12):1773–87.
11. Blixt O, Bueti D, Burford B, et al. Autoantibodies to aberrantly glycosylated MUC1 in early stage breast cancer are associated with a better prognosis. Breast Cancer Res 2011;13(2):R25.
12. Lakshminarayanan V, Supekar NT, Wei J, et al. MUC1 vaccines, comprised of glycosylated or non-glycosylated peptides or tumor-derived MUC1, can circumvent immunoediting to control tumor growth in MUC1 transgenic mice. PLoS One 2016;11(1):e0145920.
13. Wellenstein MD, de Visser KE. Cancer-cell-intrinsic mechanisms shaping the tumor immune landscape. Immunity 2018;48(3):399–416.
14. Eubank TD, Roberts RD, Khan M, et al. Granulocyte macrophage colony-stimulating factor inhibits breast cancer growth and metastasis by invoking an anti-angiogenic program in tumor-educated macrophages. Cancer Res 2009; 69(5):2133–40.
15. Lin EY, Li JF, Gnatovskiy L, et al. Macrophages regulate the angiogenic switch in a mouse model of breast cancer. Cancer Res 2006;66(23):11238–46.
16. Palucka K, Coussens LM, O'Shaughnessy J. Dendritic cells, inflammation, and breast cancer. Cancer J 2013;19(6):511–6.
17. De La Cruz LM, Nocera NF, Czerniecki BJ. Restoring anti-oncodriver Th1 responses with dendritic cell vaccines in HER2/neu-positive breast cancer: progress and potential. Immunotherapy 2016;8(10):1219–32.
18. De La Cruz LM, McDonald ES, Mick R, et al. Anti-HER2 CD4(+) T-helper type 1 immune response is superior to breast MRI for assessing response to neoadjuvant therapy in patients with HER2-positive breast cancer. Ann Surg Oncol 2017;24(4):1057–63.
19. Fracol M, Datta J, Lowenfeld L, et al. Loss of anti-HER-3 CD4+ T-helper type 1 immunity occurs in breast tumorigenesis and is negatively associated with outcomes. Ann Surg Oncol 2017;24(2):407–17.
20. Schoenborn JR, Wilson CB. Regulation of interferon-gamma during innate and adaptive immune responses. Adv Immunol 2007;96:41–101.

21. Hu X, Ivashkiv LB. Cross-regulation of signaling pathways by interferon-gamma: implications for immune responses and autoimmune diseases. Immunity 2009; 31(4):539–50.
22. Zhou F. Molecular mechanisms of IFN-gamma to up-regulate MHC class I antigen processing and presentation. Int Rev Immunol 2009;28(3–4):239–60.
23. Moroz A, Eppolito C, Li Q, et al. IL-21 enhances and sustains CD8+ T cell responses to achieve durable tumor immunity: comparative evaluation of IL-2, IL-15, and IL-21. J Immunol 2004;173(2):900–9.
24. Mittal D, Sinha D, Barkauskas D, et al. Adenosine 2B receptor expression on cancer cells promotes metastasis. Cancer Res 2016;76(15):4372–82.
25. Costa RLB, Soliman H, Czerniecki BJ. The clinical development of vaccines for HER2(+) breast cancer: current landscape and future perspectives. Cancer Treat Rev 2017;61:107–15.
26. Milani A, Sangiolo D, Aglietta M, et al. Recent advances in the development of breast cancer vaccines. Breast Cancer (Dove Med Press) 2014;6:159–68.
27. Mittendorf EA, Clifton GT, Holmes JP, et al. Clinical trial results of the HER-2/neu (E75) vaccine to prevent breast cancer recurrence in high-risk patients: from US Military Cancer Institute Clinical Trials Group Study I-01 and I-02. Cancer 2012; 118(10):2594–602.
28. Peoples GE, Gurney JM, Hueman MT, et al. Clinical trial results of a HER2/neu (E75) vaccine to prevent recurrence in high-risk breast cancer patients. J Clin Oncol 2005;23(30):7536–45.
29. Peoples GE, Holmes JP, Hueman MT, et al. Combined clinical trial results of a HER2/neu (E75) vaccine for the prevention of recurrence in high-risk breast cancer patients: U.S. Military Cancer Institute Clinical Trials Group Study I-01 and I-02. Clin Cancer Res 2008;14(3):797–803.
30. Holmes JP, Gates JD, Benavides LC, et al. Optimal dose and schedule of an HER-2/neu (E75) peptide vaccine to prevent breast cancer recurrence: from US Military Cancer Institute Clinical Trials Group Study I-01 and I-02. Cancer 2008;113(7):1666–75.
31. Benavides LC, Gates JD, Carmichael MG, et al. The impact of HER2/neu expression level on response to the E75 vaccine: from U.S. Military Cancer Institute Clinical Trials Group Study I-01 and I-02. Clin Cancer Res 2009;15(8):2895–904.
32. Galena Biopharma reports fourth quarter and year end 2016 financial results and provides a corporate update [press release]. Globe Newswire, CNBC2017. https://www.globenewswire.com/news-release/2017/03/15/939867/0/en/Galena-Biopharma-Reports-Fourth-Quarter-and-Year-End-2016-Financial-Results-and-Pr ovides-a-Corporate-Update.html. Accessed July 10, 2018.
33. Schneble E, Perez SA, Murray J, et al. Primary analysis of the prospective, randomized, phase II trial of GP2+GM-CSF vaccine versus GM-CSF alone administered in the adjuvant setting to high-risk breast cancer patients. J Clin Oncol 2014;32(Suppl 26) [abstract 134].
34. Holmes JP, Benavides LC, Gates JD, et al. Results of the first phase I clinical trial of the novel II-key hybrid preventive HER-2/neu peptide (AE37) vaccine. J Clin Oncol 2008;26(20):3426–33.
35. Miles D, Roché H, Martin M, et al, Theratope® Study Group. Theratope study group. Phase III multicenter trial of the sialyl-TN (STn)-keyhole limpet hemocyanin (KLH) vaccine for metastatic breast cancer. Oncologist 2011;16(8):1092–100.
36. Ibrahim NK, Murray JL, Zhou D, et al. Survival advantage in patients with metastatic breast cancer receiving endocrine therapy plus Sialyl Tn-KLH vaccine: post hoc analysis of a large randomized trial. J Cancer 2013;4(7):577–84.

37. Apostolopoulos V, Pietersz GA, Tsibanis A, et al. Pilot phase III immunotherapy study in early-stage breast cancer patients using oxidized mannan-MUC1 [ISRCTN71711835]. Breast Cancer Res 2006;8(3):R27.

38. Heery CR, Ibrahim NK, Arlen PM, et al. Docetaxel alone or in combination with a therapeutic cancer vaccine (PANVAC) in patients with metastatic breast cancer: a randomized clinical trial. JAMA Oncol 2015;1(8):1087–95.

39. Berinstein NL, Karkada M, Morse MA, et al. First-in-man application of a novel therapeutic cancer vaccine formulation with the capacity to induce multi-functional T cell responses in ovarian, breast and prostate cancer patients. J Transl Med 2012;10:156.

40. Kurtz SL, Ravindranathan S, Zaharoff DA. Current status of autologous breast tumor cell-based vaccines. Expert Rev Vaccines 2014;13(12):1439–45.

41. Ahlert T, Sauerbrei W, Bastert G, et al. Tumor-cell number and viability as quality and efficacy parameters of autologous virus-modified cancer vaccines in patients with breast or ovarian cancer. J Clin Oncol 1997;15:1354–66.

42. McArthur HL, Page DB. Immunotherapy for the treatment of breast cancer: checkpoint blockade, cancer vaccines, and future directions in combination immunotherapy. Clin Adv Hematol Oncol 2016;14(11):922–33.

43. Elliott RL, Head JF. Adjuvant breast cancer vaccine improves disease specific survival of breast cancer patients with depressed lymphocyte immunity. Surg Oncol 2013;22(3):172–7.

44. Norell H, Poschke I, Charo J, et al. Vaccination with a plasmid DNA encoding HER-2/neu together with low doses of GM-CSF and IL-2 in patients with metastatic breast carcinoma: a pilot clinical trial. J Transl Med 2010;8:53.

45. Zhang Y, Toh L, Lau P, et al. Human telomerase reverse transcriptase (hTERT) is a novel target of the Wnt/beta-catenin pathway in human cancer. J Biol Chem 2012; 287(39):32494–511.

46. Domchek SM, Recio A, Mick R, et al. Telomerase-specific T-cell immunity in breast cancer: effect of vaccination on tumor immunosurveillance. Cancer Res 2007;67(21):10546–55.

47. Cintolo JA, Datta J, Mathew SJ, et al. Dendritic cell-based vaccines: barriers and opportunities. Future Oncol 2012;8(10):1273–99.

48. Sharma A, Koldovsky U, Xu S, et al. HER-2 pulsed dendritic cell vaccine can eliminate HER-2 expression and impact ductal carcinoma in situ. Cancer 2012; 118(17):4354–62.

49. Lowenfeld L, Mick R, Datta J, et al. Dendritic cell vaccination enhances immune responses and induces regression of HER2(pos) DCIS independent of route: results of randomized selection design trial. Clin Cancer Res 2017;23(12):2961–71.

50. Jaini R, Loya MG, Eng C. Immunotherapeutic target expression on breast tumors can be amplified by hormone receptor antagonism: a novel strategy for enhancing efficacy of targeted immunotherapy. Oncotarget 2017;8(20): 32536–49.

51. Jaini R, Kesaraju P, Johnson JM, et al. An autoimmune-mediated strategy for prophylactic breast cancer vaccination. Nat Med 2010;16(7):799–803.

52. Tuohy VK, Jaini R, Johnson JM, et al. Targeted vaccination against human alpha-lactalbumin for immunotherapy and primary immunoprevention of triple negative breast cancer. Cancers (Basel) 2016;8(6) [pii:E56].

53. Sas S, Chan T, Sami A, et al. Vaccination of fiber-modified adenovirus-transfected dendritic cells to express HER-2/neu stimulates efficient HER-2/neu-specific humoral and CTL responses and reduces breast carcinogenesis in transgenic mice. Cancer Gene Ther 2008;15(10):655–66.

54. Allen SD, Garrett JT, Rawale SV, et al. Peptide vaccines of the HER-2/neu dimer- ization loop are effective in inhibiting mammary tumor growth in vivo. J Immunol 2007;179(1):472–82.

55. Gil EY, Jo UH, Lee HJ, et al. Vaccination with ErbB-2 peptides prevents cancer stem cell expansion and suppresses the development of spontaneous tumors in MMTV-PyMT transgenic mice. Breast Cancer Res Treat 2014;147(1):69–80.

56. Yamano T, Kaneda Y, Hiramatsu SH, et al. Immunity against breast cancer by TERT DNA vaccine primed with chemokine CCL21. Cancer Gene Ther 2007; 14(5):451–9.

57. Nguyen-Hoai T, Baldenhofer G, Sayed Ahmed MS, et al. CCL21 (SLC) improves tumor protection by a DNA vaccine in a Her2/neu mouse tumor model. Cancer Gene Ther 2012;19(1):69–76.

58. Taube JM, Klein A, Brahmer JR, et al. Association of PD-1, PD-1 ligands, and other features of the tumor immune microenvironment with response to anti-PD-1 therapy. Clin Cancer Res 2014;20(19):5064–74.

59. Loi S, Giobbe-Hurder A, Gombos A, et al. Phase Ib/II study evaluating the safety and efficacy of pembrolizumab and trastuzumab in patients with trastuzumab-resistant HER2-positive metastatic breast cancer: results from the PANACEA study. Cancer Res 2017;78(4 Suppl). GS2-06.

60. Hanahan D, Weinberg RA. Hallmarks of cancer: the next generation. Cell 2011; 144(5):646–74.

61. Dickson MA. Molecular pathways: CDK4 inhibitors for cancer therapy. Clin Can- cer Res 2014;20(13):3379–83.

62. Klein ME, Dickson MA, Antonescu C, et al. PDLIM7 and CDH18 regulate the turn- over of MDM2 during CDK4/6 inhibitor therapy-induced senescence. Oncogene 2018;37(37):5066–78.

The Current Landscape of Immune Checkpoint Inhibition for Solid Malignancies

Emily Z. Keung, MD, Jennifer A. Wargo, MD, MMSc*

KEYWORDS

- CTLA-4 • Immune checkpoint • Melanoma • Non–small cell lung carcinoma • PD-1
- PD-L1 • Renal cell carcinoma • Urothelial carcinoma

KEY POINTS

- The introduction of immune checkpoint inhibitors has resulted in unprecedented gains in the treatment and prognosis of advanced/metastatic solid malignancies.
- Initially evaluated in advanced/metastatic melanoma, immune checkpoint inhibitors have also demonstrated efficacy in other malignancies including non–small cell lung cancer, urothelial carcinoma, and MSI-high cancers.
- More recent clinical trials evaluating the use of immune checkpoint inhibitors in the adjuvant and neoadjuvant settings have shown promising results.
- Elucidating predictors of response and resistance to immunotherapies is critically important and depends on biospecimen collection and correlative analysis.

OVERVIEW OF IMMUNE CHECKPOINT BLOCKADE

The landscape of available treatment options for patients with advanced and metastatic solid malignancies has changed dramatically in recent years. Nowhere is this better highlighted than in the management of advanced and metastatic melanoma with the introduction of molecularly targeted therapies and immune checkpoint inhibitors.

Disclosure statement: J.A. Wargo is an inventor on a US patent application (PCT/US17/53,717) submitted by The University of Texas MD Anderson Cancer Center that covers methods to enhance checkpoint blockade therapy by the microbiome. J.A. Wargo is a clinical and scientific advisor at Microbiome DX and a consultant at Biothera Pharma, Merck Sharp and Dohme. J.A. Wargo has honoraria from speakers' bureau of Dava Oncology, Bristol-Myers Squibb, and Illumina, Omniprex, Imedex and is an advisory board member for GlaxoSmithKline, Novartis, and Roche/Genentech, Astra-Zeneca. E.Z. Keung is supported by National Institutes of Health grant T32 CA009599.

Department of Surgical Oncology, The University of Texas MD Anderson Cancer Center, 1515 Holcombe Boulevard, Unit 1484, Houston, TX 77030, USA
* Corresponding author.
E-mail address: JWargo@mdanderson.org

Surg Oncol Clin N Am 28 (2019) 369–386
https://doi.org/10.1016/j.soc.2019.02.008
1055-3207/19/© 2019 Elsevier Inc. All rights reserved.

Following their success in melanoma, immunotherapies have also been evaluated and their use approved in the management across a variety of other solid malignancies in the advanced and metastatic setting, including non–small cell lung carcinoma (NSCLC), urothelial carcinoma, renal cell carcinoma (RCC), and microsatellite instability-high/mismatch-repair–deficient cancers. This review provides an overview of the current landscape of immune checkpoint inhibition for solid malignancies (**Table 1**).

IMMUNE CHECKPOINT BLOCKADE FOR MELANOMA
Immune Checkpoint Blockade for Unresectable/Metastatic Melanoma

In 2011, ipilimumab (anti-CTLA-4) became the first immune checkpoint inhibitor to gain Food and Drug Administration (FDA) approval based on results of a landmark study by Hodi and colleagues.[1] In this study of 676 patients with unresectable stage III and IV melanoma who had progressed on prior therapy, those treated with ipilimumab demonstrated improved overall survival (OS) and durable responses. This was followed by the approval of the PD-1 inhibitors pembrolizumab[2] and nivolumab[3] in 2014 for the treatment of patients with unresectable or metastatic melanoma who progressed following ipilimumab treatment.

Adjuvant Immune Checkpoint Blockade for Resectable Stage III/Oligometastatic Stage IV Melanoma

Adjuvant ipilimumab
The role of adjuvant therapy for high-risk resected melanoma has historically been limited to interferon (IFN) therapy and, in select clinically appropriate settings, potential radiation therapy to the involved regional lymph node basins and/or primary melanoma site. Following the success and approval of ipilimumab for patients with metastatic melanoma, its potential as adjuvant therapy for patients with high-risk resected melanoma was investigated. In 2016, ipilimumab was approved for use in the adjuvant setting for patients with metastatic melanoma (>1 mm) to regional lymph nodes following lymphadenectomy based on results from EORTC 18071.[4,5] This was a phase 3, double-blind, randomized trial comparing high-dose ipilimumab (10 mg/kg) every 3 weeks for 4 doses then every 3 months for up to 3 years versus placebo in 951 patients with completely resected stage III cutaneous melanoma, with recurrence-free survival (RFS) as the primary endpoint. Although adjuvant ipilimumab significantly improved median RFS (26.1 months vs 17.1 months, hazard ratio [HR] 0.75, 95% confidence interval [CI] 0.64–0.90, $P = .0013$), 5-year RFS (40.8% vs 30.3%, HR 0.76, 95% CI 0.64–0.89, $P<.001$), 5-year distant metastasis-free survival (DMFS) (48.3% vs 38.9%, HR 0.76, 95% CI 0.64–0.92, $P = .002$), and 5-year OS (65.5% vs 54.4%, HR 0.72, 95% CI 0.58–0.88, $P = .001$) in patients with completely resected stage III melanoma, it was associated with significant rates of immune-related adverse events and death[4,5]

Adjuvant IFN and ipilimumab are perhaps soon to be of largely historical consequence given the results of 2 recently reported and practice changing phase 3 adjuvant trials of nivolumab versus ipilimumab for resected stage IIIB/C to stage IV melanoma[6] and of combination molecular targeted therapies dabrafenib plus trametinib for resected *BRAF*-mutant stage III melanoma,[7] with likely approval for these agents in the adjuvant setting in the near future.

Adjuvant single-agent anti-PD-1 inhibition
In the EORTC 18071 trial, adjuvant ipilimumab was associated with a significant adverse-event profile, with grade 3 or 4 immune-related adverse events occurring in

Table 1
Representative clinical trials of immune checkpoint inhibitors in solid malignancies

Malignancy	Treatment Setting	ClinicalTrials.gov Identifier	Study Description	References
Melanoma	Unresectable/metastatic	NCT00094653	A randomized, double-blind, multicenter study comparing MDX-010 monotherapy (ipilimumab), MDX-010 in combination with a melanoma peptide vaccine, and melanoma vaccine monotherapy in HLA-A2*0201-positive patients with previously treated unresectable stage III or IV melanoma	1
	Unresectable/metastatic	NCT01866319	A multicenter, randomized, controlled, 3-arm, phase 3 study to evaluate the safety and efficacy of 2 dosing schedules of pembrolizumab (MK-3475) compared with ipilimumab in patients with advanced melanoma	2
	Unresectable/metastatic	NCT01721772	A phase 3 randomized, double-blind study of BMS-936558 (nivolumab) vs dacarbazine in subjects with previously untreated, unresectable, or metastatic melanoma	3
	Adjuvant	NCT00636168	Adjuvant immunotherapy with anti-CTLA-4 monoclonal antibody (ipilimumab) vs placebo after complete resection of high-risk stage III melanoma: a randomized, double-blind phase 3 trial of the EORTC melanoma group (EORTC18071)	4,5
	Adjuvant	NCT02388906	A phase 3 randomized, double-blind study of adjuvant immunotherapy with nivolumab vs ipilimumab after complete resection of stage IIIb/c or stage IV melanoma in subjects who are at high risk for recurrence (CheckMate-238)	6

(continued on next page)

Table 1
(continued)

Malignancy	Treatment Setting	ClinicalTrials.gov Identifier	Study Description	References
	Adjuvant	NCT02362594	Adjuvant immunotherapy with anti-PD-1 monoclonal antibody pembrolizumab (MK-3475) vs placebo after complete resection of high-risk stage III melanoma: a randomized, double-blind phase 3 trial of the EORTC melanoma group (KEYNOTE-054)	[8]
	Neoadjuvant	NCT02306850	A phase 2b single-site, open-label, nonrandomized study evaluating the efficacy of neoadjuvant pembrolizumab for unresectable stage III and unresectable stage IV melanoma (NeoPembroMel)	[14]
	Neoadjuvant	NCT02519322	Neoadjuvant and adjuvant checkpoint blockade in patients with clinical stage III or oligometastatic stage IV melanoma	[15]
	Neoadjuvant	NCT02977052	A multicenter phase 2 study to identify the optimal neoadjuvant combination scheme of ipilimumab and nivolumab (OpACIN-neo)	[16]
NSCLC	Metastatic/refractory	NCT01642004	An open-label randomized phase 3 trial of BMS-936558 (nivolumab) vs docetaxel in previously treated advanced or metastatic squamous cell NSCLC (CheckMate-017)	[17]
	Metastatic/refractory	NCT01673867	An open-label randomized phase 3 trial of BMS-936558 (nivolumab) vs docetaxel in previously treated advanced or metastatic nonsquamous NSCLC (CheckMate-057)	[18]

Metastatic/refractory	NCT02578680	A randomized, double-blind, phase 3 study of platinum + pemetrexed chemotherapy with or without pembrolizumab (MK-3475) in first-line metastatic nonsquamous NSCLC subjects (KEYNOTE-189)	19
Metastatic/refractory	NCT01295827	A phase 1 study of single-agent pembrolizumab (MK-3475) in patients with progressive locally advanced or metastatic carcinoma, melanoma, and NSCLC (KEYNOTE-001)	20
Metastatic/refractory	NCT01905657	A phase 2/3 randomized trial of 2 doses of MK-3475 (pembrolizumab) vs docetaxel in previously treated subjects with NSCLC (KEYNOTE-010)	21
Metastatic/refractory	NCT01903993	A phase 2, open-label, multicenter, randomized study to investigate the efficacy and safety of MPDL3280A (anti-PD-L1 antibody, atezolizumab) compared with docetaxel in patients with NSCLC after platinum failure	22
Metastatic, treatment-naive	NCT02039674	A phase 1/2 study of MK-3475 (pembrolizumab) in combination with chemotherapy or immunotherapy in patients with locally advanced or metastatic NSCLC (KEYNOTE-021)	23
Neoadjuvant	NCT02259621	Neoadjuvant nivolumab or nivolumab in combination with ipilimumab in resectable NSCLC	24
Metastatic/refractory	NCT02108652	A phase 2, multicenter, single-arm study of atezolizumab in patients with locally advanced or metastatic urothelial bladder cancer	26,27
Metastatic/refractory	NCT01693562	A phase 1/2 study to evaluate the safety, tolerability, and pharmacokinetics of MEDI4736 (durvalumab) in subjects with advanced solid tumors	28

RCC

(continued on next page)

Table 1
(continued)

Malignancy	Treatment Setting	ClinicalTrials.gov Identifier	Study Description	References
	Metastatic/refractory	NCT01772004	A phase 1, open-label, multiple-ascending dose trial to investigate the safety, tolerability, pharmacokinetics, and biological and clinical activity of avelumab (MSB0010718 C) in subjects with metastatic or locally advanced solid tumors and expansion to selected indications (JAVELIN)	[29]
	Metastatic/refractory	NCT02387996	A phase 2 single-arm clinical trial of nivolumab (BMS-936558) in subjects with metastatic or unresectable urothelial cancer who have progressed or recurred following treatment with a platinum agent (CheckMate-275)	[30]
	Metastatic/refractory	NCT01928394	A phase 1/2, open-label study of nivolumab monotherapy or nivolumab combined with ipilimumab in subjects with advanced or metastatic solid tumors (CheckMate-032)	[31]
	Metastatic/refractory	NCT01848834	A phase 1b multicohort study of MK-3475 (pembrolizumab) in subjects with advanced solid tumors (KEYNOTE-012)	[33]
	Metastatic/refractory	NCT02256436	A phase 3 randomized clinical trial of pembrolizumab (MK-3475) vs paclitaxel, docetaxel or vinflunine in subjects with recurrent or progressive metastatic urothelial cancer (KEYNOTE-045)	[34]
	Metastatic/first-line	NCT02335424	A phase 2 clinical trial of pembrolizumab (MK-3475) in subjects with advanced/unresectable or metastatic urothelial cancer (KEYNOTE-052)	[35]

HNSCC			
Recurrent/metastatic/refractory	NCT01848834	A phase 1b multicohort study of MK-3475 (pembrolizumab) in subjects with advanced solid tumors (KEYNOTE-012)	37
Recurrent/metastatic/refractory	NCT02255097	A phase 2 clinical trial of single-agent pembrolizumab (MK-3475) in subjects with recurrent or metastatic HNSCC who have failed platinum and cetuximab (KEYNOTE-055)	39
Recurrent/metastatic/refractory	NCT02105636	An open-label, randomized phase 3 clinical trial of nivolumab vs therapy of investigator's choice in recurrent or metastatic platinum-refractory squamous cell carcinoma of the head and neck (CheckMate-141)	40
Recurrent/metastatic/refractory	NCT01693562	A phase 1/2 study to evaluate the safety, tolerability, and pharmacokinetics of MEDI4736 (durvalumab) in subjects with advanced solid tumors	41
Gastric and GEJ adenocarcinoma Recurrent locally advanced/metastatic/refractory	NCT02335411	A phase 2 clinical trial of pembrolizumab as monotherapy and in combination with cisplatin + 5-fluorouracil in subjects with recurrent or metastatic gastric or GEJ adenocarcinoma (KEYNOTE-059)	43
MCC Metastatic	NCT02267603	A phase 2 study of MK-3475 (pembrolizumab) in patients with advanced Merkel cell carcinoma	46
Metastatic	NCT02155647	A phase 2, open-label, multicenter trial to investigate the clinical activity and safety of avelumab (MSB0010718 C) in subjects with Merkel cell carcinoma	47,50–53
Patients with virus-associated tumors and measureable disease by computed tomography or MRI	NCT02488759	A noncomparative, open-label, multiple-cohort, phase 1/2 study of nivolumab monotherapy and nivolumab combination therapy in subjects with virus-positive and virus-negative solid tumors (CheckMate-358)	49

(continued on next page)

Table 1
(continued)

Malignancy	Treatment Setting	ClinicalTrials.gov Identifier	Study Description	References
MSI-H/dMMR malignancies		NCT01876511	A phase 2 study of MK-3475 (pembrolizumab) in patients with microsatellite unstable tumors (KEYNOTE-016)	[56]
		NCT01848834	A phase 1b multicohort study of MK-3475 (pembrolizumab) in subjects with advanced solid tumors (KEYNOTE-012)	[37]
		NCT02054806	A phase 1b study of pembrolizumab (MK-3475) in subjects with select advanced solid tumors (KEYNOTE-028)	[54,61]
		NCT02628067	A clinical trial of pembrolizumab (MK-3475) evaluating predictive biomarkers in subjects with advanced solid tumors (KEYNOTE-158)	[58]
		NCT02460198	A phase 2 study of pembrolizumab (MK-3475) as monotherapy in subjects with previously treated locally advanced unresectable or metastatic (stage IV) mismatched-repair–deficient or microsatellite instability-high colorectal carcinoma (KEYNOTE-164)	[62]

Abbreviations: GEJ, gastroesophageal junction; HNSCC, head and neck squamous cell carcinoma; MCC, merkel cell carcinoma; MSI-H/dMMR, microsatellite instability-high/mismatch repair deficient; NSCLC, non–small cell lung cancer; RCC, renal cell carcinoma.

41.6% of patients in the ipilimumab group, 52% of patients requiring discontinuation of treatment because of ipilimumab-associated adverse events, and 5 patients (1%) who died of drug-related adverse events.[4,5] In the unresectable advanced/metastatic melanoma setting, anti-PD-1 monotherapy has typically demonstrated better tolerability and adverse-event profiles.

Anti-PD-1 monotherapy (nivolumab) was first compared with ipilimumab in the adjuvant setting for stage III and IV melanoma in CheckMate-238 (NCT02388906).[6] Results of this study led to FDA approval of nivolumab for use in the adjuvant setting in December 2017. In this double-blind randomized controlled trial (RCT), 906 patients who underwent complete resection of stage IIIB/C or IV melanoma were randomized to receive either nivolumab (3 mg/kg every 2 weeks) or ipilimumab (10 mg/kg every 3 weeks for 4 doses and then every 12 weeks) for up to 1 year. Patients in the adjuvant nivolumab arm experienced not only significantly longer RFS at 1 year (70.5% vs 60.8%, HR 0.65, 97.56% CI 0.51–0.83, $P<.001$) but also lower rates of grade 3 or 4 adverse events (14.4% vs 45.9%). On subgroup analyses, adjuvant nivolumab was associated with improved RFS compared with adjuvant ipilimumab for stage IIIB, IIIC, and IVa/b disease but not for stage IVc disease and regardless of (1) whether ulceration was present or absent in the primary melanoma, (2) *BRAF* mutational status, (3) PD-L1 expression, or (4) whether regional lymph node involvement was microscopic or macroscopic.

More recently, Eggermont and colleagues[8] reported results of KEYNOTE-054 (NCT02362594), a phase 3 trial of 1019 patients demonstrating significantly longer RFS in patients receiving pembrolizumab versus placebo following resection of high-risk stage III melanoma (75.4% vs 61%).

Additionally there are now several clinical trials investigating the role of adjuvant nivolumab in combination with ipilimumab (NCT02437279, NCT02941744, NCT02656706, NCT02523313, and NCT03068455).

Neoadjuvant Immune Checkpoint Blockade for Resectable Stage III/Oligometastatic Stage IV Melanoma

There is also increasing enthusiasm for evaluating immune checkpoint inhibitors in the neoadjuvant setting for locally and regionally advanced melanoma. For patients with locally advanced disease, upfront surgery may not be feasible or may be technically challenging and associated with considerable morbidity with a high likelihood of incomplete resection or positive margins. A neoadjuvant therapy approach with conventional chemotherapy and chemoradiation therapy to downstage disease and improve local disease control has been shown to improve survival and/or improve surgical outcomes in other solid malignancies.[5–18] Importantly, the neoadjuvant approach allows evaluation of treatment efficacy because tumor response can be monitored preoperatively clinically/radiographically, and postoperatively by pathologic evaluation of the resected tumor tissue (**Fig. 1**).

There are currently 3 ongoing phase 2 clinical trials to evaluate either anti-PD-1 antibody alone (NCT02306850)[14] or in combination with anti-CTLA-4 antibody in the neoadjuvant setting for patients with stage III or stage IV oligometastatic melanoma (NCT02519322, NCT02977052).[15,16] The largest of these is OpACIN-neo (NCT02977052), an open-label, 3-arm phase 2 trial in which 90 stage III melanoma patients will be randomized 1:1:1 to receive either: (1) 2 courses of ipilimumab 3 mg/kg + nivolumab 1 mg/kg every 3 weeks; (2) 2 courses of ipilimumab 1 mg/kg + nivolumab 3 mg/kg every 3 weeks; or (3) 2 courses of ipilimumab 3 mg/kg, directly followed by 2 courses of nivolumab 3 mg/kg every 2 weeks. All 3 treatment arms then undergo surgery. Primary outcome measures include response rate by

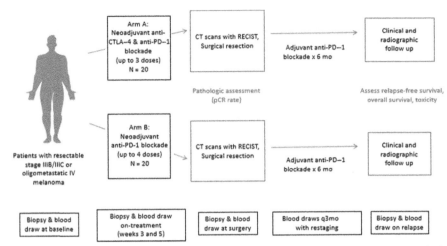

Fig. 1. Study schema of phase 2 clinical trial of neoadjuvant immune checkpoint blockade for patients with high-risk resectable metastatic melanoma (NCT02519322).

RECIST1.1 (Response Evaluation Criteria in Solid Tumors 1.1), safety, and pathologic response. Secondary outcome measus include RFS, late adverse events, and correlatives. These studies should help establish the benefit of and delineate optimal regimens for neoadjuvant immunotherapy for high-risk melanoma.

IMMUNE CHECKPOINT BLOCKADE FOR NON–SMALL CELL LUNG CANCER

Although first approved in melanoma, immune checkpoint blockade was subsequently tested in NSCLC in the metastatic setting after progression on platinum-based chemotherapy or tyrosine kinase inhibitors. CheckMate-017 was a phase 3 randomized trial of patients with advanced squamous NSCLC and disease progression during or after first-line platinum-based chemotherapy in which 272 patients were randomized to either nivolumab or docetaxel.[17] In this study, nivolumab was associated with significant OS benefit (9.2 vs 6 months, P<.001) and an objective response rate (ORR) of 20%. CheckMate-057 was a phase 3 randomized trial of patients with non-squamous NSCLC and disease progression during or after platinum-based chemotherapy in which 582 patients were randomized to either nivolumab or docetaxel.[18] Again, nivolumab was associated with significant OS benefit (12.2 vs 9.4 months, P<.002) and 17.2 months' median duration of response. Based on these data, nivolumab received FDA approval in October 2015 for use in patients with advanced NSCLC whose disease had progressed during or after platinum-based chemotherapy. In addition to results of these 2 phase 3 studies, Gandhi and colleagues[19] recently published 5-year follow-up results from an early phase 1 study of nivolumab in a similar population of patients with pretreated advanced NSCLC, reporting unprecedented 5-year OS rates of 16% compared with historical rates of 1% to 8%.

Pembrolizumab was first approved for NSCLC in October 2015 when it received accelerated approval in patients with advanced NSCLC who failed previous treatments and whose tumors expressed PD-L1. This decision was based on data from KEYNOTE-001, a large phase 1 study of 495 patients with previously treated and untreated NSCLC who received pembrolizumab at doses of either 2 or 10 mg/kg every 3 weeks or 10 mg/kg every 2 weeks.[20] ORR in this study was 19.4% and often durable. In contrast to CheckMate-017 and CheckMate-057, KEYNOTE-001 prospectively evaluated PD-L1 expression as a predictive biomarker for pembrolizumab and re-ported improved ORR among patients with membranous PD-L1 expression on 50% or more tumor cells (proportion score [PS] $\geq$50%).

In October 2016, pembrolizumab was also approved as a single-agent therapy for patients with metastatic NSCLC as (1) first-line treatment of patients whose tumors have high PD-L1 expression (tumor proportion score [TPS] $\geq$50%) as determined by an FDA-approved test and (2) treatment of patients whose tumors express PD-L1 (TPS $\geq$1%) with disease progression on or after platinum-containing chemo-therapy. Patients with EGFR or ALK genomic tumor aberrations should have disease progression on FDA-approved therapy for these aberrations before receiving pembro-lizumab.[20,21] This approval was based on data from KEYNOTE-010, a phase 2/3 trial of 1034 patients randomized to pembrolizumab 2 or 10 mg/kg or docetaxel every 3 weeks.[21] Patients with high PD-L1 expression (PS $\geq$50%) treated with either dose of pembrolizumab experienced improved OS.

Atezolizumab (anti-PD-L1) is approved for patients with metastatic NSCLC with dis-ease progression on or after platinum-containing chemotherapy and in patients with *EGFR* or *ALK* genomic tumor aberrations after disease progression on FDA-approved therapy for these aberrations.[22]

The use of immune checkpoint therapy in combination with chemotherapy as first-line therapy has also been investigated for advanced metastatic NSCLC in the phase 2 KEYNOTE-21 study. On the basis of this study, pembrolizumab received FDA approval in combination with pemetrexed and carboplatin as first-line treatment of patients with metastatic nonsquamous NSCLC in May 2017.[23] Results of the larger phase 3 KEYNOTE-189 trial confirmed the efficacy of this combination in treatment-naïve patients with advanced NSCLC without *EGFR* or *ALK* mutations and demonstrated improved survival with the addition of pembrolizumab regardless of tumor PD-L1 status.[19] In this study, patients randomized to combination pembrolizumab + chemotherapy had significantly higher OS at 1 year compared with those who received chemotherapy alone (69.2% vs 49.4%).

As in melanoma, there is growing interest in the utility of immune checkpoint blockade for patients with earlier-stage NSCLC. Forde and colleagues[24] recently re-ported data from a phase 1 study evaluating nivolumab monotherapy in the neoadju-vant setting for patients with stage I, II, or IIIa NSCLC. In this study, neoadjuvant therapy was safe, did not significantly delay surgery, and was associated with major pathologic response (defined as <10% viable tumor cells in the surgical specimen) in 45% of patients.

IMMUNE CHECKPOINT BLOCKADE FOR OTHER SOLID MALIGNANCIES

Beyond their efficacy in melanoma and NSCLC, immune checkpoint inhibitors have also demonstrated encouraging activity in other advanced and metastatic malignancies.

Locally Advanced or Metastatic Urothelial Carcinoma and Renal Cell Carcinoma

Bladder cancer is the most common malignancy involving the genitourinary system, with the most common risk factor being related to smoking and infection with *Schistosoma haematobium* in select populations.[25] The current standard of care for muscle-invasive bladder cancer remains cisplatin-based systemic chemotherapy reg-imens; however, anti-PD-1 and anti-PD-L1 therapies have recently become available for patients who are ineligible to receive cisplatin or who had disease progression after receiving platinum-based chemotherapy.

Atezolizumab,[26,27] an anti-PD-L1 inhibitor, was the first immune checkpoint inhibitor to receive FDA approval based on results of IMvigor 210, a multicenter, single-arm, 2-cohort, phase 2 trial in patients with metastatic urothelial cancer who had disease progression after receiving platinum-based chemotherapy. Compared with a historical control response rate of 10% in the second-line setting, atezolizumab showed significantly improved ORR of 26% in patients with high PD-L1 expression and 15% ORR in all patients with durable responses. Patients in this study who were ineligible to receive platinum-based therapy and who received atezolizumab in the first-line setting had an ORR of 23%.

Subsequently, 2 additional anti-PD-L1 antibodies (durvalumab[28] and avelumab[29]) have also been approved for the treatment of patients with locally advanced or metastatic urothelial carcinoma who have disease progression during or following platinum-containing chemotherapy or have disease progression within 12 months of neoadjuvant or adjuvant treatment with platinum-containing chemotherapy.

Both pembrolizumab and nivolumab have also been approved for use in the setting of locally advanced or metastatic urothelial carcinoma in patients who have disease progression during or following platinum-containing chemotherapy or within 12 months of neoadjuvant or adjuvant treatment with platinum-containing chemotherapy.[30,31] Nivolumab received FDA approval in the second-line setting for metastatic urothelial carcinoma in early 2017 based on results of CheckMate-032, a multicenter, open-label, 2-stage, multi-arm phase 1/2 study in patients with urothelial carcinoma.[31] CheckMate-275 was a larger phase 2 trial that demonstrated an ORR of 28.4% among patients who were positive for PD-L1 expression and an overall ORR of 20%.[30] Nivolumab is also approved in patients with advanced RCC who have received prior antiangiogenic therapy.[32] Pembrolizumab was approved by the FDA for use in the second-line setting based on KEYNOTE-012[33] and KEYNOTE-045[34] and in the first-line setting for patients with locally advanced or metastatic urothelial carcinoma not eligible for cisplatin-containing chemotherapy based on KEYNOTE-052.[35]

Recurrent or Metastatic Squamous Cell Carcinoma of the Head and Neck

There are numerous clinical trials evaluating the efficacy of immune checkpoint modulators in head and neck squamous cell carcinoma (HNSCC) in both the curative and recurrent/metastatic setting.[36] However, to date the 4 studies that have been reported all investigated the role of PD-1/PD-L1 inhibition in HNSCC[36–41] in the recurrent/metastatic setting. KEYNOTE-012 (NCT01848834)[37,38] and KEYNOTE-055 (NCT02255097)[39] were phase 1b and phase 2 studies of pembrolizumab, respectively, while CheckMate-141 (NCT02105636)[40] was a phase 3 study of nivolumab and (NCT01693562)[41] was a phase 1/2 study of durvalumab (anti-PD-L1). KEYNOTE-012 enrolled a total of 192 recurrent or metastatic HNSCC patients; 7 achieved complete response (CR) and 27 achieved partial response (PR) for an ORR of 17.7% and progression-free survival of 25% at 6 months. CheckMate-141 is a multicenter, randomized phase 3 study comparing nivolumab with therapy of the investigator's choice (IC) in patients with recurrent or metastatic HNSCC that demonstrated a 30% reduction in risk of death in the nivolumab-treated patients (median OS for nivolumab 7.5 months vs 5.1 months for IC). Based on the results of KEYNOTE-012 and CheckMate-141, pembrolizumab and nivolumab received FDA approval in 2016 for the treatment of patients with recurrent or metastatic HNSCC with disease progression on or after a platinum-containing chemotherapy.

Advanced Gastric and Gastroesophageal Junction Adenocarcinoma

There are multiple ongoing clinical trials investigating the role of pembrolizumab, either alone or in combination with other therapies, in the first-line and second-line settings for advanced gastric and gastroesophageal adenocarcinoma and in the third-line setting for advanced/metastatic squamous cell carcinoma of the esophagus.[42] Pembrolizumab received FDA approval in September 2017 in the third-line setting for patients with recurrent locally advanced or metastatic gastric or gastroesophageal junction (GEJ) adenocarcinoma whose tumors express PD-L1 and who have progressed on or failed 2 or more prior systemic therapies, including fluoropyrimidine- and platinum-containing chemotherapy and, if appropriate, HER2/neu-targeted therapy. Approval was based on results of KEYNOTE-059 (NCT02335411), an open-label, multicenter, noncomparative, multicohort trial that enrolled 259 patients with gastric or GEJ adenocarcinoma of whom 55% (n = 143) had tumors expressing PD-L1.[43] Among the cohort of patients whose tumors expressed PD-1, the ORR was 13.3%, with 58% having response durations of 6 months or longer and 26% having response durations of 12 months or longer.

Metastatic Merkel Cell Carcinoma

Merkel cell carcinoma (MCC) is an aggressive tumor of the skin for which surgery is the mainstay of primary treatment of localized disease and for which use of adjuvant radiation therapy has been shown to lower the risk of local and regional recurrences.[44] Five-year survival for patients with lymph node and distant metastatic disease is poor (39% and 18%, respectively), and for those who are not candidates for surgery or radiotherapy, conventional chemotherapy is unlikely to afford durative disease control or remission.[45]

The efficacy of immune checkpoint blockade for advanced MCC have been evaluated in several clinical trials,[46–48] although mature survival data are not yet available. ORR to pembrolizumab, nivolumab, and avelumab in the first-line setting were 56%,[46] 71%,[49] and 69%,[50] respectively. In the second-line setting, ORR for avelumab was 33% (11% had CR, n = 10; 22% had PR, n = 19) with durable responses.[47,51] Median OS was 12.9 months, significantly improved over histologic median OS of 4 to 6 months.[52,53] Based on these results, avelumab was approved in 2017 for the treatment of metastatic MCC at 10 mg/kg every 2 weeks until disease progression or unacceptable toxicity.

Microsatellite Instability-High or Mismatch-Repair–Deficient Cancers

Although immune checkpoint blockade has demonstrated significant and durable responses in patients with advanced melanoma and other malignancies, most patients fail to respond or have short-lived response. Investigations toward identifying predictors of response and mechanisms of resistance to immunotherapy revealed that mismatch repair deficiency (dMMR) results in characteristically high mutational burden and accumulation of mutations affecting microsatellites, resulting in the generation of immunogenic neoantigens. The so-called microsatellite instability-high (MSI-H) phenotype has been shown to be strongly associated with response to PD-1 blockade across tumor types.[37,54–62] In May 2017, pembrolizumab received accelerated approval from the FDA for the treatment of adult and pediatric patients with unresectable or metastatic MSI-H or dMMR solid tumors that have progressed after prior treatment and who have no satisfactory alternative treatment options, as well as for patients with MSI-H or dMMR colorectal cancer (CRC) following progression on a fluoropyridine, oxaliplatin, and irinotecan. This was unprecedented as the first histology-agnostic treatment approval by the FDA and was based on data from 5 uncontrolled, multicohort, multicenter, single-arm clinical trials (KEYNOTE-016, NCT01876511[56,57]; KEYNOTE-164, NCT02460198[62]; KEYNOTE-012, NCT01848834[37]; KEYNOTE-028, NCT02054806[37,54,55,61]; KEYNOTE-158, NCT02628067[58]). Of the 149 patients with MSI-H or dMMR cancers enrolled across these trials, 90 had CRC and 59 had 1 of 14 other cancer types. ORR was 40% with 11 CRs and 48 PRs, and lasted at least 6 months for 78% of responders.[63]

FUTURE LANDSCAPE OF IMMUNE CHECKPOINT BLOCKADE FOR SOLID MALIGNANCIES

The treatment landscape for advanced and metastatic solid malignancies has changed dramatically in recent years with the introduction and success of immune checkpoint inhibitors. Since their earliest successes and FDA approvals in the advanced and metastatic melanoma setting, immune checkpoint inhibitors have now demonstrated efficacy not only in other solid malignancies such as NSCLC, HNSCC, and urothelial carcinomas in the advanced and metastatic setting but also in the adjuvant and neoadjuvant settings in high-risk stage III resectable melanoma. With the plethora of ongoing clinical trials (ClinicalTrials.gov) of immune checkpoint inhibitors across tumor types, for earlier-stage disease, and in novel combinations with other therapies and treatment modalities (such as radiation therapy and targeted therapies), the future landscape of immune checkpoint inhibition in solid malignancies is bright and will likely continue to expand. Despite these advances for patients with advanced and metastatic solid malignancies in recent years, however, there remain many areas of unmet need including ongoing efforts to identify predictors of response and overcome mechanisms of primary and secondary resistance to immunotherapies.

REFERENCES

1. Hodi FS, O'Day SJ, McDermott DF, et al. Improved survival with ipilimumab in patients with metastatic melanoma. N Engl J Med 2010;363(8):711–23.
2. Robert C, Schachter J, Long GV, et al. Pembrolizumab versus Ipilimumab in Advanced Melanoma. N Engl J Med 2015;372(26):2521–32.
3. Robert C, Long GV, Brady B, et al. Nivolumab in previously untreated melanoma without BRAF mutation. N Engl J Med 2015;372(4):320–30.
4. Eggermont AMM, Chiarion-Sileni V, Grob J-J, et al. Prolonged survival in stage III melanoma with ipilimumab adjuvant therapy. N Engl J Med 2016;375(19): 1845–55.
5. Eggermont AMM, Chiarion-Sileni V, Grob JJ, et al. Adjuvant ipilimumab versus placebo after complete resection of high-risk stage III melanoma (EORTC 18071): a randomised, double-blind, phase 3 trial. Lancet Oncol 2015;16(5): 522–30.
6. Weber J, Mandala M, Del Vecchio M, et al. Adjuvant nivolumab versus ipilimumab in resected stage III or IV melanoma. N Engl J Med 2017;377(19):1824–35.
7. Long GV, Hauschild A, Santinami M, et al. Adjuvant dabrafenib plus trametinib in stage III BRAF-mutated melanoma. N Engl J Med 2017;377(19):1813–23.
8. Eggermont AMM, Blank CU, Mandala M, et al. Adjuvant pembrolizumab versus placebo in resected stage III melanoma. N Engl J Med 2018;378(19):1789–801.
9. Fisher B, Brown A. Effect of preoperative chemotherapy on local-regional disease in women with operable breast cancer: findings from National Surgical Adjuvant Breast and Bowel. J Clin Oncol 1997;15(7):2483–93.

10. Rastogi P, Anderson SJ, Bear HD, et al. Preoperative chemotherapy: updates of national surgical adjuvant breast and bowel project protocols B-18 and B-27. J Clin Oncol 2008;26(5):778–85.

11. Von Minckwitz G, Untch M, Blohmer JU, et al. Definition and impact of pathologic complete response on prognosis after neoadjuvant chemotherapy in various intrinsic breast cancer subtypes. J Clin Oncol 2012;30(15):1796–804.

12. Cortazar P, Zhang L, Untch M, et al. Pathological complete response and long-term clinical benefit in breast cancer: the CTNeoBC pooled analysis. Lancet 2014;384(9938):164–72.

13. Mauri D, Pavlidis N, Ioannidis JPA. Neoadjuvant versus adjuvant systemic treatment in breast cancer: a meta-analysis. J Natl Cancer Inst 2005;97(3):188–94.

14. Neoadjuvant pembrolizumab for unresectable stage III and unresectable stage IV melanoma (NeoPembroMel). Available at: https://clinicaltrialsgov/show/ NCT02306850. Accessed May 30, 2018.

15. Neoadjuvant and adjuvant checkpoint blockade in patients with clinical stage III or oligometastatic stage IV melanoma. Available at: https://clinicaltrialsgov/ct2/ show/study/NCT02519322. Accessed May 30, 2018.

16. Optimal neo-adjuvant combination scheme of ipilimumab and nivolumab (OpA-CIN-neo). Available at: https://clinicaltrialsgov/ct2/show/study/NCT02977052. Accessed May 30, 2018.

17. Brahmer J, Reckamp KL, Baas P, et al. Nivolumab versus docetaxel in advanced squamous-cell non-small-cell lung cancer. N Engl J Med 2015;373(2):123–35.

18. Borghaei H, Paz-Ares L, Horn L, et al. Nivolumab versus docetaxel in advanced nonsquamous non–small-cell lung cancer. N Engl J Med 2015;373(17):1627–39.

19. Gandhi L, Rodríguez-Abreu D, Gadgeel S, et al. Pembrolizumab plus chemotherapy in metastatic non-small-cell lung cancer. N Engl J Med 2018;378(22): 2078–92.

20. Garon EB, Rizvi NA, Hui R, et al. Pembrolizumab for the treatment of non-small-cell lung cancer. N Engl J Med 2015;372(21):2018–28.

21. Herbst RS, Baas P, Kim DW, et al. Pembrolizumab versus docetaxel for previously treated, PD-L1-positive, advanced non-small-cell lung cancer (KEYNOTE-010): a randomised controlled trial. Lancet 2016;387(10027):1540–50.

22. Fehrenbacher L, Spira A, Ballinger M, et al. Atezolizumab versus docetaxel for patients with previously treated non-small-cell lung cancer (POPLAR): a multicentre, open-label, phase 2 randomised controlled trial. Lancet 2016; 387(10030):1837–46.

23. Langer CJ, Gadgeel SM, Borghaei H, et al. Carboplatin and pemetrexed with or without pembrolizumab for advanced, non-squamous non-small-cell lung cancer: a randomised, phase 2 cohort of the open-label KEYNOTE-021 study. Lancet Oncol 2016;17(11):1497–508.

24. Forde PM, Chaft JE, Smith KN, et al. Neoadjuvant PD-1 blockade in resectable lung cancer. N Engl J Med 2018;378(21):1976–86.

25. Katz H, Wassie E, Alsharedi M. Checkpoint inhibitors: the new treatment paradigm for urothelial bladder cancer. Med Oncol 2017;34(10):1–11.

26. Rosenberg JE, Hoffman-Censits J, Powles T, et al. Atezolizumab in patients with locally advanced and metastatic urothelial carcinoma who have progressed following treatment with platinum-based chemotherapy: a single-arm, multicentre, phase 2 trial. Lancet 2016;387(10031):1909–20.

27. Balar AV, Galsky MD, Rosenberg JE, et al. Atezolizumab as first-line treatment in cisplatin-ineligible patients with locally advanced and metastatic urothelial carcinoma: a single-arm, multicentre, phase 2 trial. Lancet 2017;389(10064):67–76.

28. Massard C, Gordon MS, Sharma S, et al. Safety and efficacy of durvalumab (MEDI4736), an anti-programmed cell death ligand-1 immune checkpoint inhibitor, in patients with advanced urothelial bladder cancer. J Clin Oncol 2016;34(26): 3119–25.

29. Heery CR, O'Sullivan-Coyne G, Madan RA, et al. Avelumab for metastatic or locally advanced previously treated solid tumours (JAVELIN Solid Tumor): a phase 1a, multicohort, dose-escalation trial. Lancet Oncol 2017;18(5):587–98.

30. Sharma P, Retz M, Siefker-Radtke A, et al. Nivolumab in metastatic urothelial carcinoma after platinum therapy (CheckMate 275): a multicentre, single-arm, phase 2 trial. Lancet Oncol 2017;18(3):312–22.

31. Sharma P, Callahan MK, Bono P, et al. Nivolumab monotherapy in recurrent metastatic urothelial carcinoma (CheckMate 032): a multicentre, open-label, two-stage, multi-arm, phase 1/2 trial. Lancet Oncol 2016;17(11):1590–8.

32. Motzer RJ, Escudier B, McDermott DF, et al. Nivolumab versus everolimus in advanced renal-cell carcinoma. N Engl J Med 2015;373(19):1803–13.

33. Plimack ER, Bellmunt J, Gupta S, et al. Safety and activity of pembrolizumab in patients with locally advanced or metastatic urothelial cancer (KEYNOTE-012): a non-randomised, open-label, phase 1b study. Lancet Oncol 2017;18(2): 212–20.

34. Bellmunt J, de Wit R, Vaughn DJ, et al. Pembrolizumab as second-line therapy for advanced urothelial carcinoma. N Engl J Med 2017;376(11):1015–26.

35. Balar AV, Catellano D, O'Donnell PH, et al. Pembrolizumab as first-line therapy in cisplatin-ineligible advanced urothelial cancer: results from the total KEYNOTE-052 study population. J Clin Oncol 2017;35(suppl) [abstract: 284].

36. Dogan V, Rieckmann T, Münscher A, et al. Current studies of immunotherapy in head and neck cancer. Clin Otolaryngol 2018;43(1):13–21.

37. Seiwert T, Burtness B, Mehra R, et al. Safety and clinical activity of pembrolizumab for treatment of recurrent or metastatic squamous cell carcinoma of the head and neck (KEYNOTE-012): an open-label, multicentre, phase 1b trial. Lancet Oncol 2016;17(7):956–65.

38. Laura Q, Robert H, Shilpa G, et al. Antitumor activity of pembrolizumab in biomarker-unselected patients with recurrent and/or metastatic head and neck squamous cell carcinoma: results from the phase Ib KEYNOTE-012 expansion cohort. J Clin Oncol 2016;34:3838–45.

39. Bauml J, Seiwert TY, Pfister DG, et al. Pembrolizumab for platinum- and cetuximab-refractory head and neck cancer: results from a single-arm, phase II study. J Clin Oncol 2017;35(14):1542–9.

40. Ferris RL, Blumenschein G, Fayette J, et al. Nivolumab for recurrent squamous-cell carcinoma of the head and neck. N Engl J Med 2016;375(19):1856–67.

41. Segal N, Oui S-H, Balmanoukian A, et al. Updated safety and efficacy of durvalumab (MEDI4736), an anti-PD-L 1 antibody, in patients from a squamous cell carcinoma of the head and neck (SCCHN) expansion cohort. Ann Oncol 2016; 27(suppl 6):949O.

42. Joshi SS, Maron SB, Catenacci DV. Pembrolizumab for treatment of advanced gastric and gastroesophageal junction adenocarcinoma. Future Oncol 2018; 14(5):417–30.

43. Fuchs C, Doi T, Jang R, et al. KEYNOTE-059 cohort 1: efficacy and safety of pembrolizumab (pembro) monotherapy in patients with previously treated advanced gastric cancer. J Clin Oncol 2017;35(15 Suppl):4003.

44. National Comprehensive Cancer Network. NCCN guidelines version 1.2017. Merkel cell carcinoma. Plymouth Meeting (PA): NCCN; 2016.

45. Terheyden P, Becker JC. New developments in the biology and the treatment of metastatic Merkel cell carcinoma. Curr Opin Oncol 2017;29(3):221–6.
46. Nghiem PT, Bhatia S, Lipson EJ, et al. PD-1 blockade with pembrolizumab in advanced merkel-cell carcinoma. N Engl J Med 2016;374(26):2542–52.
47. Kaufman HL, Russell J, Hamid O, et al. Avelumab in patients with chemotherapy-refractory metastatic Merkel cell carcinoma: a multicentre, single-group, open-label, phase 2 trial. Lancet Oncol 2016;17(10):1374–85.
48. Paulson KG, Bhatia S. Advances in immunotherapy for metastatic Merkel cell carcinoma: a clinician's guide. J Natl Compr Canc Netw 2018;16(6):782–90.
49. Topalian SL, Bhatia S, Hollebecque A, et al. Non-comparative, open- label, multiple cohort, phase 1/2 study to evaluate nivolumab (NIVO) in patients with virus-associated tumors (CheckMate 358): efficacy and safety in Merkel cell carcinoma (MCC). Cancer Res 2017;77(Suppl 13). https://doi.org/10.1158/1538-7445. AM2017-CT074 [abstract: CT074].
50. D'Angelo SP, Russell J, Hassel JC, et al. First-line (1L) avelumab treatment in patients (pts) with metastatic Merkel cell carcinoma (mMCC): preliminary data from an ongoing study. J Clin Oncol 2017;35(Suppl 15) [abstract: 9530].
51. Kaufman HL, Russell JS, Hamid O, et al. Updated efficacy of avelumab in patients with previously treated metastatic Merkel cell carcinoma after ≥1 year of follow-up: JAVELIN Merkel 200, a phase 2 clinical trial. J Immunother Cancer 2018;6(1):7.
52. Cowey CL, Mahnke L, Espirito J, et al. Real-world treatment outcomes in patients with metastatic Merkel cell carcinoma treated with chemotherapy in the USA. Future Oncol 2017;13(19):1699–710.
53. Becker JC, Lorenz E, Ugurel S, et al. Evaluation of real-world treatment outcomes in patients with distant metastatic Merkel cell carcinoma following second-line chemotherapy in Europe. Oncotarget 2017;8(45):79731–41.
54. Ott PA, Bang YJ, Berton-Rigaud D, et al. Safety and antitumor activity of pembrolizumab in advanced programmed death ligand 1–positive endometrial cancer: results from the KEYNOTE-028 study. J Clin Oncol 2017;35(22):2535–41.
55. Ott PA, Piha-Paul SA, Munster P, et al. Safety and antitumor activity of the anti-PD-1 antibody pembrolizumab in patients with recurrent carcinoma of the anal canal. Ann Oncol 2017;28(5):1036–41.
56. Le DT, Uram JN, Wang H, et al. PD-1 blockade in tumors with mismatch-repair deficiency. N Engl J Med 2015;372(26):2509–20.
57. Le D, Durham J, Smith K, et al. Mismatch repair deficiency predicts response of solid tumors to PD-1 blockade. Science 2017;357(6349):409–13.
58. Schellens J, Marabelle A, Zeigenfuss S, et al. Pembrolizumab for previously treated advanced cervical squamous cell cancer: preliminary results from the phase 2 KEYNOTE-158 study. J Clin Oncol 2017;35l(15 Suppl):5514.
59. Overman MJ, McDermott R, Leach JL, et al. Nivolumab in patients with metastatic DNA mismatch repair-deficient or microsatellite instability-high colorectal cancer (CheckMate 142): an open-label, multicentre, phase 2 study. Lancet Oncol 2017; 18(9):1182–91.
60. Czink E, Kloor M, Goeppert B, et al. Successful immune checkpoint blockade in a patient with advanced stage microsatellite-unstable biliary tract cancer. Cold Spring Harb Mol Case Stud 2017;3(5) [pii:a001974].
61. Hsu C, Lee S-H, Ejadi S, et al. Safety and antitumor activity of pembrolizumab in patients with programmed death-ligand 1-positive nasopharyngeal carcinoma: results of the KEYNOTE-028 study. J Clin Oncol 2017;35(36):4050–6.

62. Le D, Yoshino T, Jager D, et al. KEYNOTE-164: phase II study of pembrolizumab (MK-3475) for patients with previously treated, microsatellite instability- high advanced colorectal carcinoma. J Clin Oncol 2016;34(Suppl):TPS787.

63. Nebot-Bral L, Brandao D, Verlingue L, et al. Hypermutated tumours in the era of immunotherapy: the paradigm of personalised medicine. Eur J Cancer 2017;84: 290–303.

Immunotherapy Toxicities

Katherine Sanchez, MD*, David B. Page, MD, Walter Urba, MD, PhD

KEYWORDS

- Immune-related adverse events (irAE) • Immune checkpoint inhibitors side effects
- T cell mediated toxicity • Mechanisms of irAE

KEY POINTS

- Distinct classes of immunotherapy have unique mechanisms of action and distinct irAEs.
- The most common irAEs associated with ICIs include rash, diarrhea/colitis, pneumonitis, and endocrinopathies, although any organ system can be involved.
- Proposed mechanisms for irAEs may be related to collateral effector functions of activated T cells, modulation of other immune cell types such as B cells or the innate immune system, or by other mechanisms.
- Clinical factors—including the microbiome, timing of treatment, and pre-existing autoimmunity—may influence irAEs.

INTRODUCTION

Immunotherapy is a class of antineoplastic therapy aimed at modulating the immune system to facilitate control or elimination of cancer. Immune checkpoint inhibitors (ICIs) are therapeutic antibodies that target regulatory molecules on T cells, and represent the most widely used US Food and Drug Administration (FDA)-approved class of immunotherapy. ICIs are associated with unique immune-mediated toxicities, called immune-related adverse events (irAEs). These toxicities may affect any organ system, and the precise mechanisms of action are still under investigation. Current evidence suggests that activation of T cells are involved; however, other components of the immune response have been implicated. Other host factors may affect immune-mediated toxicities, including the microbiome, pre-existing autoimmune disease, and timing of treatment. This article summarizes toxicities

Disclosure Statement: D.B. Page receives research support from Merck Biopharmaceuticals, Bristol-Myers Squibb, and IRX Therapeutics, and has served on advisory boards for the following related companies: Merck Biopharmaceuticals, Bristol-Myers Squibb, Nektar. W. Urba is an investigator for BMS and receives grant support, a consultant for MedImmune and Celldex, receives honoraria for serving on data safety boards, and is a consultant for Oncosec and NewLink for which he receives honoraria. K. Sanchez has nothing to disclose.
Earle A. Chiles Research Institute, 4805 Northeast Glisan Street, North Pavilion, 2N, Portland, OR 97213, USA
* Corresponding author. 4805 Northeast Glisan Street, North Pavilion, Portland, OR 97213.
E-mail address: katherine.sanchez@providence.org

associated with ICIs and discusses potential mechanisms of action, management strategies, and other clinical considerations. Also reviewed are the unique mechanisms of action and immune-related toxicities of other FDA-approved classes of immunotherapy, including cellular adoptive T cell therapy, cancer vaccines, and cytokine therapies.

TOXICITIES OF IMMUNE CHECKPOINT INHIBITORS
Proposed Mechanisms of Immune Checkpoint Antibody-Related Toxicities

The mechanistic differences of anti-CTLA4 versus anti-PD-1/L1 may contribute to distinct patterns of immune-related toxicity, which was first demonstrated in murine models. Mice with CTLA-4 knockout experienced fatal lymphoproliferation,[1] whereas mice with PD-1 knockout had more limited adverse events related to autoimmunity, with toxicities such as arthritis or lupus-like glomerulonephritis.[2] In humans, anti-CTLA-4 therapy is generally more toxic relative to anti-PD-1/L1, with higher rates of adverse events and treatment-associated mortality. Furthermore, toxicities are more dose dependent with anti-CTLA-4, whereas toxicities are relatively stable across doses for anti-PD-1/L1.[3]

The specific mechanisms of checkpoint antibody-related toxicity are still under investigation. However, recent preclinical and clinical data support the notion that toxicities are manifestations of disturbed immunologic homeostasis, and are primarily mediated by T cells, although other immune cell types may be involved. Under normal physiologic conditions, immune checkpoint signals prevent autoimmunity via a process of T cell tolerance, whereby autoreactive T cells are suppressed. ICIs interfere with T cell tolerance, facilitating a desired effect of reinvigorating T cell responses against tumor antigens, but may also activate T cells against self-antigens. The proposed mechanisms for immune-related toxicities are best demonstrated by considering activated T cells and their effector functions, and how activated T cells may interface with other components of immunologic homeostasis, including regulatory T cells (Tregs), B cells, cytokines released by T cells, innate immune cells/complement, and granulocytes (**Fig. 1**).

Effector T cell–mediated toxicities

ICIs likely cause aberrant activation of autoreactive T cells and/or activation of tumor-reactive T cells against antigens that are shared by tumor and normal tissue. One example was seen in 2 patients following combination therapy with nivolumab and ipilimumab who developed fatal myocarditis caused by refractory cardiac electrical instability. Postmortem evaluation of the myocardium showed dense $CD3^+CD8^+$ T-lymphocytic infiltration in cardiac muscle. Quantitative DNA sequencing of the T cell receptor demonstrated that clonal, high-frequency, T cell receptor sequences were shared in the tumor, cardiac muscle, and striated muscle, suggesting a shared antigen across the tissues.[4] Another example is vitiligo, a clinical manifestation of depigmentation caused by immunologic destruction of melanocytes. It is proposed that melanoma cells share antigen with normal melanocytes, leading to T cell–mediated activation against both melanoma cells and melanocytes. One study performed immunohistochemistry (IHC) staining of melanoma, which showed $CD4^+$ and melan-A–specific $CD8^+$ T cells in close proximity to apoptotic melanocytes following treatment with anti-CTLA-4 antibody.[5]

Regulatory T cell–mediated toxicities

CTLA-4 is constitutively expressed by Tregs, and there are multiple proposed mechanisms of anti-CTLA-4 mediated toxicities via its effects on Tregs. In some studies,

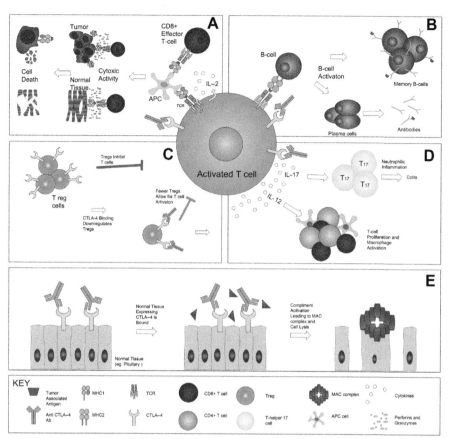

Fig. 1. Proposed mechanism for immune-related adverse events (irAEs). The specific mechanisms for irAEs are still under investigation; they are thought to be primarily T cell mediated, but other immune cell types have been proposed. The figure depicts many of the proposed mechanisms. (*A*) When activated by ICIs, tumor-reactive T cells may also recognize shared antigen expressed by normal tissue, leading to unwanted cytotoxic activity. (*B*) PD-1 is expressed on IgM-secreting memory B cells; anti-PD1/L1 may modulate antibody production by these B cells, leading to unmasked autoimmunity, especially antibody-mediated thyroid disease. (*C*) CTLA-4 is constitutively expressed on regulatory T cells, and anti-CTLA-4 blockade may lead to macrophage-dependent depletion of regulatory T cells; this may deregulate homeostasis leading to irAEs, most notably thyroid dysfunction. (*D*) IrAEs may also be mediated by cytokine release, further potentiating T cell activation. One example is increased IL-17 leading to colitis. (*E*) CTLA-4 has also been shown to be expressed on normal tissues, such as pituitary, and with treatment of CTLA-4 blockade complement-mediated inflammation and destruction is activated. APC, antigen-presenting cell; CTLA-4, cytotoxic T lymphocyte–associated protein 4; IL, interleukin; MAC, membrane attack complex; MHC, major histocompatibility complex; T17, T-helper 17 cells; TCR, T cell receptor; Treg, regulatory T cell.

ipilimumab (anti-CTLA-4) is associated with an increase in the ratio of effector T cells to regulatory T cells within the tumor microenvironment, which is thought to be mediated by Fc-γ receptor and macrophage-dependent depletion of Tregs.[6] Other data suggest that anti-CTLA4 may bind Tregs and deregulate Treg homeostasis driven by CTLA-4, allowing the recognition of self-antigens.[7] In preclinical models, deletion of CLTA-4 on Tregs leads to fatal autoimmune disease affecting multiple organs, especially myocarditis.[8] In other preclinical models, anti-CTLA-4 was administered to suppress Tregs in mice that were then administered thyroglobulin, leading to thyroiditis.[9] This mechanism may partially explain why patients treated with anti-CTLA-4 have an increased susceptibility to thyroid dysfunction following treatment.

B cell–mediated and antibody-mediated toxicity

PD-1 is expressed on all B cell subsets and plays an integral role in regulation of the humoral immune response. PD-1 is highly expressed in immunoglobulin M (IgM)-secreting memory B cells, which develop via a T cell–independent mechanism. Thus, anti-PD-1/L1 may indirectly modulate antibody production by facilitating downstream B cell immunoglobulin production. This mechanism is believed to mediate antibody-mediated thyroid dysfunction following anti-PD-1/L1. In non–small cell lung cancer (NSCLC), 21% of patients treated with pembrolizumab developed thyroid dysfunction. Of these patients, 80% developed antithyroid antibodies after treatment. These autoantibodies became clinically detectable shortly after initiation of treatment, suggesting that anti-PD-1 results in rapid activation of memory B cells and unmasking of quiescent autoimmunity.[10] In another study, patients with detectable antithyroglobulin or anti-TPO antibodies at baseline were more likely to develop destructive thyroiditis while receiving anti-PD-1/L1.[11] Bullous pemphigoid has been reported following anti-PD-1/L1 therapy, with a proposed mechanism of B cell–mediated auto-antibody production against the hemidesmosomal protein BP180, which is present in melanoma and NSCLCs, but also present in the basement membrane of normal skin.[12]

Cytokine-mediated toxicity

IrAEs are also thought to be mediated via noncellular immune components, including cytokines and complement. Interleukin (IL)-17, a proinflammatory cytokine produced by T-helper cells, has been shown to be increased in both preclinical models of colitis and patients with ipilimumab-induced colitis.[13] On resolution of clinical colitis, IL-17 levels decreased to levels comparable with those in patients without colitis. In another study, IL-17 levels were predictive of immune checkpoint-related colitis, whereas increased serum levels of IL-10 and transforming growth factor β1 were associated with improved progression-free survival but were not predictive of irAEs.[14] Several antibodies that block IL-17 are being used currently for treatment of rheumatologic conditions of psoriasis and ankylosing spondylitis. In a case report of ICI colitis and severe psoriasis, both resolved following treatment with the IL-17 inhibitor, secukinumab.[15] IL-6 is also under investigation as a biomarker for immune-related toxicities. In patients treated with ipilimumab, those with lower baseline serum levels had an increased risk of irAEs.[16]

Complement-mediated toxicity

Complement-mediated type 2 hypersensitivity reactions have been proposed in anti-CTLA-4–associated hypophysitis. Patients who developed ipilimumab-induced hypopituitarism were shown to express pituitary antibodies after being negative before treatment. In preclinical models of anti-CTLA-4, CTLA-4/anti-CTLA-4 immune complexes were found in excised pituitary glands. Subsequent binding of complement and activation of the classical complement cascade was noted.[17] This observation was also noted in patients treated with anti-CTLA-4. Patients negative for pituitary antibodies at baseline developed antibodies to thyrotropin, follicle-stimulating hormone, and corticotropin-secreting cells, and had complement activation and increased immune infiltration.[18]

Histamine-mediated toxicity

Acute infusion reactions are common with monoclonal antibodies. The proposed mechanism of infusion-related reactions includes drug binding cell-bound immuno-globulin E, stimulating the release of histamine. Although the mechanism of infusion reactions for ICIs has not been formally studied, it is thought to be a hypersensitivity reaction similar to that of monoclonal antibodies. In patients treated with PD-1/L1 therapy across tumor types, grades 1 to 3 infusion reactions are reported in 3% to 10% of patients.[19] In cases of grade 3 infusion reactions, patients received antihistamine and corticosteroids, and no dose reductions or interruptions were necessary. With future infusions patients were pretreated safely with diphenhydramine and/or corticosteroids.[20]

Influence of Histology on Immune-Related Adverse events

As ICIs start being used for indications beyond melanoma, patterns of irAEs related to tumor histology have been described. Early characterization of these patterns in the most studied tumor types from PD-1 trials suggests some distinct differences. The most obvious and widely reported example is vitiligo, which is more common in patients with melanoma than in patients with other tumor types. Similarly, melanoma patients treated with anti-PD-1 agents are more likely to experience pruritus and colitis than patients with renal cell carcinoma (RCC).[3] In a meta-analysis of patients treated with anti-PD-1 agents, pneumonitis was observed more often in patients with NSCLC than in patients with melanoma.[21] Other associations observed were myasthenia gravis in patients treated with pembrolizumab for thymic epithelial tumors, and cytopenias in patients treated for lymphoma.[22,23] One challenge of documenting these associations is the small study populations of phase 2 and phase 2 clinical trials. The signal of these rare (<5%) irAEs may be underappreciated in small cohorts of usually 10 to 100 patients. The model of shared antigens may explain why some irAEs seem to be histology driven.

Involved Organ Systems

Although any organ system can be affected, phase 3 studies suggest that the most common irAEs occur in the skin, gastrointestinal tract, and endocrine, hepatic, pulmonary, or renal organs. The most serious irAEs have been cardiac, pulmonary, and neurologic toxicities.[24] **Table 1** provides a noninclusive list of the spectrum of irAEs observed with ICIs, organized by organ system (see **Table 1**).

Timing of Occurrence of Immune-Related Adverse Events

Early and late immune-related toxicities are thought to be mechanistically distinct. Early irAEs are common and are often related to skin/mucosa (colitis, rash, and pneumonitis). It is proposed that these irAEs are related to global disturbances in immunologic homeostasis causing activation of effector T cells, leading to the recruitment of proinflammatory cells including neutrophils in the mucosa.[25] Delayed irAEs generally occur between 8 and 12 weeks and affect specific organs (hypophysitis, vitiligo, hepatitis). They are proposed to be related to a breakdown of organ-specific tolerance leading to the activation of tumor-specific T cells that may recognize shared antigens. Clinical trial data support this model: dermatologic toxicities are common irAEs and typically occur early, usually after the second cycle of treatment, whereas hypophysitis and liver toxicities usually occur after 8 weeks.[26] Hepatitis and hypophysitis have been reported up to 1 year after discontinuation of therapy.[27] As duration of therapy increases from months to years, it is unknown whether this prolonged drug exposure is associated with different immune-related toxicities or mechanisms of toxicity.

Table 1
Immune-related toxicities by organ system

Dermatologic Toxicity	Cardiac Toxicity
Rash	Myocarditis
Inflammatory dermatitis	Pericarditis
Bullous dermatosis	Arrhythmias
SCARs (severe cutaneous adverse reactions)	Heart failure
Stevens-Johnson Syndrome	Vasculitis
Toxic epidermal necrolysis	Venous thromboembolism
Lichenoid drug reactions	Coronary artery disease
Endocrinopathies	Rheumatologic Toxicity
Primary hypothyroidism	Inflammatory arthritis
Hyperthyroidism	Myositis
Hypophysitis	Polymyalgia-like syndrome
Primary adrenal insufficiency	Renal Toxicity
Type 1 diabetes mellitus	Nephritis
Hepatotoxicity	Ocular Toxicity
Gastrointestinal Toxicity	Uveitis/iritis
Diarrhea	Episcleritis
Colitis	Blepharitis
Pulmonary Toxicity	Vision changes
Pneumonitis	Hematologic Toxicity
Neurologic Toxicity	Autoimmune hemolytic anemia
Myasthenia gravis	Acquired thrombotic
Guillain-Barré syndrome	thrombocytopenic purpura
Peripheral neuropathy	Hemolytic uremic syndrome
Aseptic meningitis	Aplastic anemia
Encephalitis	Lymphopenia
Transverse myelitis	Immune thrombocytopenia
	Acquired hemophilia

Immune checkpoint inhibitors can result in toxicity involving any organ. Listed are irAEs by organ system across tumor types and grades.

Cumulative toxicities have not been observed in melanoma patients with prolonged drug exposure treated with nivolumab.[28]

Influence of Combination Therapy on Immune-Related Adverse events

Combination immunotherapy with CTLA-4 and PD-1/L1 blockade is currently approved by the FDA for metastatic melanoma and advanced RCC, and is being evaluated in many other tumor types. Generally irAEs associated with combination checkpoint therapy affect more patients, and toxicities are of higher grade and occur more quickly. In large cohorts, grade 3 to 4 treatment-related adverse events occur in 59% of melanoma patients receiving nivolumab/ipilimumab, versus 21% or 28% for nivolumab or ipilimumab, respectively.[29] Increased toxicity of combination therapy is the limiting factor in clinical use of this strategy, with some clinicians opting to treat patients with sequential monotherapy. irAEs with combination therapy leading to discontinuation of treatment currently occur in nearly 40% of patients.[30]

Another evolving theory is that the timing of ICIs may influence toxicity and efficacy. In preclinical models, mice treated with concurrent combination administration of the T cell agonist antibody, anti-OX40, with anti-PD-1 had increased cytokine release and immune-related toxicity, whereas mice treated with sequential combination administration of anti-OX40 followed by anti-PD-1 had reduced but sustained cytokine production, enhanced antitumor activity, and reduced immune-related toxicity. These preliminary data suggest that the timing of various immunotherapy modalities may influence immune-related toxicity as well as efficacy.[31]

Influence of Prior Therapies on Immune-Related Adverse Events

Patients experiencing immune-related toxicity with monotherapy with either anti-CTLA-4 or PD-1/L1 therapy are at risk of developing irAEs when receiving subsequent immunotherapy.[32] Despite the increased risk, subsequent treatment has been shown to be safe. In a large study of patients previously treated with anti-CTLA-4 therapy, treatment with anti-PD-1 was safely tolerated, even when grade 3 toxicity had occurred.[33] A retrospective analysis of melanoma patients who received high-dose IL-2 following ipilimumab suggested that prior ipilimumab did not influence response rate and did not increase the risk of ipilimumab-related toxicities.[34] Another clinical consideration is rechallenging patients following dose-limiting toxicity. In a study evaluating NSCLC patients discontinuing anti-PD-L1 following grade 3 to 4 toxicity, 50% of the rechallenged patients had no subsequent irAEs, 25% had recurrence of the initial irAE, and the other 25% had a new irAE.[35] These data suggest that retreatment may be an option, especially in cases with clear clinical response and no other safe therapeutic alternatives.

Biomarkers and Host Factors to Predict Immune-Related Adverse Events

Despite provocative preliminary data, no genetic, biomarker, or microbiological risk factors of immune-related toxicity have been validated for routine clinical use. Despite well-known associations with smoking status and clinical benefit following anti-PD-1/L1 in NSCLC, former or current smoking status did not increase the risk of pneumonitis with anti-PD-1/L1 or combination immunotherapy. In the same study, chest radiation therapy was not a risk factor either.[36] Genetic studies have failed to demonstrate human leukocyte antigen (HLA) as a significant predictive factor for toxicity. Serum cytokine levels, such as IL-6 and IL-17, may serve as predictive biomarkers of toxicity.[16,37]

Pre-existing Autoimmunity as a Predictor of Immune-Related Adverse Events

The safety and efficacy of treatment of patients with pre-existing autoimmune conditions is still unclear because most of these patients have been excluded from clinical trials. Patients with a history of autoimmune diseases may have antibodies to self-antigen or disturbances in peripheral tolerance. As described earlier, ICIs can lead to irAEs, which are similar to autoimmune disease in patients without a history of autoimmune disease. Inflammatory arthritis, synovitis, and sicca syndrome are all irAE events reported following ICIs that mirror symptoms of autoimmune diseases.[38] ICIs, including PD-1/L1 and CTLA-4, have been described in the pathophysiology of some autoimmune diseases.[39] One clinical series reported antibody-positive rheumatoid arthritis (anti-CCP) following treatment with ICIs, frequently requiring systemic immunosuppression for treatment of the disease.[40] In a registry of patients experiencing grade 2+ irAEs, only 11 of 20 of subjects with pre-existing autoimmune disease experienced a flare of their conditions and only 25% required treatment discontinuation.[41] In another study, 42% of patients with pre-existing autoimmune disease experienced flare during treatment, whereas 16% developed an unrelated irAE. All flares or new irAEs were managed successfully with immunosuppression and symptom management, and no patients required termination of anti-PD-1 treatment without affecting response rates.[42] In these patients it is important for clinicians to balance the risk of possible worsening of treatable autoimmune disease with certain death from stage IV disease.

The safety of ICIs in organ transplant patients has not been evaluated because these patients are generally excluded from clinical trials. In preclinical models, treatment with anti-CTLA-4 has led to rejection in a murine model of cardiac transplant.[43] PD-1/L1 is thought to have a stronger role in peripheral tolerance than CTLA-4, suggesting that anti-PD-1/L1 therapies may lead to increased organ rejection.[44] Currently only 12 organ transplant cases have been reported in the literature, the majority being renal transplant patients with melanoma. Of the 12 cases, 4 renal transplant patients developed graft rejection that was reversible with immunosuppressive treatment. Despite the possible rejection, 8 of the 12 patients had a response or stabilization of their disease with ICIs.[45]

Influence of Microbiome on Immune-Related Adverse Events

The intestinal microbiome is a complex microbial community that contributes to host health, with certain bacterial species being important for modulating the immune environment of the colon. Bacterial genera such as Bacteroides, *Clostridium*, and *Faecalibacterium* have been shown to induce expansion of Tregs, creating an anti-inflammatory environment.[46] Anti-CTLA-4 is thought to cause a disruption of mucosal immune regulation leading to colitis. One study suggested a protective role of the Bacteroidetes phylum.[47] This study also found underrepresentation of Bacteroidetes in patients with new-onset immune-mediated colitis. This finding is supportive of the previous studies that classified Bacteroidetes as a phyla of the colonic microbiota that can limit inflammation by stimulating Treg differentiation.[48]

Recent studies have evaluated the role of the microbiome on efficacy and toxicity associated with ICI therapy, raising the question about the impact of antibiotic therapy on such therapies. The impact of antibiotic use in humans was explored in a cohort of patients receiving anti-PD-1/L1. Subjects treated with antibiotics before, during, or shortly after anti-PD-1/L1 treatment had significantly lower progression-free survival and overall survival compared with the no-antibiotic group.[49] In another cohort, responding patients were more likely to have high levels of *Akkermansia muciniphila*.[50] These preliminary data suggest that certain bacterial species may be associated with response or toxicity and may be modulated by antibiotic therapy. These observations of the stool microbiome have led to the current recommendation that antibiotics should be avoided in patients treated with anti-PD-1.[49] These preliminary data suggest that the microbiome may also have future implications for fecal transplants or treatment with probiotics before or during treatment. Other future directions of research are investigation of other microbiomes—oral, pulmonary, urinary, vaginal, and skin—that are only now being examined and may also be important for ICI treatment in the future.

Association of Clinical Benefit with Immune-Related Toxicity

Across multiple tumor types, development of toxicities has been associated with increased response rate or survival, in particular in NSCLC. In NSCLC patients, the development of thyroid dysfunction following pembrolizumab or nivolumab correlates with increased survival compared with similar patients without thyroid dysfunction.[10,51] In melanoma, vitiligo and rash correlated with overall survival, whereas other toxicities, such as thyroid dysfunction, diarrhea, or pneumonitis did not.[52] It may be difficult to confirm prospectively the association of immune-related toxicity with clinical benefit, because subjects who benefit from ICIs are more likely to receive ongoing therapy and therefore have greater exposure to the drug relative to subjects who do not benefit from ICIs.

Guidelines for Management of Immune-Related Adverse Events

To maximize both clinical benefit and safety, it is imperative that clinicians are knowledgeable about irAEs and their management because early intervention is often the key. Although there are no prospective studies to validate management of irAEs, expert consensus recommendations have been compiled and published by organizations such as the Society for Immunotherapy of Cancer (SITC), the American Society for Clinical Oncology (ASCO), and the European Society for Medical Oncology (ESMO). These recommendations define toxicity syndromes by organ system, outline the diagnostic workup, grade irAEs, and give appropriate treatment recommendations. Recommended treatments generally consist of topical or systemic steroids as first-line treatment with dose and route of administration depending on the severity of the toxicity. With steroid treatment slow tapers are key to avoiding exacerbations. In specific situations, the use of other agents such as infliximab, mycophenolate mofetil, or cyclophosphamide may be recommended. For example, for grade I toxicities ASCO recommends continued ICI dosing, with topical steroids or low-dose systemic steroids (<20 mg oral prednisone daily). For grade 2 irAEs, ASCO recommends temporary treatment discontinuation, moderate systemic steroids (eg, 1–2 mg/kg of oral prednisone), and restarting ICIs after symptoms resolve. For grade 3/4 irAEs, ASCO recommends permanent ICI discontinuation, high-dose systemic steroids intravenously (eg, methylprednisolone 1 mg/kg/d tapered over weeks). Retrospective studies of patients with melanoma have shown that patients treated with steroids did not have worse outcomes, leading to the current practice of liberal use of steroids.[53] Ancillary immunosuppression is specific to the nature of the toxicity. For example, infliximab is recommended for grade 3/4 pneumonitis, whereas mycophenolate mofetil is recommended for grade 3/4 nephritis, hepatitis, and myocarditis, among others. Another example of infliximab use is in ICI-mediated colitis, whereby patients with grade 3/4 colitis treated with infliximab have a significantly shorter time to resolution compared with patients treated with steroids. As discussed earlier, IL-17 antagonists have also been proposed as an additional method of managing severe immune-related colitis.[15] Beyond these treatment recommendations, review articles can be consulted for recommendations, especially for rare irAEs (eg, myocarditis, bullous dermatitis, myasthenia gravis).

UNIQUE TOXICITIES OF OTHER IMMUNOTHERAPY CLASSES

Other classes of immunotherapy may carry their own distinct toxicity profile. Classes include cancer vaccines, cytokine therapy, and adoptive cellular therapies. Specific proposed mechanisms and clinical data are reported here.

Cancer Vaccines

Cancer vaccines generally have minimal toxicities, in part because of their mechanism of action being directed to eliciting immune responses against a narrow range of tumor-associated antigens. Vaccine target antigens ideally are highly expressed in cancer cells but are minimally expressed or not expressed in normal cells. Synthetic vaccines are similar to infectious disease vaccines, and use a vector to deliver the antigen(s). Toxicity can be related to the antigen or the vector. Vaccine vectors may be viral or bacterial, which introduces the potential for vector-based toxicity. Cases of disseminated *Listeria* infection have been reported with the cancer vaccine CRS-207, which uses live attenuated *Listeria* as a vector.[54]

Sipuleucel-T (Provenge), the first cellular FDA-approved vaccine, is an autologous cellular vaccine generated from autologous dendritic cells for advanced prostate cancer. This vaccine was well tolerated in the phase 3 trials where grade 4 adverse events were reported in less than 4% of patients, and included catheter-associated bacteremia and cardiovascular events.[55]

Cytokine Therapy

The use of cytokine therapies has been limited by the modest efficacy and the severe toxicities associated with therapeutic doses. High-dose IL-2 and interferon-α are the only approved cytokine therapies; however, other cytokines are being evaluated in ongoing clinical trials. The acute toxicity of high-dose IL-2 requires inpatient hospital administration because of capillary leak syndrome causing hypotension. The complex mechanism of IL-2 capillary leak syndrome involves induction of circulating proinflammatory cytokines, generation of complement-activation products, neutrophil activation, and activation of vascular endothelial cell antigen. Complement activation and capillary leak may lead to acute organ dysfunction (cardiac, renal, and hepatic), although this is rapidly reversible on discontinuation of IL-2.[56] The PROCLAIM registry is a database of patients treated with high-dose IL-2 over 10 years for metastatic melanoma and metastatic RCC. The most common irAEs occurring in greater than 70% were vitiligo and thyroid dysfunction. Overall, less than 5% of irAEs (other than acute toxicity) related to IL-2 required cycles to be held. The most serious irAEs reported occurred during treatment and included myocarditis, hepatitis, myasthenia gravis, and Guillain-Barré syndrome. Patients developing irAEs had significantly improved responses, tumor control, and overall survival.[57] IL-2 has been used in combination with ICIs and has been shown to be tolerated with similar additional toxicity as expected with checkpoint monotherapy. In an attempt to reduce toxicity related to cytokine therapy, pegylated cytokine therapies are in development. A phase 1 trial of pegylated IL-2 demonstrated encouraging preliminary safety, with treatment-related grade 3 irAEs in only 14% of patients, with the most common irAEs being hypotension and rash.[58]

Cellular Therapy

Adoptive T cell therapy

Tumor-infiltrating lymphocytes (TILs) are more likely to be tumor-reactive than peripheral blood lymphocytes. Adoptive T cell therapy isolates endogenous TILs, which are then expanded in vitro before being administered to the patient. Often, adoptive T cell therapy is combined with chemotherapy, high-dose IL-2, and ICIs. Many of the toxicities associated with TIL therapy are related to chemotherapy and/or IL-2 therapy. Preliminary data suggest that these combinations are safely tolerated, with irAEs additive but not synergistic to combination therapy.[59]

T cell therapy with affinity-enhanced T cell receptors

The affinity of T cell receptors (TCRs) for antigens expressed in tumors is generally low, and in response T cells have been engineered to express high-affinity TCRs to antigen expressed on tumors. Modified T cells engineered to express an affinity-enhanced TCR to the cancer testis antigens NY-ESO and LAGE-1 have been shown to be safe and have progression-free survival in patients with advanced myeloma.[60] Although this is a powerful strategy, clinical use has been limited by toxicity caused by the on-target but off-tumor effects. Despite extensive testing in preclinical molecular, biophysical, and immunologic testing in vitro and in mouse models for MAGE-A3/HLA-A*01, a peptide expressed on many tumor types, treatment resulted in severe cardiac toxicity caused by on-target but off-tumor antigen recognition of a similar epitope on a cardiac protein called titin.[61] Severe irAEs have also been reported in melanoma patients treated with T cells with modified TCRs directed against MART-1(AAG)/HLA-A2, whereby severe melanocyte destruction led to uveitis and hearing loss.[62] Other severe and unexpected irAEs occurred in melanoma patients receiving TCRs directed against MAGE-A39(KVA)/HLA-A2, resulting in severe mental status changes and coma in 2 patients.[63]

Chimeric antigen receptor T cell therapy
Chimeric antigen receptor (CAR) T cell therapy is a type of adoptive cellular therapy whereby autologous T cells are genetically modified to express a cell surface receptor that may bind tumor cells directly, allowing the T cell to be activated in a TCR-independent fashion. Infused CAR T cells are directly cytotoxic to tumor cells, and may also promote immune surveillance through antigen release and epitope spread. Toxicities associated with CAR T cells can be related to cytokine release/T cell activation, or to on-target effects that depend on the specificity of the single-chain variable fragment causing T cell activation. CD19, a B cell marker, is one of the most common CARs, and is designed to treat B cell leukemias and lymphomas. B cell aplasia resulting from CD19 CAR T cell therapy is an expected, on-target toxicity related to depletion of nonneoplastic B cells that also express CD19. This irAE is reversible over time after CAR T cells are ablated.[64]

The use of CAR T cell therapy has been limited in solid tumors because of the potent cytotoxic effect on shared antigens in normal tissue. This effect was radically demonstrated in a patient who experienced fatal cytokine storm following administration of CAR T cells recognizing ERBB2 in a patient with HER2-positive breast cancer. Despite safe treatment of this target with a monoclonal antibody, trastuzumab, CAR T treatment resulted in systemic signs of ischemia and hemorrhagic microangiopathic injury of multiple organs seen at autopsy.[65] Despite these severe events, other targets and strategies are in development for use in solid tumors, including incorporation of suicide genes to permit rapid ablation of CAR T cells.

Another common toxicity associated with CAR T cells is cytokine release syndrome, which manifests as fever, hypotension, hypoxia, and neurologic changes. Cytokine release syndrome is most common with patients who have a high tumor burden, as measured by blasts in the bone marrow.[66] New strategies for treatment of this cytokine release syndrome include administration of anti-IL-6-receptor antagonist, tocilizumab, which has been approved by the FDA for CAR T cell–induced cytokine release syndrome.[67] As with vaccines, integration of viral vectors has been a potential safety concern, although in more than 1000 patients treated with CAR T cell therapy no occurrence has been reported.

SUMMARY

The irAEs associated with ICIs and toxicities of other classes of immunotherapy are still under investigation. The mechanisms outlined herein demonstrate our early understanding of the side effects of these medications. As additional clinical trials and treatments emerge, interesting and unexpected associations such as the effect of antibiotics on microbiome and response will help clinicians gain a greater understanding about the immune system and immunotherapy. Currently available treatment guidelines from ASCO, SITC, and ESMO rest on expert consensus and trials data to guide clinicians on appropriate and expeditious management of irAEs.

REFERENCES

1. Tivol EA, Borriello F, Schweitzer AN, et al. Loss of CTLA-4 leads to massive lymphoproliferation and fatal multiorgan tissue destruction, revealing a critical negative regulatory role of CTLA-4. Immunity 1995;3(5):541–7.

2. Nishimura H, Nose M, Hiai H, et al. Development of lupus-like autoimmune diseases by disruption of the PD-1 gene encoding an ITIM motif-carrying immunoreceptor. Immunity 1999;11(2):141–51.

3. Khoja L, Day D, Wei-Wu Chen T, et al. Tumour- and class-specific patterns of immune-related adverse events of immune checkpoint inhibitors: a systematic review. Ann Oncol 2017;28(10):2377–85.

4. Johnson DB, Balko JM, Compton ML, et al. Fulminant myocarditis with combination immune checkpoint blockade. N Engl J Med 2016;375(18):1749–55.

5. Weber JS, Kahler KC, Hauschild A. Management of immune-related adverse events and kinetics of response with ipilimumab. J Clin Oncol 2012;30(21):2691–7.

6. Romano E, Kusio-Kobialka M, Foukas PG, et al. Ipilimumab-dependent cell-mediated cytotoxicity of regulatory T cells ex vivo by nonclassical monocytes in melanoma patients. Proc Natl Acad Sci U S A 2015;112(19):6140–5.

7. Kavanagh B, O'Brien S, Lee D, et al. CTLA4 blockade expands FoxP3+ regulatory and activated effector CD4+ T cells in a dose-dependent fashion. Blood 2008;112(4):1175–83.

8. Wing K, Onishi Y, Prieto-Martin P, et al. CTLA-4 control over Foxp3+ regulatory T cell function. Science 2008;322(5899):271–5.

9. Wei WZ, Jacob JB, Zielinski JF, et al. Concurrent induction of antitumor immunity and autoimmune thyroiditis in CD4+ CD25+ regulatory T cell-depleted mice. Cancer Res 2005;65(18):8471–8.

10. Osorio JC, Ni A, Chaft JE, et al. Antibody-mediated thyroid dysfunction during T-cell checkpoint blockade in patients with non-small-cell lung cancer. Ann Oncol 2017;28(3):583–9.

11. Kobayashi T, Iwama S, Yasuda Y, et al. Patients with antithyroid antibodies are prone to develop destructive thyroiditis by nivolumab: a prospective study. J Endocr Soc 2018;2(3):241–51.

12. Naidoo J, Schindler K, Querfeld C, et al. Autoimmune bullous skin disorders with immune checkpoint inhibitors targeting PD-1 and PD-L1. Cancer Immunol Res 2016;4(5):383–9.

13. Callahan M, Yang A, Tandon S, et al. Evaluation of serum IL-17 levels during ipilimumab therapy: correlation with colitis. J Clin Oncol 2011;29(15_suppl):2505.

14. Tarhini AA, Zahoor H, Lin Y, et al. Baseline circulating IL-17 predicts toxicity while TGF-β1 and IL-10 are prognostic of relapse in ipilimumab neoadjuvant therapy of melanoma. J Immunother Cancer 2015;3(1):39.

15. Esfahani K, Miller WH Jr. Reversal of autoimmune toxicity and loss of tumor response by interleukin-17 blockade. N Engl J Med 2017;376(20):1989–91.

16. Valpione S, Pasquali S, Campana LG, et al. Sex and interleukin-6 are prognostic factors for autoimmune toxicity following treatment with anti-CTLA4 blockade. J Transl Med 2018;16(1):94.

17. Iwama S, De Remigis A, Callahan MK, et al. Pituitary expression of CTLA-4 mediates hypophysitis secondary to administration of CTLA-4 blocking antibody. Sci Transl Med 2014;6(230):230ra245.

18. Sharma A, Subudhi SK, Blando J, et al. Anti-CTLA-4 immunotherapy does not deplete FOXP3+ regulatory T cells (Tregs) in human cancers. Clin Cancer Res 2019;25(4):1233–8.

19. Garon EB, Rizvi NA, Hui R, et al. Pembrolizumab for the treatment of non–small-cell lung cancer. N Engl J Med 2015;372(21):2018–28.

20. Momtaz P, Park V, Panageas KS, et al. Safety of infusing ipilimumab over 30 minutes. J Clin Oncol 2015;33(30):3454–8.

21. Wu J, Hong D, Zhang X, et al. PD-1 inhibitors increase the incidence and risk of pneumonitis in cancer patients in a dose-independent manner: a meta-analysis. Sci Rep 2017;7:44173.

22. Cho J, Ahn M-J, Yoo KH, et al. A phase II study of pembrolizumab for patients with previously treated advanced thymic epithelial tumor. J Clin Oncol 2017; 35(15_suppl):8521.

23. Moskowitz CH, Zinzani PL, Fanale KH, et al. Pembrolizumab in relapsed/refractory classical Hodgkin lymphoma: primary end point analysis of the phase 2 Keynote-087 study. Blood 2016;128:1107.

24. Weber JS, Hodi FS, Wolchok JD, et al. Safety profile of nivolumab monotherapy: a pooled analysis of patients with advanced melanoma. J Clin Oncol 2017;35(7): 785–92.

25. Curry JL, Tetzlaff MT, Nagarajan P, et al. Diverse types of dermatologic toxicities from immune checkpoint blockade therapy. J Cutan Pathol 2017;44(2):158–76.

26. Naidoo J, Page D, Li BT, et al. Toxicities of the anti-PD-1 and anti-PD-L1 immune checkpoint antibodies. Ann Oncol 2015;26(12):2375–91.

27. Parakh S, Cebon J, Klein O. Delayed autoimmune toxicity occurring several months after cessation of anti-PD-1 therapy. Oncologist 2018;23(7):849–51.

28. Topalian SL, Sznol M, McDermott DF, et al. Survival, durable tumor remission, and long-term safety in patients with advanced melanoma receiving nivolumab. J Clin Oncol 2014;32(10):1020.

29. Wolchok JD, Chiarion-Sileni V, Gonzalez R, et al. Overall survival with combined nivolumab and ipilimumab in advanced melanoma. N Engl J Med 2017;377(14): 1345–56.

30. Larkin J, Chiarion-Sileni V, Gonzalez R, et al. Combined nivolumab and ipilimumab or monotherapy in untreated melanoma. N Engl J Med 2015;373(1):23–34.

31. Messenheimer DJ, Jensen SM, Afentoulis ME, et al. Timing of PD-1 blockade is critical to effective combination immunotherapy with anti-OX40. Clin Cancer Res 2017;23(20):6165–77.

32. Bowyer S, Prithviraj P, Lorigan P, et al. Efficacy and toxicity of treatment with the anti-CTLA-4 antibody ipilimumab in patients with metastatic melanoma after prior anti-PD-1 therapy. Br J Cancer 2016;114(10):1084.

33. Weber JS, D'Angelo SP, Minor D, et al. Nivolumab versus chemotherapy in patients with advanced melanoma who progressed after anti-CTLA-4 treatment (CheckMate 037): a randomised, controlled, open-label, phase 3 trial. Lancet Oncol 2015;16(4):375–84.

34. Buchbinder EI, Gunturi A, Perritt J, et al. A retrospective analysis of High-Dose Interleukin-2 (HD IL-2) following Ipilimumab in metastatic melanoma. J Immunother Cancer 2016;4(1):52.

35. Santini FC, Rizvi H, Plodkowski AJ, et al. Safety and efficacy of retreating with immunotherapy after immune-related adverse events in patients with NSCLC. Cancer Immunol Res 2018;6(9):1093–9.

36. Naidoo J, Wang X, Woo KM, et al. Pneumonitis in patients treated with anti–programmed death-1/programmed death ligand 1 therapy. J Clin Oncol 2017; 35(7):709.

37. Wolchok JD, Weber JS, Hamid O, et al. Ipilimumab efficacy and safety in patients with advanced melanoma: a retrospective analysis of HLA subtype from four trials. Lancet Oncol 2010;10(1):9.

38. Cappelli LC, Gutierrez AK, Baer AN, et al. Inflammatory arthritis and sicca syndrome induced by nivolumab and ipilimumab. Ann Rheum Dis 2017;76(1):43–50.

39. Guo Y, Walsh AM, Canavan M, et al. Immune checkpoint inhibitor PD-1 pathway is down-regulated in synovium at various stages of rheumatoid arthritis disease progression. PLoS One 2018;13(2):e0192704.

40. Belkhir R, Le Burel S, Dunogeant L, et al. Rheumatoid arthritis and polymyalgia rheumatica occurring after immune checkpoint inhibitor treatment. Ann Rheum Dis 2017;76(10):1747–50.

41. Danlos F-X, Voisin A-L, Dyevre V, et al. Safety and efficacy of anti-programmed death 1 antibodies in patients with cancer and pre-existing autoimmune or inflammatory disease. Eur J Cancer 2018;91:21–9.

42. Kähler KC, Eigentler TK, Gesierich A, et al. Ipilimumab in metastatic melanoma patients with pre-existing autoimmune disorders. Cancer Immunol Immunother 2018;67(5):825–34.

43. Zhang T, Fresnay S, Welty E, et al. Selective CD28 blockade attenuates acute and chronic rejection of murine cardiac allografts in a CTLA-4-dependent manner. Am J Transplant 2011;11(8):1599–609.

44. Herz S, Höfer T, Papapanagiotou M, et al. Checkpoint inhibitors in chronic kidney failure and an organ transplant recipient. Eur J Cancer 2016;67:66–72.

45. Kittai AS, Oldham H, Cetnar J, et al. Immune checkpoint inhibitors in organ transplant patients. J Immunother 2017;40(7):277–81.

46. Atarashi K, Tanoue T, Shima T, et al. Induction of colonic regulatory T cells by indigenous Clostridium species. Science 2011;331(6015):337–41.

47. Dubin K, Callahan MK, Ren B, et al. Intestinal microbiome analyses identify melanoma patients at risk for checkpoint-blockade-induced colitis. Nat Commun 2016;7:10391.

48. Round JL, Mazmanian SK. Inducible Foxp3+ regulatory T-cell development by a commensal bacterium of the intestinal microbiota. Proc Natl Acad Sci U S A 2010; 107(27):12204–9.

49. Matson V, Fessler J, Bao R, et al. The commensal microbiome is associated with anti–PD-1 efficacy in metastatic melanoma patients. Science 2018;359(6371): 104–8.

50. Routy B, Le Chatelier E, Derosa L, et al. Gut microbiome influences efficacy of PD-1–based immunotherapy against epithelial tumors. Science 2018; 359(6371):91–7.

51. Toi Y, Sugawara S, Kawashima Y, et al. Association of immune-related adverse events with clinical benefit in patients with advanced non-small-cell lung cancer treated with nivolumab. Oncologist 2018;23(11):1358–65.

52. Freeman-Keller M, Kim Y, Cronin H, et al. Nivolumab in resected and unresectable metastatic melanoma: characteristics of immune-related adverse events and association with outcomes. Clin Cancer Res 2016;22(4):886–94.

53. Horvat TZ, Adel NG, Dang TO, et al. Immune-related adverse events, need for systemic immunosuppression, and effects on survival and time to treatment failure in patients with melanoma treated with ipilimumab at Memorial Sloan Kettering Cancer Center. J Clin Oncol 2015;33(28):3193.

54. Denham JD, Lee DH, Castro M, et al. Two cases of disseminated infection following live organism anti-cancer vaccine administration in cancer patients. Int J Infect Dis 2018;72:1–2.

55. Kantoff PW, Higano CS, Shore ND, et al. Sipuleucel-T immunotherapy for castration-resistant prostate cancer. N Engl J Med 2010;363(5):411–22.

56. Dutcher JP, Schwartzentruber DJ, Kaufman HL, et al. High dose interleukin-2 (Aldesleukin)—expert consensus on best management practices—2014. J Immunother Cancer 2014;2(1):26.

57. Curti B, Daniels GA, McDermott DF, et al. Improved survival and tumor control with Interleukin-2 is associated with the development of immune-related adverse events: data from the PROCLAIM SM registry. J Immunother Cancer 2017;5(1): 102.

58. Diab A, Hurwitz M, Cho DC, et al. NKTR-214 (CD-122-biased agonist) plus nivolumab in patients with advanced solid tumors: preliminary phase 1/2 results of PIVOT. J Clin Oncol 2018;36(15_suppl):3006.

59. Leidner R, Sukari A, Chung C, et al. Abstract CT170: A phase II, multicenter study to evaluate the efficacy and safety of autologous tumor infiltrating lymphocytes (LN-145) for the treatment of patients with recurrent and/or metastatic squamous cell carcinoma of the head and neck. Cancer Res 2018;78(13 suppl). https://doi. org/10.1158/1538-7445.AM2018-CT170.

60. Rapoport AP, Stadtmauer EA, Binder-Scholl GK, et al. NY-ESO-1-specific TCR-engineered T cells mediate sustained antigen-specific antitumor effects in myeloma. Nat Med 2015;21(8):914.

61. Linette GP, Stadtmauer EA, Maus MV, et al. Cardiovascular toxicity and titin cross-reactivity of affinity enhanced T cells in myeloma and melanoma. Blood 2013; 122(6):863–71.

62. Johnson LA, Morgan RA, Dudley ME, et al. Gene therapy with human and mouse T cell receptors mediates cancer regression and targets normal tissues expressing cognate antigen. Blood 2009;114(3):535–46.

63. Morgan RA, Chinnasamy N, Abate-Daga D, et al. Cancer regression and neurologic toxicity following anti-MAGE-A3 TCR gene therapy. J Immunother 2013; 36(2):133.

64. Paszkiewicz PJ, Fräßle SP, Srivastava S, et al. Targeted antibody-mediated depletion of murine CD19 CAR T cells permanently reverses B cell aplasia. J Clin Invest 2016;126(11):4262–72.

65. Morgan RA, Yang JC, Kitano M, et al. Case report of a serious adverse event following the administration of T cells transduced with a chimeric antigen receptor recognizing ERBB2. Mol Ther 2010;18(4):843–51.

66. Davila ML, Riviere I, Wang X, et al. Efficacy and toxicity management of 19-28z CAR T cell therapy in B cell acute lymphoblastic leukemia. Sci Transl Med 2014;6(224):224ra25.

67. Maude SL, Barrett D, Teachey DT, et al. Managing cytokine release syndrome associated with novel T cell-engaging therapies. Cancer 2014;20(2):119.

Current Immunotherapy Practices in Melanoma

Luke D. Rothermel, MD, MPH[a], Amod A. Sarnaik, MD[b],
Nikhil I. Khushalani, MD[b], Vernon K. Sondak, MD[b],*

KEYWORDS

- Checkpoint inhibitor • Immunotherapy • Cutaneous melanoma
- Mucosal melanoma • Uveal melanoma

KEY POINTS

- Immunotherapies demonstrate survival benefits for patients with melanoma, impacting the surgical management of this disease.
- Checkpoint inhibitor immunotherapies lead to durable responses in unresectable, advanced melanoma, improving overall survival (OS) and in some cases allowing for surgical consolidation of residual tumors.
- Adjuvant use of checkpoint inhibitors demonstrates improvements in recurrence-free survival (RFS) and OS in patients with resectable stage III - IVM1a melanoma.
- Single-agent anti-PD1 therapies demonstrate improved outcomes and toxicity profiles compared with anti-CTLA4 in metastatic and adjuvant approaches.
- Combination anti-PD1 and anti-CTLA4 demonstrates higher overall response rates than single-agent anti-PD1 in unresectable metastatic melanoma, although toxicity rates are very high and OS benefit is marginal.
- Additional therapies are being combined with checkpoint inhibitors to identify tolerable options to improve response and survival rates for unresectable metastatic melanoma.
- The use of checkpoint inhibitors in the neoadjuvant setting poses a unique opportunity and studies of efficacy are underway.
- Immunotherapies influence surgical practice for melanoma through expanded indications for resection of oligometastatic disease, and considerations for neoadjuvant and adjuvant treatments for melanoma patients.

Disclosure Statement: Dr. Sarnaik receives research funding (to the Institute) from Iovance Biotherapeutics and Provectus. He is a coinventor of intellectual property owned by the Institute and licensed to Iovance Biotherapeutics. Dr. Khushalani receives research funding (to Institute) from Bristol-Myers Squibb, Merck, Novartis, GlaxoSmithKline, HUYA, Regeneron, Amgen. He is a consultant for Bristol-Myers Squibb, EMD Serono, Regeneron, HUYA, Merck, Array, Immunocore. He is a Data Safety Monitoring Board member for AstraZeneca and also stock owner for Bellicum Pharmaceuticals, Mazor Robotics, TransEnterix, Amarin. Dr. Sondak is a consultant for Merck, Genentech/Roche, Bristol-Myers Squibb, Novartis, Regeneron. He is a Data Safety Monitoring Board member for Bristol-Myers Squibb, Array, Novartis, Polynoma, Pfizer.
[a] Moffitt Cancer Center, 12902 USF Magnolia Drive, Tampa, FL 33612, USA; [b] Department of Cutaneous Oncology, Moffitt Cancer Center, 10920 N. McKinley Drive, Tampa, FL 33612, USA
* 10920 N. McKinley Drive, Tampa, FL 33612
E-mail address: Vernon.sondak@moffitt.org

Surg Oncol Clin N Am 28 (2019) 403–418
https://doi.org/10.1016/j.soc.2019.02.001
1055-3207/19/© 2019 Elsevier Inc. All rights reserved.

INTRODUCTION

Immunotherapies have changed the landscape of melanoma treatment, and now have impacted outcomes in other cancers as well.[1–3] Before the approval of the first checkpoint inhibitor, ipilimumab, in 2011,[4] the median overall survival (OS) for patients with metastatic melanoma was less than 12 months. High-dose interleukin-2 (IL-2) was the first immunotherapy approved for the treatment of metastatic melanoma (in 1998), but its use is limited by substantial toxicities, low overall response rates, and no evidence for improved survival.[5,6] Anti-cytotoxic T-lymphocyte–associated antigen 4 (CTLA4) and anti-programmed death receptor 1 (PD1) antibody immunotherapies have now both been shown to improve survival in patients with unresectable metastatic melanoma. These agents have since been approved in the adjuvant setting for resected stage III and IV disease.[7] Indications for the use of immunotherapy for melanoma are expanding in the metastatic, adjuvant, and neoadjuvant settings, and these new indications are causing an evolution in the surgical management of this disease.

IMMUNOTHERAPY FOR METASTATIC MELANOMA

With improved understanding of the antitumor immune response, "checkpoint molecules" were identified as key therapeutic targets to regulate the activity of immune cells. CTLA4, which serves as a brake (ie, a negative regulator) on T-cell immune responses, was the first checkpoint molecule for which an inhibitory antibody (ipilimumab) was developed and approved by the Food and Drug Administration (FDA). Subsequently, antibodies against PD1 and its ligand PD-L1 have been developed and tested in a broad variety of malignancies. For patients with melanoma, anti-PD1 antibodies have increased the number of patients who respond to treatment and are more tolerable than IL-2 or ipilimumab, even in older patients (**Table 1**).[8,9] The high rates of response and/or prolonged stable disease in patients with previously unresectable tumors have led to cases in which resection of metastatic melanoma could be performed after immunotherapy treatment.[10] We review the data regarding

Table 1
Immunotherapy response rates, survival and toxicity for unresectable metastatic melanoma

Immunotherapy	High Objective Response Rate (ORR)	Longer Median Overall Survival (OS)	Less Moderate to Severe Toxicity
High-dose interleukin-2[6]	+	+	+
Anti-CTLA4 alone[13–16]	+	+	+ +
Anti-PD1 alone[20–22]	+ +	+ +	+ + +
Combination anti-CTLA4/anti-PD1[24,25]	+ + +	+ + +	+
	+ + + = >50% ORR + + = 21%–50% ORR + = <20% ORR	+ + + = >36 mo (not statistically significant vs anti-PD1 alone) + + = 20 to ~36 mo OS + = 10–20 mo OS	+ + + = <20% grade 3/4 toxicity rate + + = 20%–50% grade 3/4 toxicity rate + = >50% grade 3/4 toxicity rate

Abbreviations: +, least favorable profile; + +, intermediate profile; + + +, most favorable profile.

the current approved immunotherapies for metastatic melanoma and discuss how these impact surgical decision-making.

The patterns of treatment responses for checkpoint inhibitor immunotherapies differ from those typical of cytotoxic chemotherapies. In particular, short-term enlargement of existing lesions, or the development of new lesions during the initial weeks of therapy, may represent pseudoprogression, in which case the tumors will go on to show treatment response. Disease that is perceived to be "stable" may actually represent residual inflammatory lesions with little or no viable tumor cells remaining. Recognition of these atypical responses led to modifications of the RECIST 1.1 criteria (developed to assess chemotherapy responses) that better apply to immunotherapies.[11,12] Most publications regarding current systemic immunotherapies have used RECIST 1.1 to assess response, but this may change with the validation of immune-specific response assessment criteria.

The first immunotherapy agent approved for the treatment of unresectable metastatic melanoma was high-dose IL-2 (aldesleukin).[5] IL-2 is not a checkpoint inhibitor, but rather a cytokine that directly promotes T-cell proliferation and antitumor activity. The proof of its efficacy was durable complete responses (CRs) seen in a small percentage of patients, with some of those responses continuing for well over a decade, clearly representing cures.[5,6] Whereas this novel therapy opened a new realm of treatment for melanoma, only highly selected patients could tolerate the severe toxicities associated with its use. Even in this highly selected group, IL-2 only conferred objective response rates (ORR) of up to 16%, and a median OS of 8.9 months.

Ipilimumab was FDA approved for treatment of unresectable metastatic melanoma in 2011, based on randomized trials showing improved survival compared with treatment with a vaccine or chemotherapy.[13,14] Anti-CTLA4 therapy blocks the interaction of the negative regulator CTLA4 on effector T cells and its ligand B7 on antigen-presenting cells. ORRs using standard RECIST remain low at 12% to 19%, but a larger portion of patients derive clinical benefit, including prolonged disease stabilization in many cases. A pooled analysis of ipilimumab trials in unresectable metastatic melanoma reported a survival plateau at 3 years, with 3-year survival rates of 20% to 26%, supporting that the benefit of ipilimumab was manifest even in patients not achieving objective responses.[15] Determining the optimal dose of an immunotherapy agent can be more complex than for cytotoxic chemotherapy drugs, in which the highest tolerable dose is usually chosen. For ipilimumab, a randomized comparison of 3 mg/kg versus 10 mg/kg dosing given intravenously every 3 weeks for 4 courses demonstrated median OS of 11.5 months versus 15.7 months, suggesting that a higher dose of ipilimumab may result in improved outcome.[16] Grade 3 (severe) or grade 4 (life-threatening) toxicities, however, were noted in 18% to 28% of patients at the 3 mg/kg dose versus 34% of patients with the 10 mg/kg dose, with treatment-related death occurring in 2 (0.6%) versus 4 patients (1.1%) at the respective doses. Approved dosing of ipilimumab in the metastatic setting is 3 mg/kg every 3 weeks for a total of 4 doses, but studies of adjuvant ipilimumab largely focused on the higher (10 mg/kg) dose, using longer durations of therapy.

The PD-1/PD-L1 interaction is another immune checkpoint whereby cancer cells can suppress destruction by effector T cells. Anti-PD1 antibodies approved for treatment of unresectable metastatic melanoma include nivolumab (FDA approval 2014)[17] and pembrolizumab (FDA approval 2014).[18] These antibodies demonstrated higher response rates in comparisons against chemotherapy (27% vs 10%) and ipilimumab (36%–37% vs 13% and 44% vs 19%) in randomized trials in patients with advanced melanoma.[19–23] These higher response rates translated into superior survival: the CheckMate-067 trial showed 3-year survival of 52% versus 34% for previously untreated patients with unresectable stage III or IV melanoma receiving nivolumab or ipilimumab, respectively.[24,25] Nivolumab also had fewer grade 3 or 4 toxicities than ipilimumab (21% vs 28%). Pembrolizumab at 2 different doses was evaluated against ipilimumab in the phase III KEYNOTE-006 trial.[21,22] An update of this trial's data in 2018 noted a 4-year survival rate of 44% for pembrolizumab compared with 36% for ipilimumab in treatment-naïve patients. In this subgroup, the median progression-free survival (PFS) was 11.2 months and 3.7 months for pembrolizumab and ipilimumab, respectively.[26] Taken together, these studies substantiate that anti-PD1 treatment is the preferred initial single-agent immunotherapy treatment for patients with unresectable metastatic melanoma.

The success of single-agent anti-PD1 therapies prompted investigation into combination regimens.[27] The CheckMate-067 trial evaluated the combined use of nivolumab and ipilimumab together.[24,25] This combination therapy achieved objective responses more frequently than with either agent alone (ORR 58%). However, grade 3 and 4 toxicities were noted in 59% of patients for the combination versus 21% for nivolumab alone. Treatment discontinuation was seen in 12% of patients with nivolumab compared with 39% for the combination. Excitement about the high response rate for combination therapy was tempered not only by the high toxicity and treatment discontinuation rates, but even more so by the lack of a clear-cut demonstration that OS was improved over nivolumab alone (see **Table 1**). Nonetheless, this combination regimen is FDA approved and is preferentially used for select patients, particularly those with rapidly progressing disease or advanced brain metastases.[28] Moreover, this trial used the full approved dose of ipilimumab in the combination, which may have accounted for the high toxicity; ongoing studies are looking at whether lowering the ipilimumab dose can lessen toxicity without abrogating the efficacy of the combination.[29]

Ongoing Investigations

Although checkpoint inhibitors, as well as targeted therapies for BRAF and MEK in patients whose tumors harbor a *BRAF* mutation, have revolutionized the standard of care for metastatic melanoma, novel approaches continue to be developed.

Combination PD1/PD-L1 and targeted therapies

Ongoing studies are looking to evaluate the impact of PD1 or PD-L1 inhibitors combined with BRAF and MEK inhibitors. KEYNOTE-022 is a phase I/II study evaluating the feasibility and safety of combining pembrolizumab with the BRAF and MEK inhibitors dabrafenib and trametinib in unresectable stage III or IV *BRAF* V600-mutant melanoma.[30] Another study is a phase Ib trial of the PD-L1 inhibitor atezolizumab plus the BRAF and MEK inhibitors vemurafenib and cobimetinib.[31] Randomized phase III trials are needed to demonstrate that the combination of checkpoint blockade plus BRAF and MEK inhibition significantly improves survival compared with sequential administration of the same agents. In addition, assessment of toxicity and cost should help guide whether this combination strategy will become a future standard.

Combination PD1/IDO inhibitors

Indoleamine 2,3-dioxygenase (IDO) is an enzymatic protein used by cancer cells to suppress cytotoxic T-lymphocyte activity in the peri-tumoral microenvironment. Inhibitors of this enzyme have been developed to manipulate this immune interaction in favor of the antitumor activity of T cells. Although use of single-agent IDO inhibitors has not yet shown clinical evidence of antitumor activity, early-phase trials in combination with checkpoint inhibition suggested improved ORR. However, the first randomized phase III trial of this approach, KEYNOTE-252, failed to demonstrate improved PFS when the IDO inhibitor epacadostat was combined with pembrolizumab versus pembrolizumab alone.[32] These results cast a shadow over 2 ongoing trials of IDO inhibitor combinations with PD-1 inhibition (NCT02073123, NCT03329846), reminding us all that there is still much to learn about the various signals regulating the antitumor immune response.

Combination checkpoint inhibitors/histone deacetylase inhibitors
Histone deacetylase (HDAC) inhibitors, which effect gene expression through epigenetic modulation, have shown efficacy in boosting immunotherapy responses in preclinical studies. Inhibiting HDAC increases the expression of major histocompatibility (HLA) molecules and decreases the expression of PD-L1 and PD-L2 on tumor cells. In a phase 1 trial, the addition of panobinostat did not improve the response rate to standard-dose ipilimumab in unresectable melanoma.[33] Studies are ongoing to evaluate the use of other HDAC inhibitors in combination with ipilimumab or an anti-PD1 antibody in patients with advanced melanoma.

Combination immunotherapy with tumor-infiltrating lymphocytes
As discussed elsewhere in this issue, adoptive cell transfer of tumor-infiltrating lymphocytes (TILs) for highly selected patients with unresectable stage IV melanomas has demonstrated an overall response rate between 38% and 55%, with a significant portion of these patients achieving durable CRs.[34–37] A limitation to this therapy is the attrition rate noted during TIL generation as a result of tumor progression. The combination of checkpoint inhibition with adoptive T-cell transfer is under active investigation, as treatment administration soon after the tumor harvest could help to control the tumor during TIL generation. Moreover, it could potentially be useful prior to tumor harvest to lead to an influx of more active T cells into the tumor, resulting in more efficacious TIL. Feasibility of administering checkpoint inhibitors plus TIL was demonstrated in a pilot study of CTLA4 inhibition before and after TIL harvest (NCT03215810),[38] making this a logical area for further exploration in those centers with the capability to carry out this labor-intensive form of immunotherapy.

Combination immunotherapy/intralesional therapy
Talimogene laherparepvec (T-VEC), a genetically modified oncolytic virus FDA approved for single-agent use as an intralesional therapy, has the potential to cause activation of the immune system by lysing cancer cells and increasing antigen presentation.[39] Details of this therapy are covered elsewhere in this issue. The use of this therapy in combination with checkpoint inhibitors is under way with early-phase trials demonstrating improved OR and CR rates.[40–42] A phase III trial comparing this combination treatment with pembrolizumab alone for unresectable stage IIIB or higher disease is ongoing. Better response rates are expected from the combination of intralesional and systemic therapies, but the true test will be whether the duration of responses and survival rates are also improved.

ADJUVANT IMMUNOTHERAPY

The success of checkpoint inhibitor immunotherapies and BRAF/MEK inhibitor targeted therapy in unresectable metastatic melanoma led investigators to study their impact in the adjuvant setting. These trials have involved patients with completely resected stage III, and in some cases stage IV, melanoma. In 1995, the cytokine interferon-alfa-2b (IFNα-2b) was FDA approved as the first adjuvant treatment for high-risk melanoma.[43] Phase III studies comparing high-dose IFNα-2b versus observation or a vaccine therapy alone demonstrated improved recurrence-free survival

(RFS) and in some cases improved OS.[44,45] The OS benefit was further defined in meta-analyses of patients with stage II and III melanoma, and our institutional experience corroborates this with improved RFS, distant metastasis-free survival, and OS for patients with resected stage III disease.[46,47] The limitation to this medication was the high rate of toxicity (>67% grade 3 or 4) associated with its use. Dose reductions were required for most patients, although most toxicities were reversible after discontinuation of treatment. Pegylated IFNα-2b is another formulation that allows less-frequent administration and has somewhat fewer grade 3 and 4 toxicities (**Table 2**).[48] Despite the availability of these 2 adjuvant interferon regimens in the United States., as well as low-dose interferon in Europe, patient and physician acceptance was poor and many phase III clinical trials continued to use an observation or placebo arm as the "standard" against which newer agents were compared.

European Organisation for Research and Treatment of Cancer (EORTC) 18071 evaluated high-dose ipilimumab (10 mg/kg, higher than the approved dose for unresectable disease of 3 mg/kg) versus observation and demonstrated statistically significant improvements in RFS (median of 26.1 vs 17.1 months) and 5-year OS (65.4% vs 54.4%) for adjuvant ipilimumab.[49,50] The toxicity of this therapy was substantial (see **Table 2**), leading to discontinuation in more than half of patients, and treatment-related deaths in 1% of patients. Despite the high toxicity, high-dose ipilimumab was approved for adjuvant therapy of stage III melanoma by the FDA in 2015. A direct comparison of the adjuvant use of 3 mg/kg and 10 mg/kg ipilimumab doses against high-dose interferon as the control arm is ongoing in the E1609 trial (NCT01274338).[51]

More recently, anti-PD1 antibodies have been approved for use in the adjuvant setting. The first agent to be approved was nivolumab, which was evaluated head-to-head against high-dose ipilimumab. Preliminary results of the CheckMate-238 trial published in 2017 demonstrated a 1-year RFS of 71% with nivolumab versus 61% with ipilimumab, with lower rates of grade 3 and 4 adverse events with nivolumab (14% vs 46%) and fewer discontinuations of therapy (4% vs 30%).[52,53] As yet, no data are available regarding the OS impact of nivolumab compared with ipilimumab, but the fact that nivolumab was superior to and less toxic than an active control arm (ipilimumab) has led most oncologists to regard this therapy as the preferred option in the adjuvant setting for resected stage IIIB, IIIC, and IV disease despite the lack of survival data.

Table 2
Adjuvant immunotherapy and targeted therapy survival and toxicity for resected melanoma

Adjuvant Immunotherapy or Targeted Therapy	Improved Recurrence-Free Survival vs Comparator	Improved Overall Survival vs Comparator	Low Rates of Moderate to Severe Toxicity
Interferon-alfa-2b (HDI/Peg-IFNα)[45–48]	> Observation (HR 0.82)	> Observation (HR 0.89)	+/+ +
Anti-CTLA4 alone[50,51]	> Placebo (HR 0.75)	> Placebo (HR 0.72)	+
Anti-PD1 alone[52–54]	> Placebo (HR 0.57) > Anti-CTLA4 (HR 0.65)	(No data available)	+ + +
BRAF/MEK Inhibition[77–79]	> Placebo (HR 0.47)	> Placebo (HR 0.57, not statistically significant)	+ +

+++, <20% grade 3/4 toxicity rate; ++, 20%–50% grade 3/4 toxicity rate; +, >50% grade 3/4 toxicity rate.

Abbreviations: +, least favorable profile; ++, intermediate profile; +++, most favorable profile; HDI, high-dose interferon-alfa-2b; HR, hazard ratio from phase III trials (or meta-analysis for Interferon); Peg-IFNα, pegylated interferon-alfa-2b.

Just recently FDA approved for resected stage III melanoma adjuvant therapy, pembrolizumab is also an active agent in this setting based on the results of the KEYNOTE-054/EORTC1345 study.[54] This study compared pembrolizumab with placebo, and reported 1-year RFS rates of 75% versus 61%. Not yet known is whether OS is improved with adjuvant pembrolizumab versus the alternative of initiating pembrolizumab after disease recurrence. Grade 3 or higher adverse events were reported in 15% of patients treated with pembrolizumab, and 1 treatment-related death occurred due to myositis among 514 patients randomized to pembrolizumab. Because this trial included selected stage IIIA patients, who were not included in the CheckMate-238 trial of nivolumab versus ipilimumab, we now have broad evidence that adjuvant anti-PD1 therapy can improve RFS across the entire spectrum of high-risk patients with stage III and stage IV disease. The S1404 trial is a phase III cooperative group study comparing pembrolizumab with high-dose interferon or ipilimumab 10 mg/kg as adjuvant therapy for resected high-risk stage III (stage IIIA [American Joint Committee on Cancer (AJCC) seventh edition] with N2a disease, or stage IIIB/C) or resected stage IV disease (NCT02506153). This trial will allow for direct comparison of the survival impact of anti-PD1 adjuvant therapy with these other approved regimens in the adjuvant setting.

When initially approved, nivolumab, whether in the adjuvant or metastatic setting, was given by intravenous infusion every 2 weeks. Many patients found this to be disadvantageous compared with pembrolizumab, which is given every 3 weeks. Pharmacologic data suggested that similar blockade of PD1 could be achieved by giving twice the dose of nivolumab every 4 weeks (NCT02714218). This more convenient monthly dose received FDA approval in 2018 and has been widely adopted for adjuvant therapy, including in the phase III CheckMate-915 adjuvant trial, in which the every 4-week dose serves as the standard arm in comparison with a low-dose ipilimumab (1 mg/kg every 6 weeks) plus nivolumab (240 mg/kg every 2 weeks) combination regimen (NCT03068455).

Toxicity in Adjuvant Versus Metastatic Setting

Observed toxicity rates appear to be consistently higher with immune checkpoint inhibition in the adjuvant versus the metastatic settings. The reported rates of grade 3 and 4 toxicities for ipilimumab with the 10 mg/kg regimen were 34% in metastatic disease, and between 45% and 54% as an adjuvant therapy, with endocrinopathies reported at a higher rate in the adjuvant setting. PD-1 inhibition leads to fewer adverse events than CTLA-4 inhibition in both the adjuvant and metastatic settings, but still may have slightly more toxicity in the adjuvant setting.[55] More data are needed to determine if true biologic principles underlie reported differences in toxicity rates between the 2 treatment contexts, but it is reasonable to speculate that intense stimulation of the immune system in a patient without gross tumor is leading to more autoimmune reactivity. Other potential considerations include whether a recent surgery exposes self-antigens that are more readily targeted by the immune system than would otherwise be the case, or if the regulatory immune system is altered by the recent surgery leading to a different toxicity profile.[56,57] These observations raise the question of whether immunotherapies would be less toxic and potentially even more effective if administered before surgery (ie, in the neoadjuvant setting).

Consideration for Treatment in the Neoadjuvant Setting

In addition to the theoretic possibility of decreasing the toxicity of treatment, neoadjuvant therapy also has more clearly definable advantages, including the potential to decrease tumor burden and permit a less extensive and less morbid operation. There can also be advantages in terms of identifying patients with rapidly progressive treatment-unresponsive metastatic disease, who would not benefit from regional surgery. Other theoretic advantages of neoadjuvant immunotherapies include immune stimulation in the presence of larger quantities of tumor antigens than in the adjuvant setting, and that earlier, preoperative initiation of systemic therapy may further improve eradication of subclinical distant metastasis compared with later, postoperative initiation of treatment (**Table 3**). The optimal neoadjuvant approach will have high response rates, low rates of progression while on therapy, predictability in terms of the depth and duration of response (to facilitate timing of surgery) and low toxicity rates (especially those adverse effects that may increase surgical morbidity, **Table 4**). Theoretic disadvantages of neoadjuvant approaches include the possibility surgical intervention will become impossible, either for patients whose tumors do not respond if progression renders the disease unresectable or if toxicity of therapy is so severe that the patient becomes unfit for surgery. Even in the absence of these catastrophic outcomes, increasing surgical morbidity due to toxicities or tumor progression is a concern whenever neoadjuvant therapy is used (see **Table 3**).

An example of the neoadjuvant approach is the use of BRAF/MEK inhibitors in patients with resectable clinical stage III whose tumor harbors a susceptible *BRAF* mutation. Use of BRAF/MEK inhibitors in patients with metastatic melanoma results in frequent and rapid responses, with a very low rate of early tumor progression but a predictable development of tumor resistance in most cases, generally occurring 9 months or more after initiation of therapy. Although toxicities are not uncommon, most are quickly reversible once treatment is stopped, and the likelihood of toxicity interfering with the ability to perform subsequent surgery is therefore low. A randomized phase II study of BRAF/MEK inhibition in high-risk, resectable stage III and IV *BRAF*-mutant melanoma demonstrated improved event-free survival for neoadjuvant (2 months) plus 10 months of adjuvant dabrafenib plus trametinib therapy over standard of care treatment (resection followed by consideration of adjuvant interferon and/or radiation).[58]

Although BRAF/MEK inhibition has predictable, high response rates and manageable toxicities, it is applicable only to patients whose tumor harbors a *BRAF* mutation.

Table 3 Theoretic advantages and disadvantages of neoadjuvant versus adjuvant immunotherapy for melanoma	
PROs:	Tumor (antigens) present during treatment
	Treatment is given before the postoperative immunosuppressive state
	Ability to assess the response to treatment due to the presence of evaluable tumor burden
	Earlier treatment of subclinical disease
	Identify patients with rapidly progressive, treatment-unresponsive disease, who would not benefit from surgery
	Decreasing the tumor burden may make resection more feasible, less morbid
	Possibly fewer "off-target" toxicities due to the presence of "target" antigens
CONs:	Delays surgical intervention for resectable disease
	Progression or pseudoprogression may lead a resectable tumor to become unresectable
	Treatment toxicities may delay/prevent surgical intervention
	No proven survival benefit for neoadjuvant compared with adjuvant treatment
	Full pathologic staging not known at the time therapy is initiated

Table 4
Comparison of desired properties of neoadjuvant approaches to *BRAF*-mutant melanoma treatment between systemic immunotherapies and targeted therapy

Therapy	High Objective Response Rate (ORR)	Low Rate of Early Progression	Low Rate of Toxicity Impacting Subsequent Surgery
BRAF/MEK inhibition[77–79]	+ + +	+ + +	+ +
Combination Anti-CTLA4/Anti-PD1[24,25]	+ + +	+ + +	+
Anti-PD1 alone[20–22]	+ +	+ +	+ + +
Anti-CTLA4 alone[13–16]	+	+	+ +
	+++ = >50%	+++ = <25%	+++ = Lowest rate
	++ = 21%–50%	++ = 25%–49%	++ = Intermediate rate
	+ = <20%	+ = 50% or greater	+ = Highest rate

+++ = most favorable profile; ++ = intermediate profile; + = least favorable profile.

Combinations of ipilimumab and nivolumab also have high response rates and fairly low rates of early tumor progression, and can be used regardless of tumor mutation status, but are associated with very high rates of toxicities that could interfere with subsequent surgery. Monotherapy PD1 inhibition has lower response rates and higher rates of early progression, but with lower toxicities than the combined therapy. The ipilimumab monotherapy profile is less favorable for neoadjuvant approaches than PD1 inhibitor monotherapy, with low response rates and frequent early progression despite significant toxicity with the potential to interfere with subsequent surgery (see **Table 4**).

Although neoadjuvant immunotherapy rarely causes surgically concerning adverse hematologic effects such as thrombocytopenia or neutropenia, a more common occurrence would be the development of immune-related adverse events requiring prolonged use of high-dose steroids. Steroids were required in 35% of patients on ipilimumab monotherapy for metastatic disease in one study, and even more frequently in patients treated with both ipilimumab and a PD-1 inhibitor.[59] Operations in the context of chronic steroid use (>10 mg/d for more than 1 week) have been noted to have increased wound healing complications and surgical site infections.[60,61]

Favorable early data exist for the use of neoadjuvant nivolumab in non–small-cell lung carcinoma and Merkel cell carcinoma when 2 doses are given and surgery occurs 2 weeks after the second dose.[62,63] An ongoing phase II clinical trial is evaluating this approach in resectable, high-risk and oligometastatic melanoma (NCT02519322). These trial efforts are needed to inform the debate about advantages and disadvantages of the neoadjuvant approach, and these data will need to be clearly understood by surgeons when deciding the appropriate management of patients with resectable high-risk or oligometastatic melanoma. If neoadjuvant approaches live up to their theoretic advantages, the next step might be to determine whether immunotherapies can be used as *upfront* therapy, given until the evaluable tumors obtain the maximal response, with consolidative surgery occurring only if and when improvement is no longer seen. In cases with complete clinical responses, as well as those who progress with distant disease while the local-regional disease is controlled, surgery may never be required.

Who Do We Select for Adjuvant Therapy?

At this time, adjuvant immunotherapy treatment is indicated broadly for resected stage III and IV disease, but limited guidance exists for which patients should or should not be treated. In particular, prospective data regarding patients with stage IIIA (AJCC seventh edition) disease is limited to patients with at least 1 nodal deposit measuring 1 mm or larger, even though that threshold has never been conclusively shown to be the optimal one for defining risk of recurrence.[64] Moreover, no prospective data yet exist to define the benefits of adjuvant checkpoint inhibitor immunotherapy in patients with (node-negative) stage IIB/C disease, who can face risks of recurrence and death due to melanoma as high as or higher than stage IIIA disease. Another important consideration for surgeons is that all adjuvant therapy trials reported to date have required that node-positive patients, including those with positive sentinel lymph nodes, undergo radical lymphadenectomy before study entry. Data from the Multi-center Selective Lymphadenectomy Trial-II (MSLT-II)[65] are leading to more and more patients with positive sentinel nodes being referred for adjuvant therapy without undergoing radical lymphadenectomy. Regional recurrences will be more common in such patients, and can potentially be salvaged with surgery and adjuvant therapy at that time. So it remains an open question whether to treat all, some, or no sentinel node–positive patients with adjuvant immunotherapy if they do not first undergo a completion lymphadenectomy.

Nonetheless, recognizing the absence of data directly addressing this patient population, the evidence we do have clearly shows that many sentinel node–positive patients will manifest distant metastatic disease before or simultaneous with any type of locoregional failure.[65] These patients would obviously have lost the opportunity to receive adjuvant therapy if it was not provided after sentinel node biopsy.

Our current practice is that all patients with clinically evident resectable or borderline resectable nodal disease should first be evaluated for possible neoadjuvant therapy. BRAF mutation status is checked, and patients with BRAF-mutant resectable stage IIIB/C/D (AJCC eighth edition) are evaluated by a multidisciplinary team to consider neoadjuvant BRAF/MEK inhibition. But for most patients with resectable stage III disease, surgery remains the initial treatment step. Today, sentinel node biopsy for clinically node-negative patients represents a staging procedure, and sentinel node–positive patients generally no longer undergo completion lymphadenectomy. Patients with stage IIIA (AJCC eighth edition, ie, T1 or T2a with 1 or 2 positive sentinel nodes) disease and very small tumor deposits in the sentinel node (<1 mm and preferably <0.2 mm in maximum dimension) at our center are now routinely observed without further surgery or adjuvant therapy. But most patients with stage IIIA disease and tumor deposits ≥1 mm, as well as the overwhelming majority of sentinel node–positive patients with resected stage IIIB/C disease, are referred for consideration of clinical trial participation or adjuvant immunotherapy with nivolumab every 4 weeks for a year. Patients with clinically evident nodal disease who are not treated with a neoadjuvant approach undergo radical lymphadenectomy and are all routinely referred for consideration of clinical trial participation or adjuvant immunotherapy with nivolumab every 4 weeks for a year. BRAF testing should be considered for all patients with stage III melanoma, because patients whose tumors harbor a BRAF mutation would also have the option of adjuvant orally administered dabrafenib/trametinib for a year instead of the intravenously administered anti-PD1 immunotherapy.

Surgical Management of Recurrences

Some patients, especially those sentinel node–positive patients initially treated systemically without undergoing a completion node dissection, will develop resectable recurrent disease during the initial year of adjuvant therapy. When such resectable recurrent disease does occur, multidisciplinary planning is recommended for management. Resection followed by the completion of the remainder of the year of adjuvant therapy may be appropriate for many of these patients. For patients with *BRAF*-mutant disease who develop resectable recurrence during or after adjuvant immunotherapy, neoadjuvant and/or adjuvant dabrafenib plus trametinib represents another viable option.

UNUSUAL MELANOMA SUBTYPES

Desmoplastic melanomas, which are characterized by a fibrotic, often amelanotic appearance and locally aggressive behavior, appear to represent a highly immunogenic variant of cutaneous melanoma.[66,67] Despite a dense stromal component, these tumors are noted to have a very high mutational burden as well as high degrees of TILs, which are often considered to be markers of strong potential immunogenicity.[68,69] One recent multicenter experience noted a strikingly high 68% ORR to single-agent anti-PD1 inhibition, with nearly a third of patients achieving a complete response.[70] Southwest Oncology Group study S1512 is an ongoing pilot trial evaluating the effect of neoadjuvant pembrolizumab for resectable desmoplastic melanomas (NCT02775851). Adjuvant radiation is frequently advocated for desmoplastic melanoma,[71] unlike other types of cutaneous melanoma, but whether the indications for adjuvant immunotherapy should be different for this subtype of melanoma is currently unknown.

Melanomas arising from noncutaneous sites are rare, and differ in their clinical behaviors as well as their responses to immunotherapies from melanomas that arise on the skin. Data are limited for the use of immunotherapies, especially adjuvant therapy, in these subtypes, and ongoing clinical trials should be considered when treating patients. Nonetheless, some principles seem to be emerging from studies in patients with unresectable metastatic disease. Mucosal melanomas have low mutational burdens and low rates of TILs relative to cutaneous melanomas.[72] Objective responses to checkpoint inhibitory immunotherapies are seen somewhat less frequently for these patients than those with cutaneous melanoma, but because the great majority of these patients are *BRAF* wild-type, immunotherapy is routinely offered to patients with unresectable metastatic mucosal melanoma.[73] The role of adjuvant immunotherapy after resection of mucosal melanoma is much less clear, however.

Uveal (ocular) melanomas appear to be far less immunogenic than cutaneous melanomas.[74] Once they have metastasized, predominantly to the liver, these melanomas have very low response rates to single-agent checkpoint inhibition and even to combination treatment.[75,76] New approaches are clearly needed for treating metastatic uveal melanoma, and adjuvant immunotherapy should not be routinely used outside of a clinical trial.

SUMMARY

Immunotherapy has revolutionized the treatment of melanoma, with implications for the surgical management of this disease. The ideal immunotherapy would be one that durably stimulates the antitumor immune system beyond the ability of the cancer to resist or evade its attack, while minimizing off-target effects of the therapy. We have seen remarkable advancement in the field of immunotherapy, but significant work is still needed to achieve this goal in all patients with advanced melanoma. As our understanding of the immune system develops, additional immunotherapies will become available and the surgeon's role will continue to evolve. Surgeons must be aware of the impact of various immunotherapies on patients with resectable and unresectable disease, and how surgical decision-making should progress as a result. The indications for melanoma resection are changing. Although fewer patients will receive regional lymph node dissections after a positive sentinel node biopsy in the future, the impact of immunotherapies will increase surgeon involvement for resection of metastatic disease, whether for tumor harvests to generate autologous lymphocytes or for consolidating control of disease beyond what can be achieved with immunotherapy alone.

ACKNOWLEDGEMENT

The research was supported in part by the National Cancer Institute, part of the National Institutes of Health, under grant number P50 CA168536, Moffitt Skin Cancer SPORE.

REFERENCES

1. Chen R, Zinzani PL, Fanale MA, et al. Phase II study of the efficacy and safety of pembrolizumab for relapsed/refractory classic Hodgkin lymphoma. J Clin Oncol 2017;35(19):2125–32.
2. Gaiser MR, Bongiorno M, Brownell I. PD-L1 inhibition with avelumab for metastatic Merkel cell carcinoma. Expert Rev Clin Pharmacol 2018;11(4):345–59.
3. Reck M, Rodriguez-Abreu D, Robinson AG, et al. Pembrolizumab versus chemotherapy for PD-L1-positive non-small-cell lung cancer. N Engl J Med 2016; 375(19):1823–33.
4. Lipson EJ, Drake CG. Ipilimumab: an anti-CTLA-4 antibody for metastatic melanoma. Clin Cancer Res 2011;17(22):6958–62.
5. Atkins MB, Lotze MT, Dutcher JP, et al. High-dose recombinant interleukin 2 therapy for patients with metastatic melanoma: analysis of 270 patients treated between 1985 and 1993. J Clin Oncol 1999;17(7):2105–16.
6. Atkins MB, Kunkel L, Sznol M, et al. High-dose recombinant interleukin-2 therapy in patients with metastatic melanoma: long-term survival update. Cancer J Sci Am 2000;6(supplement 1):S11–4.
7. Ascierto PA, Palmieri G, Gogas H. What is changing in the adjuvant treatment of melanoma? Oncotarget 2017;8(67):110735–6.
8. Daste A, Domblides C, Gross-Goupil M, et al. Immune checkpoint inhibitors and elderly people: a review. Eur J Cancer 2017;82:155–66.
9. Elias R, Giobbie-Hurder A, McCleary NJ, et al. Efficacy of PD-1 & PD-L1 inhibitors in older adults: a meta-analysis. J Immunother Cancer 2018;6(1):26.
10. Bello DM, Panageas KS, Hollmann TJ, et al. Outcomes of patients with metastatic melanoma selected for surgery after immunotherapy. Ann Surg Oncol 2018; 25(supplement 1):S7.
11. Seymour L, Bogaerts J, Perrone A, et al. iRECIST: guidelines for response criteria for use in trials testing immunotherapeutics. Lancet Oncol 2017;18(3):e143–52.
12. Wolchok JD, Hoos A, O'Day S, et al. Guidelines for the evaluation of immune therapy activity in solid tumors: immune-related response criteria. Clin Cancer Res 2009;15(23):7412–20.
13. Hodi FS, O'Day SJ, McDermott DF, et al. Improved survival with ipilimumab in patients with metastatic melanoma. N Engl J Med 2010;363(8):711–23.
14. Maio M, Grob JJ, Aamdal S, et al. Five-year survival rates for treatment-naive patients with advanced melanoma who received ipilimumab plus dacarbazine in a phase III trial. J Clin Oncol 2015;33(10):1191–6.
15. Schadendorf D, Hodi FS, Robert C, et al. Pooled analysis of long-term survival data from phase II and phase III trials of ipilimumab in unresectable or metastatic melanoma. J Clin Oncol 2015;33(17):1889–94.

16. Ascierto PA, Del Vecchio M, Robert C, et al. Ipilimumab 10 mg/kg versus ipilimumab 3 mg/kg in patients with unresectable or metastatic melanoma: a randomised, double-blind, multicentre, phase 3 trial. Lancet Oncol 2017;18(5):611–22.

17. Hazarika M, Chuk MK, Theoret MR, et al. U.S. FDA approval summary: nivolumab for treatment of unresectable or metastatic melanoma following progression on ipilimumab. Clin Cancer Res 2017;23(14):3484–8.

18. Barone A, Hazarika M, Theoret MR, et al. FDA approval summary: pembrolizumab for the treatment of patients with unresectable or metastatic melanoma. Clin Cancer Res 2017;23(19):5661–5.

19. Hamid O, Puzanov I, Dummer R, et al. Final analysis of a randomised trial comparing pembrolizumab versus investigator-choice chemotherapy for ipilimumab-refractory advanced melanoma. Eur J Cancer 2017;86:37–45.

20. Robert C, Long GV, Brady B, et al. Nivolumab in previously untreated melanoma without *BRAF* mutation. N Engl J Med 2015;372(4):320–30.

21. Robert C, Schachter J, Long GV, et al. Pembrolizumab versus ipilimumab in advanced melanoma. N Engl J Med 2015;372(26):2521–32.

22. Schachter J, Ribas A, Long GV, et al. Pembrolizumab versus ipilimumab for advanced melanoma: final overall survival results of a multicentre, randomised, open-label phase 3 study (KEYNOTE-006). Lancet 2017;390(10105):1853–62.

23. Weber JS, D'Angelo SP, Minor D, et al. Nivolumab versus chemotherapy in patients with advanced melanoma who progressed after anti-CTLA-4 treatment (CheckMate 037): a randomised, controlled, open-label, phase 3 trial. Lancet Oncol 2015;16(4):375–84.

24. Larkin J, Chiarion-Sileni V, Gonzalez R, et al. Combined nivolumab and ipilimumab or monotherapy in untreated melanoma. N Engl J Med 2015;373(1):23–34.

25. Wolchok JD, Chiarion-Sileni V, Gonzalez R, et al. Overall survival with combined nivolumab and ipilimumab in advanced melanoma. N Engl J Med 2017;377(14):1345–56.

26. Long GV, Schachter J, Ribas A, et al. 4-year survival and outcomes after cessation of pembrolizumab (pembro) after 2-years in patients (pts) with ipilimumab (ipi)-naive advanced melanoma in KEYNOTE-006. J Clin Oncol 2018;36(supplement):9503.

27. Weber JS, Gibney G, Sullivan RJ, et al. Sequential administration of nivolumab and ipilimumab with a planned switch in patients with advanced melanoma (CheckMate 064): an open-label, randomised, phase 2 trial. Lancet Oncol 2016;17(7):943–55.

28. Tawbi HA, Forsyth PA, Algazi A, et al. Combined nivolumab and ipilimumab in melanoma metastatic to the brain. N Engl J Med 2018;379(8):722–30.

29. Olson D, Luke JJ, Hallmeyer S, et al. Phase II trial of pembrolizumab (pembro) plus 1mg/kg ipilimumab (ipi) immediately following progression on anti-PD-1 Ab in melanoma (mel). J Clin Oncol 2018;36(supplement):9514.

30. Ribas A, Hodi FS, Lawrence DP, et al. KEYNOTE-022 update: phase 1 study of first-line pembrolizumab (pembro) plus dabrafenib (D) and trametinib (T) for *BRAF*-mutant advanced melanoma. Ann Oncol 2017;28(supplement 5):12160.

31. Sullivan RJ, Gonzalez R, Lewis KD, et al. Atezolizumab (A) + cobimetinib (C) + vemurafenib (V) in *BRAF*V600-mutant metastatic melanoma (mel): updated safety and clinical activity. J Clin Oncol 2017;35(supplement 15):3063.

32. Long GV, Dummer R, Hamid O, et al. Epacadostat (E) plus pembrolizumab (P) versus pembrolizumab alone in patients (pts) with unresectable or metastatic melanoma: results of the phase 3 ECHO-201/KEYNOTE-252 study. J Clin Oncol 2018;36(supplement):108.

33. Khushalani N, Markowitz J, Eroglu Z, et al. A phase I trial of panobinostat with ipilimumab in advanced melanoma. J Clin Oncol 2017;35(supplement 15):9547.

34. Besser MJ, Shapira-Frommer R, Itzhaki O, et al. Adoptive transfer of tumor-infiltrating lymphocytes in patients with metastatic melanoma: intent-to-treat analysis and efficacy after failure to prior immunotherapies. Clin Cancer Res 2013; 19(17):4792–800.

35. Pilon-Thomas S, Kuhn L, Ellwanger S, et al. Efficacy of adoptive cell transfer of tumor-infiltrating lymphocytes after lymphopenia induction for metastatic melanoma. J Immunother 2012;35(8):615–20.

36. Radvanyi LG, Bernatchez C, Zhang M, et al. Specific lymphocyte subsets predict response to adoptive cell therapy using expanded autologous tumor-infiltrating lymphocytes in metastatic melanoma patients. Clin Cancer Res 2012;18(24): 6758–70.

37. Rosenberg SA, Yang JC, Sherry RM, et al. Durable complete responses in heavily pretreated patients with metastatic melanoma using T-cell transfer immunotherapy. Clin Cancer Res 2011;17(13):4550–7.

38. Mullinax JE, Hall M, Prabhakaran S, et al. Combination of ipilimumab and adoptive cell therapy with tumor-infiltrating lymphocytes for patients with metastatic melanoma. Front Oncol 2018;8:44.

39. Burke EE, Zager JS. Pharmacokinetic drug evaluation of talimogene laherparepvec for the treatment of advanced melanoma. Expert Opin Drug Metab Toxicol 2018;14(4):469–73.

40. Chesney J, Puzanov I, Collichio F, et al. Randomized, open-label phase II study evaluating the efficacy and safety of talimogene laherparepvec in combination with ipilimumab versus ipilimumab alone in patients with advanced, unresectable melanoma. J Clin Oncol 2018;36(17):1658–67.

41. Long GV, Dummer R, Ribas A, et al. Efficacy analysis of MASTERKEY-265 phase 1b study of talimogene laherparepvec (T-VEC) and pembrolizumab (pembro) for unresectable stage IIIB-IV melanoma. J Clin Oncol 2016;34(supplement 15): 9568.

42. Ribas A, Dummer R, Puzanov I, et al. Oncolytic virotherapy promotes intratumoral T cell infiltration and improves anti-PD-1 immunotherapy. Cell 2017;170(6): 1109–19.e10.

43. Kirkwood JM, Manola J, Ibrahim J, et al. A pooled analysis of Eastern Cooperative Oncology Group and intergroup trials of adjuvant high-dose interferon for melanoma. Clin Cancer Res 2004;10(5):1670–7.

44. Kirkwood JM, Ibrahim JG, Sosman JA, et al. High-dose interferon alfa-2b significantly prolongs relapse-free and overall survival compared with the GM2-KLH/QS-21 vaccine in patients with resected stage IIB-III melanoma: results of intergroup trial E1694/S9512/C509801. J Clin Oncol 2001;19(9):2370–80.

45. Kirkwood JM, Strawderman MH, Ernstoff MS, et al. Interferon alfa-2b adjuvant therapy of high-risk resected cutaneous melanoma: the Eastern Cooperative Oncology Group Trial EST 1684. J Clin Oncol 1996;14(1):7–17.

46. Mocellin S, Pasquali S, Rossi CR, et al. Interferon alpha adjuvant therapy in patients with high-risk melanoma: a systematic review and meta-analysis. J Natl Cancer Inst 2010;102(7):493–501.

47. Oliver DE, Sondak VK, Strom T, et al. Interferon is associated with improved survival for node-positive cutaneous melanoma: a single-institution experience. Melanoma Manag 2018;5(1):MMT02.

48. Eggermont AM, Suciu S, Testori A, et al. Long-term results of the randomized phase III trial EORTC 18991 of adjuvant therapy with pegylated interferon alfa-

2b versus observation in resected stage III melanoma. J Clin Oncol 2012;30(31): 3810–8.

49. Eggermont AM, Chiarion-Sileni V, Grob JJ, et al. Prolonged survival in Stage III melanoma with ipilimumab adjuvant therapy. N Engl J Med 2016;375(19): 1845–55.

50. Eggermont AM, Chiarion-Sileni V, Grob JJ, et al. Adjuvant ipilimumab versus placebo after complete resection of high-risk stage III melanoma (EORTC 18071): a randomised, double-blind, phase 3 trial. Lancet Oncol 2015;16(5):522–30.

51. Tarhini AA, Lee SJ, Hodi FS, et al. A phase III randomized study of adjuvant ipilimumab (3 or 10mg/kg) versus high-dose interferon alfa-2b for resected high-risk melanoma (U.S. Intergroup E1609): preliminary safety and efficacy of the ipilimumab arms. J Clin Oncol 2017;35(supplement 15):9500.

52. Weber J, Mandala M, Del Vecchio M, et al. Adjuvant nivolumab versus ipilimumab in resected stage III or IV melanoma. N Engl J Med 2017;377(19):1824–35.

53. Weber J, Mandala M, Del Vecchio M, et al. Adjuvant therapy with nivolumab (NIVO) versus ipilimumab (IPI) after complete resection of stage III/IV melanoma: updated results from a phase III trial (CheckMate 238). J Clin Oncol 2018; 36(supplement 15):9502.

54. Eggermont AMM, Blank CU, Mandala M, et al. Adjuvant pembrolizumab versus placebo in resected stage III melanoma. N Engl J Med 2018;378(19):1789–801.

55. Gibney GT, Kudchadkar RR, DeConti RC, et al. Safety, correlative markers, and clinical results of adjuvant nivolumab in combination with vaccine in resected high-risk metastatic melanoma. Clin Cancer Res 2015;21(4):712–20.

56. Hogan BV, Peter MB, Shenoy HG, et al. Surgery induced immunosuppression. Surgeon 2011;9(1):38–43.

57. Alieva M, van Rheenen J, Broekman MLD. Potential impact of invasive surgical procedures on primary tumor growth and metastasis. Clin Exp Metastasis 2018;35(4):319–31.

58. Amaria RN, Prieto PA, Tetzlaff MT, et al. Neoadjuvant plus adjuvant dabrafenib and trametinib versus standard of care in patients with high-risk, surgically resectable melanoma: a single-centre, open-label, randomised, phase 2 trial. Lancet Oncol 2018;19(2):181–93.

59. Horvat TZ, Adel NG, Dang TO, et al. Immune-related adverse events, need for systemic immunosuppression, and effects on survival and time to treatment failure in patients with melanoma treated with ipilimumab at Memorial Sloan Kettering Cancer Center. J Clin Oncol 2015;33(28):3193–8.

60. Wang AS, Armstrong EJ, Armstrong AW. Corticosteroids and wound healing: clinical considerations in the perioperative period. Am J Surg 2013;206(3):410–7.

61. Ismael H, Horst M, Farooq M, et al. Adverse effects of preoperative steroid use on surgical outcomes. Am J Surg 2011;201(3):305–8 [discussion: 308–9].

62. Forde PM, Chaft JE, Smith KN, et al. Neoadjuvant PD-1 blockade in resectable lung cancer. N Engl J Med 2018;378(21):1976–86.

63. Topalian SL, Bhatia S, Kudchadkar R, et al. Nivolumab (Nivo) as neoadjuvant therapy in patients with resectable Merkel cell carcinoma (MCC) in CheckMate 358. J Clin Oncol 2018;36(supplement):9505.

64. Gershenwald JE, Scolyer RA, Hess KR, et al. Melanoma staging: evidence-based changes in the American Joint Committee on Cancer eighth edition cancer staging manual. CA Cancer J Clin 2017;67(6):472–92.

65. Faries MB, Thompson JF, Cochran AJ, et al. Completion dissection or observation for sentinel-node metastasis in melanoma. N Engl J Med 2017;376(23):2211–22.

66. Feng Z, Wu X, Chen V, et al. Incidence and survival of desmoplastic melanoma in the United States, 1992-2007. J Cutan Pathol 2011;38(8):616–24.

67. Han D, Han G, Zhao X, et al. Clinicopathologic predictors of survival in patients with desmoplastic melanoma. PLoS One 2015;10(3):e0119716.

68. Goodman AM, Kato S, Bazhenova L, et al. Tumor mutational burden as an independent predictor of response to immunotherapy in diverse cancers. Mol Cancer Ther 2017;16(11):2598–608.

69. Uryvaev A, Passhak M, Hershkovits D, et al. The role of tumor-infiltrating lymphocytes (TILs) as a predictive biomarker of response to anti-PD1 therapy in patients with metastatic non-small cell lung cancer or metastatic melanoma. Med Oncol 2018;35(3):25.

70. Eroglu Z, Zaretsky JM, Hu-Lieskovan S, et al. High response rate to PD-1 blockade in desmoplastic melanomas. Nature 2018;553(7688):347–50.

71. Strom T, Caudell JJ, Han D, et al. Radiotherapy influences local control in patients with desmoplastic melanoma. Cancer 2014;120(9):1369–78.

72. Ascierto PA, Accorona R, Botti G, et al. Mucosal melanoma of the head and neck. Crit Rev Oncol Hematol 2017;112:136–52.

73. D'Angelo SP, Larkin J, Sosman JA, et al. Efficacy and safety of nivolumab alone or in combination with ipilimumab in patients with mucosal melanoma: a pooled analysis. J Clin Oncol 2017;35(2):226–35.

74. Rothermel LD, Sabesan AC, Stephens DJ, et al. Identification of an immunogenic subset of metastatic uveal melanoma. Clin Cancer Res 2016;22(9):2237–49.

75. Algazi AP, Tsai KK, Shoushtari AN, et al. Clinical outcomes in metastatic uveal melanoma treated with PD-1 and PD-L1 antibodies. Cancer 2016;122(21):3344–53.

76. Maio M, Danielli R, Chiarion-Sileni V, et al. Efficacy and safety of ipilimumab in patients with pre-treated, uveal melanoma. Ann Oncol 2013;24(11):2911–5.

77. Ascierto PA, McArthur GA, Dreno B, et al. Cobimetinib combined with vemurafenib in advanced BRAF(V600)-mutant melanoma (coBRIM): updated efficacy results from a randomised, double-blind, phase 3 trial. Lancet Oncol 2016;17(9):1248–60.

78. Long GV, Flaherty KT, Stroyakovskiy D, et al. Dabrafenib plus trametinib versus dabrafenib monotherapy in patients with metastatic BRAF V600E/K-mutant melanoma: long-term survival and safety analysis of a phase 3 study. Ann Oncol 2017;28(7):1631–9.

79. Dreno B, Ribas A, Larkin J, et al. Incidence, course, and management of toxicities associated with cobimetinib in combination with vemurafenib in the coBRIM study. Ann Oncol 2017;28(5):1137–44.

Oncolytic Immunotherapy

Morgan L. Hennessy, MD, PhD[a], Praveen K. Bommareddy, MS, PhD[b],
Genevieve Boland, MD, PhD[a], Howard L. Kaufman, MD[a,c,*]

KEYWORDS

- Cancer • Immunogenic cell death • Immunotherapy • Intratumoral • Oncolytic virus
- Treatment

KEY POINTS

- Oncolytic viruses are a new class of anticancer agents that induces immunogenic cell death and host antitumor immunity.
- Preclinical models support the therapeutic benefit of oncolytic immunotherapy as single agent and in combination with other cancer therapeutics.
- Talimogene laherparepvec is the first oncolytic virus approved for the treatment of advanced melanoma with considerable interest in using other viruses against a range of different cancers.
- There are logistical and biosafety issues associated with implementing oncolytic viruses into standard clinical practice requiring minimal education and training.
- High priorities for further investigation include integrating oncolytic viruses into combination immunotherapy, other forms of intratumoral agents, and identifying predictive biomarkers of treatment.

INTRODUCTION

Oncolytic viruses are a class of viruses, either naturally occurring or genetically engineered, which preferentially infect and replicate in cancer cells, leading to cancer cell death while sparing healthy tissue.[1–3] These viruses modulate a variety of responses within the cell itself, inducing cell death via activation of antiviral pathways, triggering of cyclic GMP-AMP synthase–stimulator of interferon genes (cGAS-STING) and interferon response factors (IRF) signaling (DNA viruses), Toll-like receptor (TLR) activation (RNA viruses), and recruitment and activation of surrounding tissue macrophages, endothelial cells, dendritic cells, and lymphocytes.[4] The complex interactions of oncolytic viruses on local tumor cell death and induction of host immune response are

Disclosures: H.L. Kaufman is an employee of Replimune, Inc. The rest of the authors have nothing to disclose.
[a] Division of Surgical Oncology, Massachusetts General Hospital, 55 Fruit Street, Yawkey 7B, Boston, MA 02114, USA; [b] School of Graduate Studies, Graduate School of Biomedical Sciences, Rutgers University, 195 Little Albany Street, New Brunswick, NJ 08901, USA; [c] Replimune, Inc., Woburn, MA, USA
* Corresponding author.
E-mail address: HLKaufman@mgh.harvard.edu

shown in **Fig. 1**. These responses can lead to activation of the adaptive immune system via presentation of tumor antigens in combination with viral proteins, leading to maturation of antigen-presenting cells and subsequent activation of cytotoxic CD8$^+$ T cells. Direct activation of the innate immune system can also result from viral infection of tumor cells, enhancing the activity of natural killer (NK) cells, which may lead to cell death of infected cancer cells. Although each virus may activate specific pathways and recruit unique subsets of immune cells to the site of infection, oncolytic immunotherapy uniformly results in lymphocyte recruitment and can, thus, turn lymphocyte-poor ("cold") tumors into lymphocyte-predominant ("hot") tumors, and this could improve systemic immunotherapy, such as immune checkpoint blockade. In this review, the authors describe the rationale for oncolytic immunotherapy in which viruses and other activators of innate immunity can be used to transition "cold" tumor microenvironments into "hot" ones, discuss early phase clinical trial data, and provide insights into logistical and biosafety issues associated with intratumoral therapies.

RATIONALE FOR ONCOLYTIC IMMUNOTHERAPY

Oncolytic immunotherapy refers to treatment that is directed to intact tumor cells and results in immunogenic cell death (ICD). In the process of ICD, tumor cells are usually

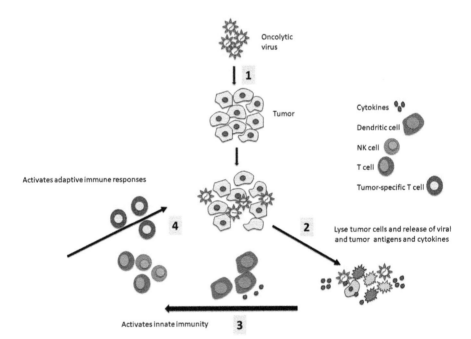

Fig. 1. Mechanisms of oncolytic virus-mediated antitumor activity. In this schematic, oncolytic viruses are injected into tumor cells (1). Following viral replication, tumor cells are lysed, releasing progeny viral particles to reinfect neighboring tumor cells, viral- and tumor-associated antigens, DAMP factors, and cytokines (2). Antigens are sampled by infiltrating dendritic cells and presented to naïve T cells generating viral- and tumor-specific T cells (3). The local cytokine milieu also drives adaptive immune responses, such as NK cell activation and adaptive immunity, with emergence of tumor-reactive T-cell responses (4). T cells are recruited to the tumor microenvironment by viral-induced chemokines and may also traffic to sites of distant metastatic disease.

killed albeit not necessarily all tumor cells, and ICD implies that a host antitumor immune response is generated. This secondary immune response is then capable of additional tumor cell eradication, which may occur locally where the oncolytic agent was injected (or delivered), and systemically at sites not treated by the oncolytic agent. This dual mechanism of antitumor activity (see **Fig. 1**) provides multiple opportunities for therapeutic manipulation using other drugs with overlapping and nonoverlapping pharmacologic mechanisms of action. Although multiple classes of agents may be considered for oncolytic immunotherapy, including cytotoxic small molecules, gene-targeted therapeutics, microRNA, molecular and antibody fragments targeting intracellular proliferative, cell-cycle, antiviral, and innate immune sensors, it is oncolytic viruses that have received the most attention to date. Because viruses have evolved to interact with intracellular signaling pathways and host immune elements and are especially lytic in cancer cells due to the frequent defects in tumor cell antiviral machinery elements, the rationale for oncolytic immunotherapy may be best demonstrated by understanding how oncolytic viruses can be used as cancer therapeutic agents.

Oncolytic viruses are defined by their ability to selectively replicate within cancer cells leading to cancer cell death. These viruses may be engineered or naturally occurring, and many subtypes of virus have been proposed as possible vectors for immunotherapy. Currently, oncolytic viruses are being developed using both RNA and DNA viruses. Oncolytic RNA viruses in development include coxsackievirus, measles virus, Maraba virus, Newcastle disease virus, polio virus, and reovirus, among others. Commonly used oncolytic DNA viruses include adenovirus, herpes simplex virus, and poxviruses. Both DNA and RNA viruses have advantages and limitations to be used as oncolytic viruses (**Table 1**). DNA viruses usually have large genomes and can be used to express transgenes encoding immune stimulatory ligands, such as cytokines or costimulatory molecules, or other anticancer agents. In contrast, the small size of most RNA viruses makes transgene expression more challenging.[2] DNA viruses are detected by the cGAS-STING and IRF pathways that promote type 1 interferon release and recruitment of dendritic cells and T cells, whereas RNA viruses activate TLRs. Preexisting antiviral antibodies may limit the ability to infect with both DNA and RNA viruses, but in general, neutralizing antibody titers are more predominant against DNA viruses than RNA viruses. Because of their small size, RNA viruses can penetrate the blood-brain barrier much more easily than RNA viruses. In addition, some viruses are susceptible to antiviral medications, which can be used in the event of uncontrolled replication. Thus, the selection of virus may depend on the tumor selected for treatment, the anatomic location of the cancer, the need to express various transgenes, and the potential safety profile of the virus.

Table 1 Key characteristics of DNA and RNA oncolytic viruses		
Feature	**DNA Viruses**	**RNA Viruses**
Viral genome	DNA	RNA
Host genome integration	Moderate to low	Low
Transgene expression	High capacity	Limited capacity
Replication in tumor cells	High	High
Preexisting neutralizing antibody response	High	Low to moderate
Ability to cross BBB	Low	High
Intracellular sensors	cGAS-STING; IRF	TLR

Abbreviation: BBB, blood-brain barrier.

Most oncolytic viruses enter host cells via surface receptors following viral binding. In many cases, the viral receptors are present at normal or higher levels on cancer cells allowing viral entry. Following entry, viral genetic material is released from the capsid, and replication proceeds. In some cases, viruses will replicate entirely within the cytoplasm of infected cells (eg, poxviruses), whereas in others, the virus must migrate into the nucleus to complete the replicative process (eg, herpes viruses). Certain viruses may also block host cell transcription and/or translation that can also cripple tumor cells. Once viral replication is completed, oncolytic viruses will orchestrate cell lysis with release of viral progeny that can then further infect neighboring cells. In this respect, a single virion can be expanded and result in significant tumor cell killing provided the virus is not eradicated by the intracellular antiviral machinery or by the host antiviral immune response. The antiviral machinery differs for DNA and RNA viruses, and the status of these antiviral factors may influence the outcome of infection with specific viruses. In general, DNA viruses are detected by cGAS-STING, PKR, and NLRP3 pathways, whereas RNA viruses are detected by TLR7, RIG1, and MDA pathways. Following lysis, in addition to releasing new virions, tumor cells will also release soluble tumor-associated antigens and various danger-associated molecular pattern (DAMP) factors that can serve as antigens and activating signals for the adaptive immune response.

In addition to inducing ICD and tumor cell lysis, oncolytic viruses attract dendritic cells via innate sensing and induction of type 1 interferons by infected cells. These dendritic cells are able to sample soluble viral- and tumor-associated antigens for presentation to T cells. In addition, local chemokine gradients are induced by the local viral infection, and this helps promote T-cell trafficking back to the tumor. In this way, oncolytic viruses both induce direct tumor cell death and induce host antitumor immunity. Furthermore, some viruses may induce expression of immune checkpoints, such as the programmed cell death ligand 1 (PD-L1), which can block programmed cell death 1 (PD-1)[+] activated T cells; this is 1 strategy through which the virus may protect itself from immune recognition. This finding, however, may also make tumors more susceptible to treatment with immune checkpoint blockade (ICB).[5]

Another advantage of oncolytic virus therapy is the ability to engineer vectors for enhanced antitumor activity and gene delivery. The therapeutic potential of an oncolytic virus can be further augmented in several ways, including alteration of the viral surface chemistry to target specific receptors that may be found on cancer cells or, more commonly, through expression of eukaryotic transgenes by the viral genome. This can include genes that promote more efficient cell killing, such as be encoding cytosine deaminase, which can then convert the prodrug, 5-fluorocytosine, to 5-fluorouracil (5-FU) within the tumor cell. Other strategies have encoded immune potentiating genes, such as cytokines or costimulatory molecules, in oncolytic viruses to enhance antitumor immunity. In addition, specific nonessential viral genes may be deleted from therapeutic viruses to reduce pathogenicity, enhance tumor cell selective replication, and provide room for foreign transgene expression. A more thorough review of how modifications can enhance oncolytic immunotherapy can be found elsewhere.[4]

CLINICAL TRIALS SUPPORTING ONCOLYTIC IMMUNOTHERAPY

In recent years, multiple clinical trials using intratumoral injection of oncolytic agents in melanoma, hepatocellular carcinoma, brain tumors, and bladder cancer have borne promising results. The diversity of disease tested highlights the possible broad applicability of this strategy across many tumor types. Furthermore, a broad array of agonistic ligands and viruses has been used in these studies, including herpes viruses, poxviruses, adenoviruses, and retroviruses. Globally, 3 oncolytic viruses have been approved for the treatment of cancer. H101 (also called oncorine) is an E1B-deleted adenovirus that is adapted for replication in p53-deficient tumor cells and was approved for the treatment of head and neck cancer in China.[6] ECHO-7 (or rigvir) is a native, oncolytic enterovirus that has been approved for the treatment of melanoma in Latvia, Georgia, Armenia, and Uzbekistan.[7] Finally, talimogene laherparepvec (T-VEC) is an attenuated, oncolytic herpes simplex virus type 1 (HSV-1) virus encoding granulocyte-macrophage colony stimulating factor (GM-CSF) and has been approved for the treatment of advanced melanoma.[8]

Talimogene Laherparepvec

T-VEC is an HSV-1, which has been engineered to selectively replicate within tumors and produce GM-CSF. Deletion of the viral ICP34.5 genes encoding the neuroviru-lence factor reduces viral pathogenicity while enhancing tumor cell replication. T-VEC also has deletion of the ICP47 gene, which encodes a protein that normally blocks peptide loading onto major histocompatibility complex (MHC) molecules and functions to block antiviral immune responses. Deletion of ICP47 allows normal peptide loading onto MHC and allows presentation of tumor-associated antigens. The local production of GM-CSF attracts and matures antigen-presenting cells, further promoting immunogenicity. T-VEC is given by direct intratumoral injection into clinically palpable or ultrasound-defined cutaneous, subcutaneous, or nodal melanomas recurrent after initial surgery. The potential therapeutic benefit of T-VEC in melanoma was first suggested in a single-arm phase 2 clinical trial in which 50 patients with stage IIIC–IV melanoma were treated with the virus by intratumoral injection.[9] In this trial, an objective response rate of 26% was reported with side effects limited to low-grade constitutional symptoms, such as fever, fatigue, nausea, and local injection site reactions. In a subset of responding patients, biopsy of regressing lesions demonstrated an increased number of melanoma-specific CD8$^+$ T cells and a decrease in regulatory CD4$^+$FoxP3$^+$ T cells and myeloid-derived suppressor cells consistent with induction of systemic antitumor immunity.[10] Based on these results, a prospective, randomized phase 3 clinical trial was conducted.

In the phase 3 study, 436 patients with stage IIIB–IV melanoma were randomized in a 2:1 manner to treatment with T-VEC or recombinant GM-CSF. The primary endpoint of the study was an improvement in durable response rate (DRR) defined as objective response lasting 6 months or greater. Patients with T-VEC demonstrated an improvement in DRR (16.3% vs 2.1; odds ratio, 8.9; $P<.001$). The overall response rate was also higher in the T-VEC arm (26.4% vs 5.7%), and median overall survival was improved from 18.9 months for GM-CSF treatment to 23.3 months in patients treated with T-VEC (hazard ratio, 0.79; $P = .51$). T-VEC efficacy was most pronounced in patients with stage IIIB, IIIC, or IVM1a disease, whereby the hazard ratio was 0.57 ($P<.001$). The most common adverse events related to T-VEC were fatigue, fever and chills, and local injection site reactions with 2.1% experiencing grade 3 cellulitis. Based on these data, T-VEC was approved in the United States and Australia for the treatment of advanced melanoma following recurrence after initial surgery, and approval in Europe was granted for patients with stage III or IVM1a disease based on the subset analysis. In another subset analysis, T-VEC was found to be particularly effective in patients with head and neck melanoma.[11] Although head and neck melanomas are usually more aggressive than extremity melanoma, the DRR was significantly higher in patients treated with T-VEC compared with GM-CSF (36.1% vs 3.8%; $P = .001$). In addition, 29.5% of the patients with head and neck melanoma treated with T-VEC had a complete response compared with no complete responses in patients treated with GM-CSF. The probability of remaining in objective response at 12 months was 73% for patients treated with T-VEC, and the median overall survival had not been reached in this subset of patients.

T-VEC has also been evaluated in combination with ICB in patients with melanoma. In a phase 1B study of T-VEC and ipilimumab in patients with advanced melanoma, an initial response rate of 50% was reported, and 18-month overall survival was 67%.[12] An important detail of this study was that, although single-agent adverse events were observed, no increase or unexpected toxicities were seen in patients receiving both drugs. These data led to a randomized phase 2 clinical study in which 198 melanoma patients were randomized to treatment with T-VEC and ipilimumab or ipilimumab alone.[13] In this study, combination treatment was associated with a significantly improved response rate (39% vs 18%; odds ratio, 2.9; $P = .002$). In addition, this trial reported regression of visceral (uninjected) disease in 52% of the patients treated with T-VEC and ipilimumab compared with 23% in those treated with ipilimumab alone. A similar toxicity profile was reported as seen in the phase 1B trial. More recently, a phase 1 study of T-VEC and pembrolizumab, an anti-PD-1 monoclonal antibody, resulted in an objective response in 62% of advanced melanoma patients treated with both agents, including a 33% complete response rate.[14] Responses were associated with an increase in local $CD8^+$ T-cell infiltration and increased expression of PD-L1, but patients without baseline T-cell responses or PD-L1 expression were able to achieve complete responses, suggesting T-VEC could enhance pembrolizumab activity in "cold" tumors. A larger randomized phase 3 clinical trial comparing T-VEC and pembrolizumab to pembrolizumab alone in melanoma has enrolled more than 700 patients, and results are anticipated shortly. Collectively, these data strongly support an important therapeutic benefit for combining T-VEC with ICB in patients with melanoma and suggest a favorable therapeutic window.

Other Oncolytic Viruses

CG0070 is a replication competent oncolytic adenovirus encoding GM-CSF that has been developed to target retinoblastoma-defective tumor cells. This agent was tested in a phase 1 clinical trial in patients with Bacillus Calmette-Guerin-refractory non-muscle-invasive bladder cancer where a complete response rate of 48.6% was reported with a tolerable safety profile.[15] In a follow-up phase 2 clinical trial, 45 patients with BCG-refractory, residual high-grade Ta, T1, or carcinoma in situ bladder tumors were treated with intravesical CG0070.[16] The 6-month complete response rate was 47% for all patients and 58% in patients with pure carcinoma in situ, although no patients had a complete response with pure T1 lesions. Treatment-related side effects included bladder spasm, hematuria, dysuria, urinary urgency, flulike symptoms, and fatigue. Grade III dysuria and hypotension occurred in 3% and 1.5% of the patients, respectively. Based on these data, a randomized phase 3 clinical trial is in progress.

Pexastimogene devacirepvec (JX-594 or Pexa-Vec) is an oncolytic vaccinia virus genetically engineered with a deleted thymidine kinase gene to promote replication in tumor cells and encoding human GM-CSF to promote immune responses. In a phase 1 trial in 22 patients with advanced solid tumors, JX-594 was associated with constitutional symptoms, thrombocytopenia, and hyperbilirubinemia with 3 of 22 patients demonstrating a partial response.[17] This study was followed by a randomized phase 2 dose finding trial in 30 patients with advanced hepatocellular carcinoma.[18] The virus was delivered by interventional image-guided injections, and intrahepatic disease control was reported in 50% of patients; survival appeared to be improved in patients receiving higher doses of JX-594 (14.1 vs 6,7 months; hazard ratio 0.39;

$P = .02$). Further clinical studies in HCC are planned.[19] JX-594 has also been tested in 15 patients with treatment-refractory colorectal cancer.[20] In this trial, Pexa-Vec was administered intravenously every 14 days at increasing doses. All patients received at least 2 doses, and the most common adverse events were low-grade flulike symptoms. Although no objective responses were seen, 10 patients (67%) had stable disease. The investigators concluded that further studies were warranted.

A rat parvovirus (H-1PV) is a single-stranded DNA virus that has shown activity in preclinical glioma tumor models and has recently been tested in a phase 1/2A clinical trial in patients with recurrent glioblastoma.[21] In this study, H-1PV was given by intratumoral or intravenous injection, and tumors were resected 9 days later with additional virus delivered to the resection cavity. The virus was detected within the tumor following both delivery methods, and a tolerable safety profile was reported with evidence of T-cell infiltration in resected tumors. Although no formal efficacy analysis could be performed, median survival compared favorably to published meta-analyses for patients with glioblastoma. More recently, recombinant oncolytic poliovirus PVS-RIPO was delivered by convection-enhanced, intratumoral administration to 61 patients with recurrent supratentorial malignant glioma across 7 increasing viral doses.[22] There was 1 dose-limiting complication of a grade 4 intracranial hemorrhage in the study. An overall survival of 21% was reported at 24 months, which appeared to be ongoing at 36 months.

Other RNA viruses are also under investigation as oncolytic agents. MV-NIS is an oncolytic Edmonston strain of measles virus encoding the sodium-iodide symporter, which is expressed as a method of monitoring viral replication through noninvasive radioiodine imaging. MV-NIS was evaluated through a phase 1 clinical trial in 32 patients with recurrent and treatment-refractory multiple myeloma in which MV-NIS was administered intravenously in combination with cyclophosphamide.[23] Adverse events included neutropenia, leukopenia, and thrombocytopenia. Viral RNA was detected in sputum, blood, and urine specimens, and Iodine 123 scans were positive in 8 subjects. Although transient decreases in serum-free light chains were observed in some patients, 1 patient underwent a complete response. Another RNA virus, coxsackievirus A21, has been tested by both intratumoral and intravenous delivery in patients with melanoma and other solid tumors with evidence of tumor regression in some patients.[4]

Retroviruses used in clinical trials include vocimagene amiretrorepvec (Toca 511), studied in the preclinical trials mentioned above, which expresses cytosine deaminase and converts prodrug 5-fluorocytosine into the active chemotherapeutic 5-FU intracellularly. This virus has been studied with administration into the tumor directly, intravenously, and into tumor resection cavities. In a phase 1 trial of Toca 511 in recurrent high-grade glioma, patients underwent resection and had virus injected into the cavity wall. They then received oral fluorocytosine. Multiyear durable responses were observed in a proportion of patients.[24]

Other Intratumoral Agents in Clinical Development

The TLR family represents an interesting target for immune manipulation because TLR agonists will activate local innate immunity and can help to initiate adaptive immune responses. Thus, TLR agonists alone and in combination with other therapeutic strategies have begun clinical testing. The first such agent to gain attention was imiquimod 5% cream, which is a TLR7 agonist and was initially approved for the treatment of genital warts. Later, imiquimod demonstrated activity in actinic keratoses, a premalignancy cutaneous tumor and superficial basal cell carcinoma.[25] There have also been reports demonstrating therapeutic activity of imiquimod for superficial lentigo malignant melanoma, although this has not been confirmed in larger studies.[26,27] As a topical agent, imiquimod is not directly injected but can be placed over the skin of epidermal, dermal, and soft tissue lesions. In a recent single-arm phase 2 clinical study, imiquimod was given for 4 consecutive days every 4 weeks to patients with treatment-refractory chest wall breast cancer.[28] The patients were also treated with intravenous nab-paclitaxel once every 3 weeks. Of the 15 patients treated, 14 were evaluable, 5 had a complete response (36%), and 5 had a partial response (36%). Therapy was well tolerated with largely low-grade expected adverse events reported. Further studies of imiquimod and related TLR7 and TLR8 agonists are currently in progress.

TLR9 is another therapeutic target under investigation. TLR (CD289) is expressed in dendritic cells, macrophages, NK cells, and other immune cells and functions to sense bacterial and viral DNA resulting in signaling cascades that release proinflammatory cytokines.[29] Synthetic agonists of TLR9 have been developed by linking short single-stranded, unmethylated CpG oligodinucleotides (ODNs) together. These CpG ODNs can be directly injected into the subcutaneous skin where they can augment vaccines against infectious diseases and cancer.[30] In addition, CpG ODNs can be injected into tumors alone or in combination with other agents, such as ICB for cancer immunotherapy. Indeed, several trials have reported acceptable safety profiles, and further clinical efficacy studies are underway. Preliminary data from a phase 1b clinical trials recently reported that CpG ODN (SD-101) given with pembrolizumab to patients with unresectable or metastatic melanoma had an objective response rate of 78% in 9 patients who were naïve to prior pembrolizumab therapy but was only 15% in 13 patients whose tumors were refractory to pembrolizumab.[31] Treatment was well tolerated with transient mild to moderate flulike symptoms and was associated with recruitment of immune cells to the tumor microenvironment, including T cells, dendritic cells, NK cells, and B cells. In another small single-arm trial, 29 patients with untreated indolent lymphoma were treated with low-dose radiation followed by 5 weekly injections of CpG ODN (SD-101) into a single lymphoma tumor.[32] All patients demonstrated tumor regression with 25 of the 29 patients showing regression in uninjected tumors as well. Overall, 5 patients achieved an objective partial response, and 1 patient had a complete response. Treatment was associated with an accumulation of CD8+ effector cells in the injected tumors, and a decrease in follicular and regulatory helper CD4+ T cells was also reported. Other TLR agonists, such as polyinosinic:polycytidylic acid or poly(I:C), is similar to viral RNA and serves as a TLR3 agonist. Poly(I:C) has been studied as a therapeutic agent for cancer with limited evidence of therapeutic benefit (PMID:2402994). Overall, the safety of these agents and a better understanding of how these agonists can help reprogram the immune response may suggest their role in future clinical studies, especially for patients with immunologically "cold" tumors.

As discussed above, activation of the cGAS-STING pathway has been associated with recruitment of lymphocytes and increased sensitivity to immunotherapy.[33] Studies of a synthetic cyclic dinucleotide that activated STING (ADU-S100) has been developed and is entering clinical trials alone and with pembrolizumab in patients with advanced melanoma. Results from these studies are anticipated in the near future. A more comprehensive discussion for intratumoral approaches can be found in a review by Bommareddy and colleagues.[34]

LOGISTICAL ISSUES ASSOCIATED WITH ONCOLYTIC IMMUNOTHERAPY

The clinical administration of intratumoral agents and live viruses may be associated with special logistical and biosafety issues. Logistical issues involved with oncolytic virus therapy can be easily managed by early education and training of hospital administration and health care provider staff with attention to certain details (**Table 2**). Although oncolytic immunotherapy represents a departure from routine oncology practice for many ambulatory clinics, most institutions and large clinical practices should be able to provide seamless integration by adopting a few best practices to accommodate the management of patients electing treatment or clinical trial participation with oncolytic agents. Live viruses, in particular, may require additional biosafety review by local infection control boards before clinical use. Physicians need to be educated about these agents and understand how specific oncolytic agents are attenuated and/or retain susceptibility to antiviral medications. The storage and preparation of these agents are usually comparable to the management of BCG and live influenza vaccine preparations, which are often well established at most oncology clinics.

For some oncolytic viruses, storage in −70°C to −80°C freezers may represent a significant barrier if such freezers are not available, and, thus, it is important to note the storage requirements for any new agents before delivery. For most oncolytic agents, as for all oncology drug preparation, assembly in a dedicated biosafety cabinet in a secure pharmacy is advisable. General recommendations for preparation and handling of viral agents should include appropriate use of universal precautions throughout the preparations and administration process. A double container delivery system may also be useful if the oncolytic drug needs to travel to other parts of the health care facility, such as radiology suites. Developing standard operating procedures for each agent with information on proper handling, disposal, and treatment of spills or inadvertent injections should be prepared ahead of time, and there are now published guidelines for successful policies used at other institutions.[35,36] In general, the use of universal precautions, including gowns, gloves, masks, and eye protection, is sufficient for health care providers during injections. Depending on the biosafety

Table 2
Logistical considerations in clinical administration of oncolytic immunotherapy

Logistical Issue	Solutions
Drug storage	• May require −70°C freezer
Drug preparation	• Dedicated biosafety cabinet and universal precautions for pharmacists • Direct tumor measurement and drug orders delayed until day of treatment
Biosafety and contact transmission	• Universal precautions when handling and administering agent • Education for health care providers • Education for patients and patient families
Lesion access	• Image guidance through portable ultrasound or computed tomographic imaging to access challenging lesion
Contamination	• Establish procedures for dealing with biohazard waste and spills • Terminal cleaning of examination room where patients are injected
Clinic logistics	• Care coordinator, especially when patients are receiving more than 1 treatment per visit
Technical issues	• Staff training to perform intratumoral injections • Integration with interventional radiology for deep/visceral lesions
Reimbursement	• Expertise in charge capture for multiple components of OI delivery

Abbreviation: OI, Oncolytic immunotherapy.

level of the agent, disposal of soiled materials, including needles and sharps, can be in hospital or clinic biohazard waste and sharps disposal units. Health care workers involved in the injection program should be educated about the agents, proper procedure for administration and waste disposal, interventions available for inadvertent exposures (eg, antiviral medications) and be advised to avoid handling during time of potential immune suppression.

In addition to educating health care providers, patients and their families also require additional time to receive education around managing the injection site. Typically, the site can be covered with dry gauze and transparent dressing, such as a Tegaderm bandage. Patients should be instructed to leave the bandage on as long as possible (usually around 5–7 days is sufficient). Patients can be given extra dressings and a small biohazard waste bag to collect used bandages for return to the site. Patients should also be instructed to wash their hands before and after dressings are handled and to use gloves whenever possible. To date, there have been no reports of household contact transmission for any oncolytic agent.

Finally, the use of oncolytic immunotherapy can cause some shift in the normal ambulatory clinic flow. For many agents, dosing is based on the day of treatment diameter of the tumor, and this requires patients to be seen for measurement before ordering the drug, which can delay the clinic process and necessitate a longer wait by patients. In some centers, a single room is used allowing all patients needing measurements to come in early and then allowing them a break to return later for injections. Terminal cleaning of the examination suite should occur after the last patient and requires use of 10% bleach solution. A similar procedure can be used in radiology suites for patients needing image-guided injections. Although requiring some initial education and training, most centers can easily establish and manage a busy oncolytic immunotherapy program.

SUMMARY

Although oncolytic viruses have led the field with approval of T-VEC for the treatment of melanoma, other immune targets, such as TLRs, and innate agonists, such as cGAS-STING, are gaining interest for therapeutic drug development. Clinical trials are exploring numerous oncolytic agents, and combination studies appear especially promising with improved therapeutic responses without considerable added toxicity being reported. Despite the enthusiasm, logistical and biosafety issues are important considerations for clinicians electing to offer oncolytic immunotherapy to their patients. Future studies will likely focus on expanding treatment to a wider range of cancers, use of image-guided injections for visceral tumors, and extending treatment into the neoadjuvant setting. Oncolytic immunotherapy offers patients with melanoma another therapeutic option and may be useful for patients with other types of cancer.

REFERENCES

1. Kaufman HL, Kohlhapp FJ, Zloza A. Oncolytic viruses: a new class of immunotherapy drugs. Nat Rev Drug Discov 2015;14:642–62.
2. Bommareddy PK, Patel A, Hossain S, et al. Talimogene laherparepvec (T-VEC) and other oncolytic viruses for the treatment of melanoma. Am J Clin Dermatol 2017;18:1–15.
3. Jhawar SR, Thandoni A, Bommareddy PK, et al. Oncolytic viruses-natural and genetically engineered cancer immunotherapies. Front Oncol 2017;7:202.
4. Bommareddy PK, Shettigar M, Kaufman HL. Integrating oncolytic viruses in combination cancer immunotherapy. Nat Rev Immunol 2018;18:498–513.

5. Bommareddy PK, Kaufman HL. Unleashing the therapeutic potential of oncolytic viruses. J Clin Invest 2018;128:1258–60.

6. Garber K. China approves world's first oncolytic virus therapy for cancer treatment. J Natl Cancer Inst 2006;98:298–300.

7. Donina S, Strēle I, Proboka G, et al. Adapted ECHO-7 virus Rigvir immunotherapy (oncolytic virotherapy) prolongs survival in melanoma patients after surgical excision of the tumour in a retrospective study. Melanoma Res 2015;25:421–6.

8. Andtbacka RH, Kaufman HL, Collichio F, et al. Talimogene laherparepvec improves durable response rate in patients with advanced melanoma. J Clin Oncol 2015;33:2780–8.

9. Senzer NN, Kaufman HL, Amatruda T, et al. Phase II clinical trial of a granulocyte-macrophage colony-stimulating factor-encoding, second-generation oncolytic herpesvirus in patients with unresectable metastatic melanoma. J Clin Oncol 2009;27:5763–71.

10. Kaufman HL, Kim DW, DeRaffele G, et al. Local and distant immunity induced by intralesional vaccination with an oncolytic herpes virus encoding GM-CSF in patients with stage IIIc and IV melanoma. Ann Surg Oncol 2010;17:718–30.

11. Andtbacka RH, Agarwala SS, Ollila DW, et al. Cutaneous head and neck melanoma in OPTiM, a randomized phase 3 trial of talimogene laherparepvec versus granulocyte-macrophage colony-stimulating factor for the treatment of unresected stage IIIB/IIIC/IV melanoma. Head Neck 2016;38:1752–8.

12. Puzanov I, Milhem MM, Minor D, et al. Talimogene laherparepvec in combination with ipilimumab in previously untreated, unresectable stage IIIB-IV melanoma. J Clin Oncol 2016;34:2619–26.

13. Chesney J, Puzanov I, Collichio F, et al. Randomized, open-label phase II study evaluating the efficacy and safety of talimogene laherparepvec in combination with ipilimumab versus ipilimumab alone in patients with advanced, unresectable melanoma. J Clin Oncol 2018;36:1658–67.

14. Ribas A, Dummer R, Puzanov I, et al. Oncolytic virotherapy promotes intratumoral T cell infiltration and improves anti-PD-1 immunotherapy. Cell 2017;170: 1109–19.e10.

15. Burke JM, Lamm DL, Meng MV, et al. A first in human phase 1 study of CG0070, a GM-CSF expressing oncolytic adenovirus, for the treatment of nonmuscle invasive bladder cancer. J Urol 2012;188:2391–7.

16. Packiam VT, Lamm DL, Barocas DA, et al. An open label, single-arm, phase II multicenter study of the safety and efficacy of CG0070 oncolytic vector regimen in patients with BCG-unresponsive non-muscle-invasive bladder cancer: Interim results. Urol Oncol 2018;36:440–7.

17. Park BH, Hwang T, Liu TC, et al. Use of a targeted oncolytic poxvirus, JX-594, in patients with refractory primary or metastatic liver cancer: a phase I trial. Lancet Oncol 2008;9:533–42.

18. Heo J, Reid T, Ruo L, et al. Randomized dose-finding clinical trial of oncolytic immunotherapeutic vaccinia JX-594 in liver cancer. Nat Med 2013;19:329–36.

19. Breitbach CJ, Moon A, Burke J, et al. A phase 2, open-label, randomized study of pexa-vec (JX-594) administered by intratumoral injection in patients with unresectable primary hepatocellular carcinoma. Methods Mol Biol 2015;1317:343–57.

20. Park SH, Breitbach CJ, Lee J, et al. Phase 1b trial of biweekly intravenous Pexa-Vec (JX-594), an oncolytic and immunotherapeutic vaccinia virus in colorectal cancer. Mol Ther 2015;23:1532–40.

21. Geletneky K, Hajda J, Angelova AL, et al. Oncolytic H-1 parvovirus shows safety and signs of immunogenic activity in a first phase I/IIa glioblastoma trial. Mol Ther 2017;25:2620–34.
22. Desjardins A, Patel NV, Kwan K, et al. Recurrent glioblastoma treated with recombinant poliovirus. N Engl J Med 2018;379:150–61.
23. Dispenzieri A, Tong C, LaPlant B, et al. Phase I trial of systemic administration of Edmonston strain of measles virus genetically engineered to express the sodium iodide symporter in patients with recurrent or refractory multiple myeloma. Leukemia 2017;31:2791–8.
24. Cloughesy TF, Landolfi J, Hogan DJ, et al. Phase 1 trial of vocimagene amiretrorepvec and 5-fluorocytosine for recurrent high-grade glioma. Sci Transl Med 2016; 8:341ra375.
25. Hanna E, Abadi R, Abbas O. Imiquimod in dermatology: an overview. Int J Dermatol 2016;55:831–44.
26. Kai AC, Richards T, Coleman A, et al. Five-year recurrence rate of lentigo maligna after treatment with imiquimod. Br J Dermatol 2016;174:165–8.
27. Marsden JR, Fox R, Boota NM, et al. Effect of topical imiquimod as primary treatment for lentigo maligna: the LIMIT-1 study. Br J Dermatol 2017;176:1148–54.
28. Salazar LG, Lu H, Reichow JL, et al. Topical imiquimod plus nab-paclitaxel for breast cancer cutaneous metastases: a phase 2 clinical trial. JAMA Oncol 2017;3:969–73.
29. Ntoufa S, Vilia MG, Stamatopoulos K, et al. Toll-like receptors signaling: a complex network for NF-kappaB activation in B-cell lymphoid malignancies. Semin Cancer Biol 2016;39:15–25.
30. Huang X, Yang Y. Targeting the TLR9-MyD88 pathway in the regulation of adaptive immune responses. Expert Opin Ther Targets 2010;14:787–96.
31. Ribas A, Medina T, Kummar S, et al. SD-101 in combination with pembrolizumab in advanced melanoma: results of a phase Ib, multicenter study. Cancer Discov 2018;8:1250–7.
32. Frank MJ, Reagan PM, Bartlett NL, et al. In situ vaccination with a TLR9 agonist and local low-dose radiation induces systemic responses in untreated indolent lymphoma. Cancer Discov 2018;8:1258–69.
33. Woo SR, Fuertes MB, Corrales L, et al. STING-dependent cytosolic DNA sensing mediates innate immune recognition of immunogenic tumors. Immunity 2014;41: 830–42.
34. Bommareddy PK, Silk AW, Kaufman HL. Intratumoral approaches for the treatment of melanoma. Cancer J 2017;23:40–7.
35. Harrington KJ, Michielin O, Malvehy J, et al. A practical guide to the handling and administration of talimogene laherparepvec in Europe. Onco Targets Ther 2017; 10:3867–80.
36. Collichio F, Burke L, Proctor A, et al. Implementing a program of talimogene laherparepvec. Ann Surg Oncol 2018;25:1828–35.

Immunologic Targeting of Cancer Stem Cells

Jing Zhang, MD[a,b], Qiao Li, PhD[c], Alfred E. Chang, MD[d],*

KEYWORDS

- Cancer stem cells • Immunotherapy • Tumor antigens • Vaccine
- Innate immune response

KEY POINTS

- As CSCs are intrinsically resistant to conventional chemoradiotherapy and drive tumor progression and metastasis, immunologically targeting CSCs represents a novel direction for overcoming treatment resistance in cancer.
- Increasing evidence shows that innate immune responses are involved in the regulation of CSCs and can be modulated to target CSCs.
- There is a need to identify new antigens or genetic alterations in CSCs that can serve as specific targets for immunotherapy.
- Immunologic reagents can alter the tumor microenvironment niche that contributes to the regulation of CSCs, and may serve as effective therapeutic approaches to CSCs.
- The immunotherapy of CSCs will need to be combined with other more conventional therapies (ie, chemotherapy, radiotherapy, and surgery) to fully achieve optimal outcomes.

INTRODUCTION

Despite increasing improvements in cancer treatment, disease progression and recurrence resulting from cancer stem cells (CSCs) are still main factors for cancer-related mortality. In 1937, researchers reported that a single cell from a mouse leukemia could initiate leukemia in a recipient mouse, indicating the existence of CSCs.[1] In the last 20 years, CSCs have successfully been identified in a variety of solid tumors, such as breast cancer, colorectal cancer, lung cancer, and melanoma. By definition, both

Disclosure Statement: This review was partially supported by the Gillson Longenbaugh Foundation, Houston, TX.
[a] Division of Surgical Oncology, University of Michigan Rogel Cancer Center, Room 3410, 1150 East Medical Center Drive, Ann Arbor, MI 48109, USA; [b] Department of the 2nd Thoracic Medical Oncology, Hubei Cancer Hospital, Tongji Medical College, Huazhong University of Science and Technology, No. 116 Zhuodaoquan South Road, Hongshan District, Wuhan, Hubei Province 430070, China; [c] Division of Surgical Oncology, University of Michigan Rogel Cancer Center, 3520B MSRB-1, 1150 West Medical Center Drive, Ann Arbor, MI 48109, USA; [d] Division of Surgical Oncology, University of Michigan Rogel Cancer Center, Room 3304, 1500 East Medical Center Drive, Ann Arbor, MI 48109, USA
* Corresponding author.
E-mail address: aechang@med.umich.edu

CSCs and normal tissue stem cells possess self-renewal capacity, but it is typically deregulated in CSCs. CSCs represent a distinct population that can be isolated from the remainder of the tumor cells and can be shown to have clonal long-term repopulation and self-renewal capacity, the defining features of a CSC.[2–4]

CSCs are more resistant to conventional chemotherapy and radiotherapy than non-CSCs, which has been attributed to increased expression of antiapoptotic proteins, slow proliferation rate of stem cells, increased levels of ATP-binding cassette transporters and transmembrane protein transporters, which are known to mediate drug efflux.[5–9] Furthermore, CSC-mediated immunoresistance is another crucial mechanism for treatment failure. Many antigen-processing molecules, such as β-microglobulin, and major histocompatibility complex (MHC) molecules I and II, are downregulated in CSCs compared with their non-CSCs counterparts in glioblastoma multiforme and melanoma.[10,11] Meanwhile, CSCs have also been shown to secrete inhibitive cytokines, such as transforming growth factor β (TGF-β), interleukin (IL)-6, IL-10, and IL-13 in vitro, which can promote tumor immune evasion and ultimately increase tumorigenic growth.[12]

Because CSCs drive tumor progression and metastasis, long-term benefit of cancer therapies may depend on their ability to effectively target CSCs.[13] Theoretically, conventional approaches such as surgery, chemotherapy, and/or radiation therapy are ineffective in eliminating CSCs. Thus, the immunologic targeting of CSCs represents a new direction for overcoming treatment resistance in cancer therapeutics.

CSCs were first isolated in 1997 by Bonnet and Dick,[14] who demonstrated that the $CD34^+$ $CD38^-$ cells were capable of initiating human acute myeloid leukemia in non-obese diabetic (NOD) severe combined immunodeficiency (SCID) mice. These cells possessed differentiative and proliferative capacities, and the potential for self-renewal expected of a leukemic stem cell.[14] In 2003, Al-Hajj and colleagues[15] identified and isolated the first CSCs in solid tumors, which was characterized by the surface markers $CD44^+/CD24^-/lin^-$ in breast cancer. Subsequently, CSCs have been identified in different tumor types, such as melanoma,[16] head and neck cancer,[17] lung cancer,[18] gastric cancer,[19] pancreas cancer,[20] bladder cancer,[21] and prostate cancer.[22]

The cell surface markers most commonly used in solid tumors to identify CSCs are CD133, CD44, IL-6R, CD24, epithelial cell adhesion molecule, leucine-rich repeat–containing G protein–coupled receptor 5 (Lgr5), CD166, and CD29, alone or in combination.[23] However, there are no universally accepted specific markers for different malignancies. Exploring new CSC markers will be helpful to further enhance our understanding on the biological behavior of CSCs and identify potential therapeutic targets against cancers.

As a metabolic enzyme, aldehyde dehydrogenase (ALDH) can be found in different cellular compartments, including the cytosol, nucleus, mitochondria, and endoplasmatic reticulum, and is involved in detoxifying a wide variety of endogenous and exogenous aldehydes to their corresponding weak carboxylic acids.[24,25] Interestingly, high ALDH activity is associated with both normal stem cells and CSCs. In breast cancer, high ALDH activity identified the tumorigenic cell fraction, capable of self-renewal and of generating tumors that recapitulate the heterogeneity of the parental tumor. Expression of ALDH1 detected by immunostaining correlated with poor prognosis in 577 patients with breast cancer.[26] $ALDH^{high}$ cells readily formed distant metastases with strongly enhanced tumor progression at both orthotopic and metastatic sites in preclinical models.[27] $ALDH^{high}$ cells represented a small percentage of an entire tumor (1%–8%), and are highly tumorigenic when implanted in immunocompromised NOD/SCID mice compared with non-CSCs.[28] Isolated lung cancer cells with relatively high ALDH1 activity displayed in vitro features of CSCs, including capacities for proliferation, self-renewal, and differentiation, resistance to chemotherapy, and expression of the CSC surface marker CD133; and in vivo experiments showed that ALDH1-positive cancer cells could also generate tumors that recapitulated the heterogeneity of the parental lung cancer cells.[29] ALDH3A1 was significantly upregulated in the DU145-derived prostate CSCs, and elevation of ALDH3A1 expression was clearly associated with progression and lung metastasis of prostate cancer in vivo.[30] Collectively, ALDH has been used as a promising and reliable marker for the identification and isolation of CSCs in many malignancies. A summary of CSC markers[31–47] are listed in **Table 1**.

THERAPEUTIC APPROACHES INVOLVING THE INNATE IMMUNE RESPONSE
Toll-like Receptors

Increasing evidence indicates that innate immune responses are involved in the regulation of CSCs. CSCs constitutively exhibit higher nuclear factor κB (NF-κB) activation by the ligation of the Toll-like receptor (TLR) signaling pathway, which then increases stemness in cancer cells.[48] Stimulation of TLR3 promoted breast cancer cells toward a CSC phenotype in vitro and in vivo, moreover, cardamonin, an NF-κB inhibitor, was capable of effectively abolishing TLR3 activation-enhanced CSC phenotypes in vitro and successfully controlling TLR3 stimulation-induced tumor growth in human breast cancer xenografts.[49] In another model, activation of TLR4 in breast cancer cells, resulted in enhancement of their stemness and tumorigenicity. In addition, immunohistochemistry results showed that high light chain 3/TLR4 levels predicted increased relapse rate and poor prognosis in 180 patients with luminal breast cancers.[50] Different from the results of this study, Alvarado and colleagues[51] demonstrated that TLR4 was downregulated on glioblastoma CSCs, and that its overexpression

Table 1
Summary of CSC markers in solid tumors

Tumors	CSC Markers
Breast cancer	CD44, CD24, ALDH1, CD29[31,32]
Head and neck cancer	CD44, ALDH1, CD133, c-Met[33]
Lung cancer	CD133, EpCAM[34]
Esophageal cancer	CD44, CD24[35]
Gastric cancer	CD44, CD133, ALDH1[36]
Colorectal cancer	EpCAM, Lgr5, CD133, IL-6R[37,38]
Liver cancer	EpCAM, CD133, CD90[39]
Pancreatic cancer	CD133, CXCR4, c-Met, ESA[40]
Renal cell cancer	CD105, CD133, CXCR4[41]
Prostate cancer	CD117, CD133, E-cadherin, cytokeratin 5[42]
Bladder cancer	CD44v6, laminin receptor, ALDH1[43]
Ovarian cancer	CD133, ALDH1A1, CD44[44]
Cervical cancer	ABCG2, ALDH1, CD49f, CD133[45]
Glioma	CD133, CD15, integrin-α6[46]
Melanoma	CD166, CD133, Nestin[47]

Abbreviations: ABCG2, ATP-binding cassette subfamily G member 2; CXCR4, C-X-C chemokine receptor type 4; EpCAM, epithelial cellular adhesion molecule; ESA, epithelial-specific antigen; Lgr5, leucine-rich repeat-containing G protein-coupled receptor 5.

could inhibit proliferation and maintenance of CSCs by reducing retinoblastoma binding protein 5 that was originally increased in CSCs. These findings provide a foundation for developing new strategies to target TLR and modulate the activity of CSCs.

Tumor-Associated Macrophages

New evidence has demonstrated that tumor-associated macrophages (TAMs) might contribute to the regulation and development of CSCs. TAMs can regulate the endothelial protein C receptor (a CSC marker) signaling pathway that is involved in the mammosphere cell–initiating and tumor cell–initiating activity.[52] Hyaluronan synthase 2 is upregulated in highly metastatic breast CSCs defined by the CD44$^+$CD24$^-$/ESA$^+$ phenotype, which is critical for the interaction of CSCs and TAMs, resulting in the enhanced secretion of platelet-derived growth factor from TAMs, and activation of stromal cells and enhancement of CSC self-renewal.[53] Milk-fat globule-epidermal growth factor-VIII, a downstream factor of TAMs, mainly activates Stat3 and Sonic Hedgehog pathways in CSCs and further amplifies their anticancer drug resistance in cooperation with IL-6, suggesting that TAMs can be a potential target of CSCs.[54] Wan and colleagues[55] also reported that TAMs produce IL-6 and promote the expansion of human hepatocellular carcinoma stem cells in vitro; blockade of IL-6 signaling with tocilizumab, a drug approved by the US Food and Drug Administration for treatment of rheumatoid arthritis, inhibited TAM-stimulated activity.

Natural Killer Cells

Many studies support that CSCs might be susceptible targets of natural killer (NK) cell cytotoxicity. Tseng and colleagues[56] reported increased cytotoxicity, and augmented secretion of interferon γ (IFN-γ) was observed when NK cells were coincubated with oral squamous carcinoma stem cells, human embryonic stem cells, mesenchymal stem cells, dental pulp stem cells, and human induced pluripotent stem cells, compared with their differentiated counterparts or parental lines. In another study, glioblastoma CSCs were highly susceptible to lysis mediated by both allogeneic and autologous IL-2 (or IL-15)-activated NK cells, although they were resistant to freshly isolated NK cells.[57] Another study showed that freshly purified allogeneic NK cells recognized and killed colorectal carcinoma–derived CSCs, whereas the non-CSC counterparts of the tumors (differentiated tumor cells) were less susceptible to either autologous or allogeneic NK cells; this difference in the NK cell susceptibility correlated with distinct expression of ligands for NKp30 and NKp44 on CSCs.[58] These studies suggest that adoptive cellular therapy with NK cells may play a role in the future for treating residual CSCs in a multimodal approach.

$\gamma\delta$T Cells

$\gamma\delta$T cells mediate well-established antitumor immunity, largely on the basis of their potent cytotoxicity and IFN-γ production.[59] $\gamma\delta$T cells induce upregulation of MHC-I and CD54/ICAM-1 on CSC-like cells and thereby increase their susceptibility to antigen-specific killing by CD8$^+$ T cells. Alternatively, $\gamma\delta$T-cell responses could be specifically directed against CSC-like cells using the humanized anti-GD2 monoclonal antibody hu14.18K322 A, which identifies a powerful synergism between MHC-restricted and non–MHC-restricted T cells in eradicating cancer cells, including breast CSCs.[60] Bisphosphonate zoledronate, a medication used to inhibit bone resorption and reduce skeleton-related events in patients with cancer was found to sensitize colon CSCs to Vγ9Vδ2 T cell cytotoxicity that was mediated by T cell receptor and NKG2D.[61] This role of zoledronate involving the innate immunity against CSCs was supported by another study, in which zoledronate efficiently sensitized both neuroblastoma-derived adherent cells and sphere-forming cells to γδT cell–mediated cytolysis.[62] Furthermore, a clinical trial showed that administration of Vγ9Vδ2 T cells resulted in an activated effector memory phenotype, expressed chemokine receptors predictive of homing to peripheral tissues and were cytotoxic in vitro against tumor.[63] Thus, ex vivo expanded γδT cells represent a novel cellular approach against CSCs. A summary of the cellular interactions of innate immunity and CSCs are shown in **Fig. 1**.

ANTIGEN-SPECIFIC IMMUNOTHERAPIES OF CANCER STEM CELLS
Aldehyde Dehydrogenase

In addition to ALDH being a CSC marker, much evidence indicates that it can act as an immunologic target. Visus and colleagues[64] reported a subset of tumor cells in human carcinomas identified as ALDH^{bright} cells that were recognized and eliminated in vitro by HLA-A2-restricted, ALDH1A1$_{88-96}$ peptide-specific CD8$^+$ T cells. Furthermore, adoptive transfer of ALDH1A1-specific CD8$^+$ T cells inhibited tumor growth and reduced lung metastases in human xenograft tumor models.[64] In another study, disulfiram (DSF), an irreversible pan-ALDH inhibitor, blocked in vitro and in vivo irradiation-induced conversion of nonstem breast cancer cells into breast CSCs by downregulation of the NF-κB stemness signal pathway, and enhanced the radiotherapy sensitivity of breast cancer when combined with copper (Cu^{2+}).[65] In addition, DSF/Cu inhibited ALDH-positive lung cancer cells in vitro and tumors derived from sorted ALDH-positive lung CSCs in vivo.[66] These studies demonstrate that ALDH is critical for stemness maintenance of CSCs, and it can be a promising target against CSCs.

CD133

CD133 is a common marker of CSCs. Targeting CD133 has given some promising results in preclinical studies. A genetically modified toxin conjugated to an anti-human CD133 monoclonal antibody significantly inhibited the proliferation of CD133$^+$ cells in cultures of established cell lines derived from head and neck squamous cell carcinomas in a dose-dependent manner, which provides a foundation for targeting

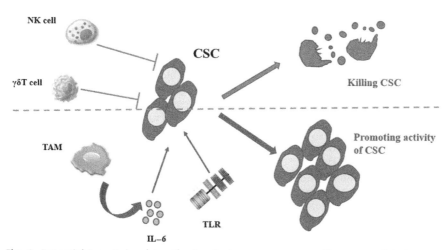

Fig. 1. Potential targets involving the innate immune responses. Tumor-associated macrophages (TAMs) and Toll-like receptors (TLRs) enhance the stemness of cancer stem cells (CSCs) by secreting IL-6 or activating NF-κB signaling. However, natural killer (NK) cells and γδT cells directly recognize and kill CSCs by cytotoxicity and secretion of IFN-γ.

CD133[+] CSCs.[67] Cytokine-induced killer (CIK) cells armed with anti-CD3/anti-CD133 bispecific antibody (BsAb-CIK) demonstrated higher killing capacity on CD133[high] pancreatic (SW1990) and hepatic (Hep3B) cancer cells, and significantly delayed CD133[high] tumor growth than the parental CIK, furthermore, BsAb-CIK cells cocultured with CD133[high] cells produced significantly higher amounts of IFN-γ.[68] One more example was that CD133 knockdown enhanced the efficacy of cisplatin chemotherapy and reduced colony-forming ability in oral squamous cell carcinoma cells.[69]

CD44

CD44, especially CD44v isoforms, are CSC markers and critical players in regulating the properties of CSCs, including self-renewal, tumor initiation, metastasis, and chemoradioresistance.[70] Administration of the activating monoclonal antibody directed to the adhesion molecule CD44 resulted in marked reduction of the leukemic burden in NOD/SCID mice transplanted with primary acute myeloid leukemia cells.[71] Absence of leukemia in serially transplanted mice demonstrated that leukemic stem cells were directly targeted.[71] Oligonucleotides coding CD44v6 shRNA downregulated the anti-apoptotic cell survival signaling and reduced colon adenoma number and growth.[72] It is encouraging that several of the new humanized anti-CD44 or anti-CD44v antibodies are under preclinical investigation for anti-CSCs therapy.

Her-2

A significant body of evidence has accumulated to support the notion that Her-2 drives tumorigenesis, invasion, and treatment resistance by regulating breast CSCs.[73–77] The effects of Her-2 amplification on mammary carcinogenesis, tumorigenicity, and invasion result from effects of this signaling pathway in mammary CSCs.[75] Unexpectedly, Her-2 also plays an important role in regulating the CSC population in luminal breast cancers that do not display Her-2 amplification and are classified as Her-2 negative.[78] Activated T cells (ATCs) armed with anti-CD3 $\times$ anti-Her-2/neu BsAb demonstrated significantly higher cytotoxicity in response to Her-2/neu[+] breast cancer cells than unarmed ATCs.[79] In a prostate cancer model (PC-3), Davol and colleagues[80] reported that ATCs armed with anti-Her-2 BsAb increased the cytotoxicity to PC-3 cells 2- to 3-fold, and increased the secretion of Th1 cytokines such as granulocyte-macrophage colony-stimulating factor (GM-CSF), tumor necrosis factor alpha, and IFN-γ, compared with unarmed ATCs or ATCs armed with an irrelevant BsAb. Intravenous administration of anti-Her-2 BsAb-armed ATCs mediated cytotoxicity in response to tumor cells and significantly delayed the PC-3 tumor growth, but not Her-2/neu[−] LS174 T colon adenocarcinoma xenografts.[80] A phase 1 trial reported by Lum and colleagues[81] demonstrated that infusions of anti-Her-2 BsAb-armed ATCs in combination with low-dose IL-2 and GM-CSF induced antitumor responses, and enhanced the Th1 cytokine and IL-12 serum levels in patients with Her-2–positive and Her-2–negative breast cancer. A randomized trial showed that vaccination with Her-2 peptide-pulsed dendritic cells (DCs) was effective in inducing immune and clinical responses in patients with invasive breast cancer.[82] This suggests that the role of anti-Her-2 therapeutic strategies in cancer treatment should be further investigated, taking into account the specific effect of Her-2 inhibition on the CSC subpopulation of tumor cells.[83]

Cancer Stem Cell–Based Vaccines

DC-based vaccines involve the administration of DCs that have been primed with tumor antigens. It has been tested in the clinic and proven to be immunogenic, but the clinical responses had been confined to a limited number of patients, which may result from the inability to target CSCs with current immunotherapies.[67] We have developed a vaccination strategy using cell lysates from ALDH[high] SCC7 (squamous cell carcinoma) or D5 (melanoma) CSCs to pulse DCs (CSC-DC), and found that CSC-DC vaccines conferred significant antitumor immunity in a tumor protection model.[84] Subsequently, we found that vaccination with ALDH[high] SCC7 CSC-DC in mice significantly inhibited SCC7 local tumor recurrence after surgical resection, compared with either ALDH[low] non–CSC-DC or unsorted tumor cells-DC vaccination, and that simultaneous programmed death-ligand 1 (PD-L1) immune checkpoint blockade further significantly enhanced the efficacy of CSC-DC vaccine in this model (**Fig. 2**).[85] Furthermore, after localized radiation therapy of established SCC7 and D5 tumors, our data also suggested that CSC-DC vaccine significantly inhibited residual tumor growth, reduced development of spontaneous metastases, and prolonged mice survival.[86] In other studies, pancreatic CSC lysate-pulsed DC vaccines effectively promoted lymphocyte proliferation, and induced significant cytotoxic effects of lymphocytes to both pancreatic CSCs and pancreatic cancer cells by secreting high levels of IFN-γ and IL-2.[87] Breast CSC lysate-pulsed DC vaccines efficiently inhibited the tumor progression and prolonged the survival of mice in a humanized breast cancer xenograft model.[88] Together, these studies offer evidence that CSC-DC vaccines can mediate significant antitumor effects. Combining CSC-DC vaccination with traditional therapies (eg, surgery, chemotherapy, or radiotherapy), and immune checkpoint inhibition represent promising multimodal treatment strategies for cancer (**Fig. 3**).[89]

IMMUNOLOGICALLY TARGETING THE CANCER STEM CELLS NICHE
Cytokines

CSCs in primary tumors reside in niches, which are anatomically distinct regions within the tumor microenvironment. These niches maintain the principal properties of CSCs. Inflammatory cytokines such as IL-6 and IL-8 activate the Stat3/NF-κB pathway in tumor and stromal cells to further secrete cytokines in a positive feedback loop that prompted CSC self-renewal, angiogenesis, and metastasis.[90,91] CXCR1 (IL-8 receptor) blockade using either a CXCR1-specific blocking antibody or repertaxin, a

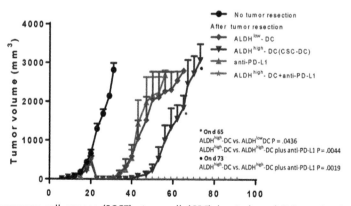

Fig. 2. Squamous cell cancer (SCC7) stem cell (CSC) lysate-based DC vaccination significantly reduced tumor recurrence after surgical resection of SCC7 tumors in a mouse model. ALDH[low]-DC is a non-CSC vaccine, and ALDH[high]-DC is a CSC vaccine. Optimal results occurred when the CSC vaccine was given in combination with anti-PD-L1 monoclonal antibody. (*From* Hu Y, Lu L, Xia Y, et al. Therapeutic efficacy of cancer stem cell vaccines in the adjuvant setting. Cancer Res 2016;76(16):4661-72; with permission.)

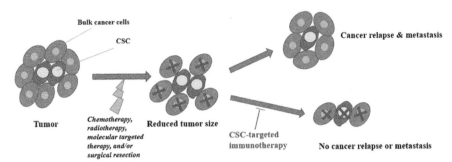

Fig. 3. Proposal for use of cancer stem cell (CSC)-targeted immunotherapy. Standard therapies generally cannot eradicate CSCs, so cancers will ultimately relapse and metastasize. CSC-targeted immunotherapy is postulated to work optimally as adjuvant treatment following standard therapy.

small-molecule CXCR1 inhibitor, selectively decreased the proportion and activity of human breast CSCs *in vitro*, as measured by a decrease in the fraction of ALDH-positive breast CSCs and mammosphere formation, respectively.[92] More importantly, repertaxin was able to decrease breast tumor growth and increase the efficacy of docetaxel chemotherapy, which was associated with decreased CSCs, as demonstrated by a reduction of tumor formation following reimplantation of breast cancer cells into recipient mices.[92] Knockdown of testicular nuclear receptor 4 in prostate cancer stem/progenitor cells led to downregulation of Oct4 expression, which in turn downregulated the IL-1 receptor antagonist expression, and led to increased drug sensitivity to 2 commonly used chemotherapeutic drugs, docetaxel and etoposide.[93] IL-6 secreted by breast non-CSCs activated the JAK1-Stat signal pathway and upregulated CSC-associated Oct4 gene expression. Inhibiting this pathway with anti-IL-6 antibody or niclosamide/LLL12 effectively downregulated Oct4 gene expression, suggesting that IL-6 plays an important role in the inducible formation of CSCs;[94] however, the exact mechanism of the conversion of non-CSCs into CSCs needs to be further clarified.

Immune Checkpoints (PD-1/PD-L1 Signaling Pathways)

Intratumoral T cells displayed a broad spectrum of dysfunctional states in murine and human cancer, shaped by the multifaceted inhibitory signaling pathways that occurred within the tumor microenvironment, in particular, the upregulation of PD-1 on T cells has emerged as a major marker of T cell dysfunction.[95–97] PD-1/PD-L1-mediated activation maintained Oct4 and Nanog in breast cancer and led to sustaining stemness of breast cancer cells. Targeting PD-L1 would decrease the pool of breast CSCs and have a beneficial consequence for improvement of efficacy in breast cancer.[98] It was observed that PD-L1 expression of CSCs was much higher in a variety of cancers, compared with their non–stem-like cancer cells, such as breast cancer, colon cancer, melanoma, and ovarian cancer.[99,100] Enriched PD-L1 expression on CSCs has been suggested to facilitate CSC immune evasion in lung, head and neck, and breast cancer.[101–103]

Etoposide was one of the few cytotoxic drugs with CSC-targeting ability, which can effectively downregulate PD-L1 expression in both breast CSCs and non-CSC populations of mesenchymal-like cancer cells.[103] Thus, it potentially provides a reasonable explanation why it is generally effective in many heavily treated advanced and metastatic cancers. Recent studies indicate that targeting the PD-1/PD-L1 pathway can

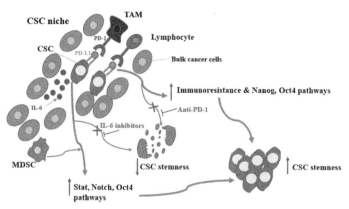

Fig. 4. The interactions between cancer stem cells (CSCs) and tumor microenvironment contribute to the stemness of CSCs by upregulation of PD-1/PD-L1, Oct4, Stat, and Notch signal pathways, and secretion of cytokines (such as IL-6). Anti-PD-1 monoclonal antibody and IL-6 inhibitors kill CSCs by overcoming immunoresistance and downregulating the stemness pathways. MDSC, myeloid-derived suppressor cells; TAMs, tumor-associated macrophages.

successfully overcome CSC-mediated immunoresistance. Silencing PD-L1 in murine B16 melanoma and ID8agg ovarian carcinoma cells reduced CSC numbers, the stemness genes Nanog and Oct4, and functions, as assessed by tumor sphere development in vivo.[100] Blockade of the PD-1/PD-L1 pathway promotes mouse NK cells to kill GL261 glioma stem cells.[104] Furthermore, the presence of TAMs correlated with poor prognosis in human cancers.[105] Both murine and human TAMs express high levels of PD-1, which correlate with decreased phagocytosis. More importantly, blockade of PD-1/PD-L1 increased TAM phagocytosis and then decreased CT26 colon cancer burden in vivo.[106] Hence, it is important to include immune checkpoint blockade with strategies to immunologically target CSCs (**Fig. 4**).

Myeloid-Derived Suppressor Cells

Myeloid-derived suppressor cells (MDSCs) contribute to immune suppression. Peng and colleagues[107] demonstrated that MDSCs promoted tumor formation by enhancing breast cancer cell stem-like properties and suppressed T cell activation. This effect relied on crosstalk between the Stat3 and Notch pathways in cancer cells, with MDSC inducing IL-6 phosphorylation of Stat3 and activating Notch through nitric oxide. In clinical specimens of breast cancer, the presence of MDSCs independently correlated with poor survival. Targeting MDSCs would provide a strategy that would adversely affect the function of CSCs.

SUMMARY

Although CSCs are a rare subpopulation within a tumor, it can self-renew, give rise to tumors, and promote recurrence and metastasis. In addition, CSCs are intrinsically resistant to conventional chemoradiotherapy. These characterizations make it difficult to eliminate the "root" of cancer with current anticancer treatments. Immunotherapy has become a major modality of cancer therapy. This review describes various immunologic approaches that can modulate the biology of CSCs for therapeutic benefit as well as elicit immunologic targeting of CSCs. These approaches represent promising advances in the treatment of cancers.

REFERENCES

1. Furth J, Kahn MC. The transmission of leukemia of mice with a single cell. Am J Cancer 1937;31:276–82.
2. Kreso A, Dick JE. Evolution of the cancer stem cell model. Cell Stem Cell 2014; 14(3):275–91.
3. Clarke MF, Dick JE, Dirks PB, et al. Cancer stem cells–perspectives on current status and future directions: AACR Workshop on cancer stem cells. Cancer Res 2006;66(19):9339–44.
4. Nguyen LV, Vanner R, Dirks P, et al. Cancer stem cells: an evolving concept. Nat Rev Cancer 2012;12(2):133–43.
5. Al-Hajj M, Becker MW, Wicha M, et al. Therapeutic implications of cancer stem cells. Curr Opin Genet Dev 2004;14(1):43–7.
6. Bouwens L, De Blay E. Islet morphogenesis and stem cell markers in rat pancreas. J Histochem Cytochem 1996;44(9):947–51.
7. Peters R, Leyvraz S, Perey L. Apoptotic regulation in primitive hematopoietic precursors. Blood 1998;92(6):2041–52.
8. Feuerhake F, Sigg W, Hofter EA, et al. Immunohistochemical analysis of Bcl-2 and Bax expression in relation to cell turnover and epithelial differentiation markers in the non-lactating human mammary gland epithelium. Cell Tissue Res 2000;299(1):47–58.
9. Zhou S, Schuetz JD, Bunting KD, et al. The ABC transporter Bcrp1/ABCG2 is expressed in a wide variety of stem cells and is a molecular determinant of the side-population phenotype. Nat Med 2001;7(9):1028–34.
10. Di Tomaso T, Mazzoleni S, Wang E, et al. Immunobiological characterization of cancer stem cells isolated from glioblastoma patients. Clin Cancer Res 2010; 16(3):800–13.
11. Schatton T, Schutte U, Frank NY, et al. Modulation of T-cell activation by malignant melanoma initiating cells. Cancer Res 2010;70(2):697–708.
12. Schatton T, Frank MH. Antitumor immunity and cancer stem cells. Ann N Y Acad Sci 2009;1176:154–69.
13. Pan Q, Li Q, Liu S, et al. Concise review: targeting cancer stem cells using immunologic approaches. Stem Cells 2015;33(7):2085–92.
14. Bonnet D, Dick JE. Human acute myeloid leukemia is organized as a hierarchy that originates from a primitive hematopoietic cell. Nat Med 1997;3(7):730–7.
15. Al-Hajj M, Wicha MS, Benito-Hernandez A, et al. Prospective identification of tumorigenic breast cancer cells. Proc Natl Acad Sci U S A 2003;100(7):3983–8.
16. Boiko AD, Razorenova OV, van de Rijn M, et al. Human melanoma-initiating cells express neural crest nerve growth factor receptor CD271. Nature 2010; 466(7302):133–7.
17. Dionne LK, Driver ER, Wang XJ. Head and neck cancer stem cells: from identification to tumor immune network. J Dent Res 2015;94(11):1524–31.
18. Sullivan JP, Minna JD. Tumor oncogenotypes and lung cancer stem cell identity. Cell Stem Cell 2010;7(1):2–4.
19. Quante M, Wang TC. Stem cells in gastroenterology and hepatology. Nat Rev Gastroenterol Hepatol 2009;6(12):724–37.
20. Fitzgerald TL, McCubrey JA. Pancreatic cancer stem cells: association with cell surface markers, prognosis, resistance, metastasis and treatment. Adv Biol Regul 2014;56:45–50.
21. Goodwin Jinesh G, Willis DL, Kamat AM. Bladder cancer stem cells: biological and therapeutic perspectives. Curr Stem Cell Res Ther 2014;9(2):89–101.

22. Wang G, Wang Z, Sarkar FH, et al. Targeting prostate cancer stem cells for cancer therapy. Discov Med 2012;13(69):135–42.
23. Codd AS, Kanaseki T, Torigo T, et al. Cancer stem cells as targets for immunotherapy. Immunology 2018;153(3):304–14.
24. Sladek NE. Human aldehyde dehydrogenases: potential pathological, pharmacological, and toxicological impact. J Biochem Mol Toxicol 2003;17(1):7–23.
25. Black WJ, Stagos D, Marchitti SA, et al. Human aldehyde dehydrogenase genes: alternatively spliced transcriptional variants and their suggested nomenclature. Pharmacogenet Genomics 2009;19(11):893–902.
26. Ginestier C, Hur MH, Charafe-Jauffret E, et al. ALDH1 is a marker of normal and malignant human mammary stem cells and a predictor of poor clinical outcome. Cell Stem Cell 2007;1(5):555–67.
27. van den Hoogen C, van der Horst G, Cheung H, et al. High aldehyde dehydrogenase activity identifies tumor-initiating and metastasis-initiating cells in human prostate cancer. Cancer Res 2010;70(12):5163–73.
28. Clay MR, Tabor M, Owen JH, et al. Single-marker identification of head and neck squamous cell carcinoma cancer stem cells with aldehyde dehydrogenase. Head Neck 2010;32(9):1195–201.
29. Jiang F, Qiu Q, Khanna A, et al. Aldehyde dehydrogenase 1 is a tumor stem cell-associated marker in lung cancer. Mol Cancer Res 2009;7(3):330–8.
30. Yan J, De Melo J, Cutz JC, et al. Aldehyde dehydrogenase 3A1 associates with prostate tumorigenesis. Br J Cancer 2014;110(10):2593–603.
31. Brescia P, Richichi C, Pelicci G. Current strategies for identification of glioma stem cells: adequate or unsatisfactory? J Oncol 2012;2012:376894.
32. Brungs D, Aghmesheh M, Vine KL, et al. Gastric cancer stem cells: evidence, potential markers, and clinical implications. J Gastroenterol 2016;51(4):313–26.
33. Burgos-Ojeda D, Rueda BR, Buckanovich RJ. Ovarian cancer stem cell markers: prognostic and therapeutic implications. Cancer Lett 2012;322(1):1–7.
34. Chan KS, Volkmer JP, Weissman I. Cancer stem cells in bladder cancer: a revisited and evolving concept. Curr Opin Urol 2010;20(5):393–7.
35. Corro C, Moch H. Biomarker discovery for renal cancer stem cells. J Pathol Clin Res 2018;4(1):3–18.
36. de Beca FF, Caetano P, Gerhard R, et al. Cancer stem cells markers CD44, CD24 and ALDH1 in breast cancer special histological types. J Clin Pathol 2013;66(3):187–91.
37. Eramo A, Lotti F, Sette G, et al. Identification and expansion of the tumorigenic lung cancer stem cell population. Cell Death Differ 2008;15(3):504–14.
38. Harris KS, Kerr BA. Prostate cancer stem cell markers drive progression, therapeutic resistance, and bone metastasis. Stem Cells Int 2017;2017:8629234.
39. Huang R, Rofstad EK. Cancer stem cells (CSCs), cervical CSCs and targeted therapies. Oncotarget 2017;8(21):35351–67.
40. Klein WM, Wu BP, Zhao S, et al. Increased expression of stem cell markers in malignant melanoma. Mod Pathol 2007;20(1):102–7.
41. Major AG, Pitty LP, Farah CS. Cancer stem cell markers in head and neck squamous cell carcinoma. Stem Cells Int 2013;2013:319489.
42. Munro MJ, Wickremesekera SK, Peng L, et al. Cancer stem cells in colorectal cancer: a review. J Clin Pathol 2018;71(2):110–6.
43. Qian X, Tan C, Wang F, et al. Esophageal cancer stem cells and implications for future therapeutics. Onco Targets Ther 2016;9:2247–54.
44. Qiu L, Li H, Fu S, et al. Surface markers of liver cancer stem cells and innovative targeted-therapy strategies for HCC. Oncol Lett 2018;15(2):2039–48.

45. Vassilopoulos A, Chisholm C, Lahusen T, et al. A critical role of CD29 and CD49f in mediating metastasis for cancer-initiating cells isolated from a Brca1-associated mouse model of breast cancer. Oncogene 2014;33(47):5477–82.

46. Vaz AP, Ponnusamy MP, Seshacharyulu P, et al. A concise review on the current understanding of pancreatic cancer stem cells. J Cancer Stem Cell Res 2014;2.

47. Ying J, Tsujii M, Kondo J, et al. The effectiveness of an anti-human IL-6 receptor monoclonal antibody combined with chemotherapy to target colon cancer stem-like cells. Int J Oncol 2015;46(4):1551–9.

48. Gu J, Liu Y, Xie B, et al. Roles of toll-like receptors: from inflammation to lung cancer progression. Biomed Rep 2018;8(2):126–32.

49. Jia D, Yang W, Li L, et al. beta-Catenin and NF-kappaB co-activation triggered by TLR3 stimulation facilitates stem cell-like phenotypes in breast cancer. Cell Death Differ 2015;22(2):298–310.

50. Zhao XL, Lin Y, Jiang J, et al. High-mobility group box 1 released by autophagic cancer-associated fibroblasts maintains the stemness of luminal breast cancer cells. J Pathol 2017;243(3):376–89.

51. Alvarado AG, Thiagarajan PS, Mulkearns-Hubert EE, et al. Glioblastoma cancer stem cells evade innate immune suppression of self-renewal through reduced TLR4 expression. Cell Stem Cell 2017;20(4):450–61.e4.

52. Schaffner F, Yokota N, Carneiro-Lobo T, et al. Endothelial protein C receptor function in murine and human breast cancer development. PLoS One 2013; 8(4):e61071.

53. Okuda H, Kobayashi A, Xia B, et al. Hyaluronan synthase HAS2 promotes tumor progression in bone by stimulating the interaction of breast cancer stem-like cells with macrophages and stromal cells. Cancer Res 2012;72(2):537–47.

54. Jinushi M, Chiba S, Yoshiyama H, et al. Tumor-associated macrophages regulate tumorigenicity and anticancer drug responses of cancer stem/initiating cells. Proc Natl Acad Sci U S A 2011;108(30):12425–30.

55. Wan S, Zhao E, Kryczek I, et al. Tumor-associated macrophages produce interleukin 6 and signal via STAT3 to promote expansion of human hepatocellular carcinoma stem cells. Gastroenterology 2014;147(6):1393–404.

56. Tseng HC, Arasteh A, Paranjpe A, et al. Increased lysis of stem cells but not their differentiated cells by natural killer cells; de-differentiation or reprogramming activates NK cells. PLoS One 2010;5(7):e11590.

57. Castriconi R, Daga A, Dondero A, et al. NK cells recognize and kill human glioblastoma cells with stem cell-like properties. J Immunol 2009;182(6):3530–9.

58. Tallerico R, Todaro M, Di Franco S, et al. Human NK cells selective targeting of colon cancer-initiating cells: a role for natural cytotoxicity receptors and MHC class I molecules. J Immunol 2013;190(5):2381–90.

59. Silva-Santos B, Serre K, Norell H. Gammadelta T cells in cancer. Nat Rev Immunol 2015;15(11):683–91.

60. Chen HC, Joalland N, Bridgeman JS, et al. Synergistic targeting of breast cancer stem-like cells by human gammadelta T cells and CD8(+) T cells. Immunol Cell Biol 2017;95(7):620–9.

61. Todaro M, D'Asaro M, Caccamo N, et al. Efficient killing of human colon cancer stem cells by gammadelta T lymphocytes. J Immunol 2009;182(11):7287–96.

62. Nishio N, Fujita M, Tanaka Y, et al. Zoledronate sensitizes neuroblastoma-derived tumor-initiating cells to cytolysis mediated by human gammadelta T cells. J Immunother 2012;35(8):598–606.

63. Nicol AJ, Tokuyama H, Mattarollo SR, et al. Clinical evaluation of autologous gamma delta T cell-based immunotherapy for metastatic solid tumours. Br J Cancer 2011;105(6):778–86.

64. Visus C, Wang Y, Lozano-Leon A, et al. Targeting ALDH(bright) human carcinoma-initiating cells with ALDH1A1-specific CD8(+) T cells. Clin Cancer Res 2011;17(19):6174–84.

65. Wang Y, Li W, Patel SS, et al. Blocking the formation of radiation-induced breast cancer stem cells. Oncotarget 2014;5(11):3743–55.

66. Liu X, Wang L, Cui W, et al. Targeting ALDH1A1 by disulfiram/copper complex inhibits non-small cell lung cancer recurrence driven by ALDH-positive cancer stem cells. Oncotarget 2016;7(36):58516–30.

67. Damek-Poprawa M, Volgina A, Korostoff J, et al. Targeted inhibition of CD133+ cells in oral cancer cell lines. J Dent Res 2011;90(5):638–45.

68. Huang J, Li C, Wang Y, et al. Cytokine-induced killer (CIK) cells bound with anti-CD3/anti-CD133 bispecific antibodies target CD133(high) cancer stem cells in vitro and in vivo. Clin Immunol 2013;149(1):156–68.

69. Yu CC, Hu FW, Yu CH, et al. Targeting CD133 in the enhancement of chemosensitivity in oral squamous cell carcinoma-derived side population cancer stem cells. Head Neck 2016;38(Suppl 1):E231–8.

70. Yan Y, Zuo X, Wei D. Concise review: emerging role of CD44 in cancer stem cells: a promising biomarker and therapeutic target. Stem Cells Transl Med 2015;4(9):1033–43.

71. Jin L, Hope KJ, Zhai Q, et al. Targeting of CD44 eradicates human acute myeloid leukemic stem cells. Nat Med 2006;12(10):1167–74.

72. Misra S, Hascall VC, De Giovanni C, et al. Delivery of CD44 shRNA/nanoparticles within cancer cells: perturbation of hyaluronan/CD44v6 interactions and reduction in adenoma growth in Apc Min/+ MICE. J Biol Chem 2009;284(18):12432–46.

73. Duru N, Fan M, Candas D, et al. HER2-associated radioresistance of breast cancer stem cells isolated from HER2-negative breast cancer cells. Clin Cancer Res 2012;18(24):6634–47.

74. Korkaya H, Wicha MS. HER2 and breast cancer stem cells: more than meets the eye. Cancer Res 2013;73(12):3489–93.

75. Korkaya H, Paulson A, Iovino F, et al. HER2 regulates the mammary stem/progenitor cell population driving tumorigenesis and invasion. Oncogene 2008;27(47):6120–30.

76. Korkaya H, Kim GI, Davis A, et al. Activation of an IL6 inflammatory loop mediates trastuzumab resistance in HER2+ breast cancer by expanding the cancer stem cell population. Mol Cell 2012;47(4):570–84.

77. Ithimakin S, Day KC, Malik F, et al. HER2 drives luminal breast cancer stem cells in the absence of HER2 amplification: implications for efficacy of adjuvant trastuzumab. Cancer Res 2013;73(5):1635–46.

78. Buzdar AU, Ibrahim NK, Francis D, et al. Significantly higher pathologic complete remission rate after neoadjuvant therapy with trastuzumab, paclitaxel, and epirubicin chemotherapy: results of a randomized trial in human epidermal growth factor receptor 2-positive operable breast cancer. J Clin Oncol 2005;23(16):3676–85.

79. Sen M, Wankowski DM, Garlie NK, et al. Use of anti-CD3 x anti-HER2/neu bispecific antibody for redirecting cytotoxicity of activated T cells toward HER2/neu+ tumors. J Hematother Stem Cell Res 2001;10(2):247–60.

80. Davol PA, Smith JA, Kouttab N, et al. Anti-CD3 x anti-HER2 bispecific antibody effectively redirects armed T cells to inhibit tumor development and growth in hormone-refractory prostate cancer-bearing severe combined immunodeficient beige mice. Clin Prostate Cancer 2004;3(2):112–21.

81. Lum LG, Thakur A, Al-Kadhimi Z, et al. Targeted T-cell therapy in stage IV breast cancer: a phase I clinical trial. Clin Cancer Res 2015;21(10):2305–14.

82. Lowenfeld L, Mick R, Datta J, et al. Dendritic cell vaccination enhances immune responses and induces regression of HER2(pos) DCIS independent of route: results of randomized selection design trial. Clin Cancer Res 2017;23(12): 2961–71.

83. Roesler R, Cornelio DB, Abujamra AL, et al. HER2 as a cancer stem-cell target. Lancet Oncol 2010;11(3):225–6.

84. Ning N, Pan Q, Zheng F, et al. Cancer stem cell vaccination confers significant antitumor immunity. Cancer Res 2012;72(7):1853–64.

85. Hu Y, Lu L, Xia Y, et al. Therapeutic efficacy of cancer stem cell vaccines in the adjuvant setting. Cancer Res 2016;76(16):4661–72.

86. Lu L, Tao H, Chang AE, et al. Cancer stem cell vaccine inhibits metastases of primary tumors and induces humoral immune responses against cancer stem cells. Oncoimmunology 2015;4(3):e990767.

87. Yin T, Shi P, Gou S, et al. Dendritic cells loaded with pancreatic cancer stem cells (CSCs) lysates induce antitumor immune killing effect in vitro. PLoS One 2014;9(12):e114581.

88. Pham PV, Le HT, Vu BT, et al. Targeting breast cancer stem cells by dendritic cell vaccination in humanized mice with breast tumor: preliminary results. Onco Targets Ther 2016;9:4441–51.

89. Lin M, Chang AE, Wicha M, et al. Development and application of cancer stem cell-targeted vaccine in cancer immunotherapy. J Vaccines Vaccin 2017;8(6) [pii:371].

90. Korkaya H, Liu S, Wicha MS. Regulation of cancer stem cells by cytokine networks: attacking cancer's inflammatory roots. Clin Cancer Res 2011;17(19): 6125–9.

91. Scheller J, Rose-John S. Interleukin-6 and its receptor: from bench to bedside. Med Microbiol Immunol 2006;195(4):173–83.

92. Ginestier C, Liu S, Diebel ME, et al. CXCR1 blockade selectively targets human breast cancer stem cells in vitro and in xenografts. J Clin Invest 2010;120(2): 485–97.

93. Yang DR, Ding XF, Luo J, et al. Increased chemosensivity via targeting testicular nuclear receptor 4 (TR4)-Oct4-interleukin 1 receptor antagonist (IL1Ra) axis in prostate cancer CD133+ stem/progenitor cells to battle prostate cancer. J Biol Chem 2013;288(23):16476–83.

94. Kim SY, Kang JW, Song X, et al. Role of the IL-6-JAK1-STAT3-Oct-4 pathway in the conversion of non-stem cancer cells into cancer stem-like cells. Cell Signal 2013;25(4):961–9.

95. Thommen DS, Schumacher TN. T cell dysfunction in cancer. Cancer Cell 2018; 33(4):547–62.

96. Chen DS, Mellman I. Oncology meets immunology: the cancer-immunity cycle. Immunity 2013;39(1):1–10.

97. Schreiber RD, Old LJ, Smyth MJ. Cancer immunoediting: integrating immunity's roles in cancer suppression and promotion. Science 2011;331(6024):1565–70.

98. Almozyan S, Colak D, Mansour F, et al. PD-L1 promotes OCT4 and Nanog expression in breast cancer stem cells by sustaining PI3K/AKT pathway activation. Int J Cancer 2017;141(7):1402–12.

99. Wu Y, Chen M, Wu P, et al. Increased PD-L1 expression in breast and colon cancer stem cells. Clin Exp Pharmacol Physiol 2017;44(5):602–4.

100. Gupta HB, Clark CA, Yuan B, et al. Tumor cell-intrinsic PD-L1 promotes tumor-initiating cell generation and functions in melanoma and ovarian cancer. Signal Transduct Target Ther 2016;1 [pii:16030].

101. Lee Y, Shin JH, Longmire M, et al. CD44+ cells in head and neck squamous cell carcinoma suppress T-cell-mediated immunity by selective constitutive and inducible expression of PD-L1. Clin Cancer Res 2016;22(14):3571–81.

102. Xu C, Fillmore CM, Koyama S, et al. Loss of Lkb1 and Pten leads to lung squamous cell carcinoma with elevated PD-L1 expression. Cancer Cell 2014;25(5): 590–604.

103. Hsu JM, Xia W, Hsu YH, et al. STT3-dependent PD-L1 accumulation on cancer stem cells promotes immune evasion. Nat Commun 2018;9(1):1908.

104. Huang BY, Zhan YP, Zong WJ, et al. The PD-1/B7-H1 pathway modulates the natural killer cells versus mouse glioma stem cells. PLoS One 2015;10(8): e0134715.

105. Pollard JW. Tumour-educated macrophages promote tumour progression and metastasis. Nat Rev Cancer 2004;4(1):71–8.

106. Gordon SR, Maute RL, Dulken BW, et al. PD-1 expression by tumour-associated macrophages inhibits phagocytosis and tumour immunity. Nature 2017; 545(7655):495–9.

107. Peng D, Tanikawa T, Li W, et al. Myeloid-derived suppressor cells endow stem-like qualities to breast cancer cells through IL6/STAT3 and NO/NOTCH crosstalk signaling. Cancer Res 2016;76(11):3156–65.

Immunotherapy in Ovarian Cancer

Weimin Wang, PhD[a], Janice Rebecca Liu, MD[b], Weiping Zou, MD, PhD[c],*

KEYWORDS

- Immunotherapy ● Ovarian cancer ● Checkpoint blockade ● Adoptive T-cell transfer
- Cancer vaccine

KEY POINTS

- The application of immunotherapy in ovarian cancer is being tested.
- Checkpoint blockade can restore the antitumor activity of effector T cells and mediate tumor regression.
- Adoptive transfer of ex vivo–expanded tumor-specific T cells can directly increase the number of CD8[+] effector T cells in tumor.
- Cancer vaccine may activate tumor-associated antigen–specific CD8[+] T-cell response through antigen presentation cells.

INTRODUCTION

Epithelial ovarian cancer (EOC) is the most common cause of gynecologic cancer–associated death in women.[1] To date, there are no effective means of screening or early detection for this disease, and consequently, most of the patients have advanced stage disease involving metastasis at the time of initial diagnosis.[2] The first-line therapy for EOC includes surgical debulking and platinum-based chemotherapy.[3] Although initial response is often excellent, patients oftentimes develop resistance to chemotherapy and succumb to their disease. Therefore, it is critical to develop novel treatment strategies to improve clinical outcomes.

Current immunotherapy, including checkpoint blockade and adoptive T-cell transfer (ACT), has become a clinically effective treatment modality for a wide variety of cancer

Disclosure Statement: This work was supported in part by research grants from the NIH/NCI R01 grants (W. Zou) (CA217648, CA123088, CA099985, CA193136 and CA152470) and the NIH through the University of Michigan Roger Cancer Center Support Grant (CA46592).
a Department of Surgery, University of Michigan School of Medicine, BSRB 5448, 109 Zina Pitcher Place, Ann Arbor, MI 48109-0669, USA; b Department of Obstetrics and Gynecology, University of Michigan School of Medicine, L4604 WH, 1500 East Medical Center, Ann Arbor, MI 48109, USA; c Department of Surgery, University of Michigan School of Medicine, BSRB 5071, 109 Zina Pitcher Place, Ann Arbor, MI 48109-0669, USA
* Corresponding author.
E-mail address: wzou@med.umich.edu

Surg Oncol Clin N Am 28 (2019) 447–464
https://doi.org/10.1016/j.soc.2019.02.002

surgonc.theclinics.com

types. However, the application of immunotherapy in EOC is still being tested in clinical trials. Tumor-infiltrating lymphocytes (TILs), positively correlating with patient survival, have now been recognized as a predictive biomarker for immunotherapy and chemotherapy responses.[3,4] In ovarian cancer, the presence of CD3[+] T cell and its correlation with improved clinical outcome had been observed in an early study, which establishes the validity of using immunotherapy for EOC management.[5] Later studies demonstrated the prognostic significance of FOXP3[+] T_{reg} cells[6] and/or the ratio of CD8[+] T cells versus FOXP3[+] T_{reg} cells in ovarian cancer and confirmed CD8[+] T cells as important antitumor effectors.[6,7] CD8[+] effector T cells, are poised to eliminate tumor cells after recognizing tumor-associated antigens (TAAs) and particularly the neoantigens presented on the surface of tumor cells.[8] However, their activation and effector functions are often held in check and attenuated by inhibitory signals in the tumor microenvironment, which include inhibitory cytokines, immunosuppressive metabolites, and immunoinhibitor B7 family members expressed on the antigen-presenting cells (APCs) and tumor cells.[9,10] Checkpoint blockade can restore the antitumor activity of effector T cells and mediate tumor regression.[11] Adoptive transfer of ex vivo–expanded tumor-specific T cells can directly increase the number of CD8[+] effector T cells in tumor.[12] Cancer vaccine may activate TAA-specific CD8[+] T-cell response through APCs.[13] These immunotherapeutic strategies have been tested or are under development in ovarian cancer. The progress of immunotherapy in EOC will be discussed in this review.

CHECKPOINT BLOCKADE

Several checkpoint molecules have been identified, including cytotoxic T-lymphocyte–associated antigen 4 (CTLA-4), programmed death cell protein 1 (PD-1), and PD ligand 1 (PD-L1, B7-H1). Antibodies targeting these checkpoints can block their inhibitory function, thus unleashing the antitumor activity of effector T cells and mediating tumor regression.[14] There are currently 6 immune checkpoint inhibitors approved by the Food and Drug Administration: one CTLA-4 antibody (Ipilimumab), two PD-1 antibodies (Pembrolizumab and Nivolumab), and three PD-L1 antibodies (Avelumab, Atezolizumab and Durvalumab). These antibodies have demonstrated remarkable clinical benefits in a wide range of tumor types, such as melanoma, non–small cell lung carcinoma (NSCLC), renal cell, and urothelial cancer.[11]

Although anti-CTLA-4 and anti-PD-1/PD-L1 enhance antitumor immune response through increasing the number of tumor-infiltrating T cells and recovering the effector function of cytotoxic T cells, their underlining cellular and molecular mechanisms are distinct. CTLA-4 is a receptor on T cells and shares the same set of ligands with costimulatory receptor CD28 but with a much higher affinity, therefore providing a competitive inhibition.[15] Antibody targeting CTLA-4 blocks the ligation of CTLA-4 with its ligands, which prevents inhibitory signal transduction and results in increased CD28-mediated costimulation. CTLA-4 blockade has been shown to directly enhance the proliferation and activation of tumor-specific CD8[+] T cells.[16]

PD-1 is another inhibitory receptor expressed on T cells. Unlike CTLA-4, which regulates T-cell activation at the priming phase, PD-1 inhibits effector T-cell activity mainly in the effector phase in peripheral tissue and tumor microenvironment.[17] On activation by its ligands PD-L1 or PD-L2, PD-1 becomes phosphorylated and recruits the inhibitory phosphatase SHP-2, which rapidly dephosphorylates CD28 and inactivates the costimulatory signaling.[18] Of the 2 ligands, PD-L1 is considered to be more relevant in the tumor microenvironment because of its expression on tumor, stromal, and immune cells.[19] Antibodies targeting either PD-1 or PD-L1 result in abrogation of the negative signal, thus restoring the function of tumor-infiltrating T cells and mediating tumor regression.[20]

Single-Agent Checkpoint Inhibitor in Ovarian Cancer

Several antibodies targeting PD-1, PD-L1, and CTLA-4 have been tested in patients with recurrent ovarian cancer. Overall, objective response (OR) (complete response [CR] + partial response [PR]) rates range from 5.9% to 15% (**Table 1**).

In an early phase I trial, 207 patients with selected advanced cancers, including 17 with EOC, received anti-PD-L1 antibody (BMS-936559). Among the 17 women, 1 (5.9%) had a PR and a total of 4 women (23%) had disease control. These data suggest immune checkpoint blockade as a potentially valuable therapeutic approach in ovarian cancer.[21] Later, a phase II trial of an anti-PD1 antibody (nivolumab) was conducted in 20 patients with platinum-resistant EOC. Two patients experienced a CR, 1 had a PR, and 6 had a stable disease (SD), leading to a disease control rate of 45%.[22] Pembrolizumab, another anti-PD1 antibody, was shown to have an OR rate of 11.5% and a disease control rate of 34.6% in 26 patients with advanced EOC. Patients were selected with a PD-L1 expression level of greater than or equal to 1% of tumor cells for trial entry, and 85% of patients were heavily pretreated.[23] Atezolizumab is a fully humanized monoclonal antibody against PD-L1 and has been approved for metastatic NSCLC treatment. In a phase I study (NCT01375842), 12 patients with recurrent ovarian cancer were treated with atezolizumab until loss of clinical benefit. Of 9 response-evaluable patients, 2 patients (22%) had a PR and 5 patients had PD. PD-L1 status on immune cells was found to correlate with response.[24] More recently, a study assessed the safety and activity of another anti-PD-L1 antibody (avelumab) in 124 women with recurrent or refractory EOC (NCT01772004). This is the largest study of anti-PD(L)1 agents in patients with EOC to date. Avelumab achieved an OR of 9.7% and a disease control rate of 54.0%. Again, in this cohort more than two-thirds of the patients had received previous lines of therapy. This study showed that single-agent avelumab was clinically active in heavily pretreated patients with EOC.[25]

In addition to PD(L)1 blockade, the activity and safety of anti-CTLA-4 antibody in EOC was studied. In a phase II trial, 40 patients with recurrent platinum-sensitive EOC received an anti-CTLA-4 antibody ipilimumab (NCT01611558). The OR rate was 10.3% and adverse events of grade greater than or equal to 3 occurred in 50% of the patients.[26]

Table 1						
Clinical studies of checkpoint blockade in epithelial ovarian cancer						
Target	Agent	Phase	Trial Identifier	Disease Status	Patients	Response
PD-1	Nivolumab	II	UMIN000005714	Platinum-resistant EOC	20	CR 2, PR 1, SD 6
PD-1	Pembrolizumab	I	NCT02054806	Recurrent EOC	26	CR 1, PR 2, SD 6
PD-L1	BMS-936559	I	NCT00729664	Recurrent EOC	17	CR 0, PR 1, SD 3
PD-L1	Avelumab	I	NCT01772004	Recurrent EOC	124	CR 0, PR 12, SD 55
PD-L1	Atezolizumab	I	NCT01375842	Recurrent EOC	9	CR 0, PR 2, SD 0
CTLA-4	Ipilimumab	I, II	NCT01611558	Recurrent EOC	40	10% best response rate

Abbreviations: NCT, national clinical trial; SD, stable disease.

In summary, these studies suggest that single-agent checkpoint inhibitor, in particular PD(L)-1 blockade, is promising in EOC, although the OR rate is much lower compared with the response rates achieved in melanoma, NSCLC, renal cell, and urothelial cancer. Although potential mechanisms of resistance toward immune checkpoint blockade are under investigation, combining checkpoint inhibitors with other biological agents to enhance the antitumor immune response has been rationally illustrated and numerous combinatorial trials have entered the clinic. The combination of 2 checkpoint blockades (nivolumab + ipilimumab) was firstly tested in melanoma.[27] In EOC, the same combination (NCT03342417) and another combination of durvalumab (anti-PD-L1) and tremelimumab (anti-CTLA-4) (NCT03026062) are both being investigated.

Combination with Poly (ATP-Ribose) Polymerase Inhibitor

Tumor mutational burden (TMB) is a recently suggested biomarker of response to PD(L)-1 blockade therapy.[28] Tumor-specific mutations can result in immunogenic neoantigens, therefore high TMB correlates with high neoantigen load. This higher neoantigen load correlated with an increased number of TILs, which is counterbalanced by PD-1/PD-L1 signaling.[29] Melanoma, lung cancer, and a subtype of colorectal cancer with mismatch repair deficiency have a significantly higher TMB, and they all have a remarkable response to PD-1 inhibition.[30] In ovarian cancer, roughly the 25% to 30% of the high-grade serous (HGS) harbor a mutation in the BRCA1 or BRCA2 genes, which have integral functions in DNA homologous recombination (HR) repair. The presence of an HR deficiency is associated to a higher mutation burden and increased TILs compared with the BRCA wild-type tumors.[31] Thus, BRCA-mutated HGS ovarian cancer could represent a subtype with potential increased response to immune checkpoint blockade alone or in combination with poly (ATP-ribose) polymerase (PARP) inhibitors. Several clinical trials evaluating the combination of olaparib (PARP inhibitor) and checkpoint blockade in patients with BRCA-mutated ovarian cancer are currently ongoing (**Table 2**). In an ongoing phase II trial (NCT02734004), the combination of olaparib and durvalumab (anti-PD-L1) was found to induce objective responses in more than 70% of patients with relapsed, platinum-sensitive, BRCA-mutated ovarian cancer.[32] Another phase I/II trial evaluating the combination of olaparib with anti-CTLA-4 and anti-PD-L1 in patients with BRCA1/BRAC2-mutated EOC (NCT02953457) is also ongoing.

Combination with Vascular Endothelial Growth Factor Inhibitor

Another interesting novel approach is to combine vascular endothelial growth factor (VEGF) inhibitor and checkpoint blockade. VEGF is primarily known as a mediator of angiogenesis; however, emerging studies have also recognized VEGF as a critical mediator of immune suppression in the tumor microenvironment.[33] Inhibitors targeting VEGF or VEGF receptors (VEGFR) have been shown to decrease the number of regulatory T cells and myeloid-derived suppressor cells and enhance the infiltration of effector T cells.[33,34] Several clinical trials are currently ongoing to evaluate the safety and efficacy of the combination of bevacizumab (anti-VEGF) and checkpoint blockade in melanoma, NSCLC, and renal cell cancer. For EOC, a phase II trial focused on platinum-resistant disease, in which atezolizumab (anti-PD-L1) is given together with bevacizumab and acetylsalicylic acid (NCT02659384). In another study, durvalumab combined with olaparib or the VEGFR inhibitor cediranib in EOC is being tested (NCT02484404).

Table 2
Ongoing trials of checkpoint inhibitors in combination with other biological agents in epithelial ovarian cancer

Combined Agents	Combination	Treatment Setting	Study Population	Phase	Trial Identifier
Checkpoint inhibitor	aCTLA-4 +aPD-1	Nivolumab vs nivolumab + ipilimumab	Recurrent or pesistent EOC	IIa	NCT02498600
	aPD-L1 +aCTLA-4	Durvalumab + tremelimumab		I	NCT02261220
PARP inhibitor	aCTLA-4 +PARPi	Tremelimumab + olaparib	BRCA-deficient Ovarian Cancer	I/II	NCT02571725
	aCTLA-4 +PARPi	Tremelimumab vs tremelimumab + olaparib	Recurrent or Persistent EOC	I/II	NCT02485990
	aPD-L1 +PARPi	Durvalumab + olaparib vs durvalumab + cediranib	Recurrent EOC and germline BRCA1 or BRCA2 mutation	I/IIa	NCT02484404
	aCTLA4 +aPD-L1 +PARPi	Durvalumab + tremelimumab + olaparib	Recurrent EOC and germline or somatic BRCA1 or BRCA2 mutation	I/II	NCT02953457
VEGF inhibitor	aPD-L1+Bev	Atezolizumab + Bev	Recurrent platinum-resistant ovarian cancer	IIa	NCT02659384
Chemotherapy	aPD-L1 +PLD	Avelumab + pegylated liposomal doxorubicin	Platinum-resistant/refractory ovarian cancer	IIIa	NCT02580058
	aPD-L1 + TC	Avelumab + carboplatin + paclitaxel	Advanced EOC with no prior treatment	III	NCT02718417
	aPDL1 +Bev + TC/PLD	Atezolizumab + Avastin + platinum-based chemotherapy (carboplatin combined with gemcitabine or paclitaxel or PLD)	Recurrent platinum-sensitive EOC	III	NCT02891824
	aPD-L1 +Bev + TC	Atezolizumab + paclitaxel, carboplatin + Bev	Newly diagnosed EOC with no prior treatment	III	NCT03038100
	aPD-L1 +Bev + PLD	Atezolizumab + pegylated liposomal doxorubicin hydrochloride + or Bev	Platinum-resistant EOC	III	NCT02839707
	aPD-L1 +PLD	Durvalumab + PLD	Recurrent, platinum-resistant ovarian cancer	I/II	NCT02431559
	aPD-1 + TC	Pembrolizumab + TC	Frontline ovarian cancer	II	NCT02520154
	aPD-1 + ddT	Pembrolizumab + ddT	Recurrent, platinum-resistant ovarian cancer	II	NCT02440425

Abbreviations: aCTLA4, anti-CTLA-4; Bev, bevacizumab; ddT, dose-dense paclitaxel; NCT, national clinical trial; PARPi, PARP inhibitor; PLD, pegylated liposomal doxorubicin; TC, paclitaxel + carboplatin.

Combination with Chemotherapy

Chemotherapy can be used in combination with checkpoint blockade to amplify the antitumor immune response. In addition to direct cytotoxic effects on tumor cells, a proportion of chemotherapy agents may actually induce immunogenic cell death, expand neoantigen repertoire, increase antigen presentation, change the inflammatory milieu of tumor microenvironment, and/or decrease the number of immunosuppressive cells, thereby inducing or enhancing the antitumoral immune response.[35,36] There are now more than 200 clinical trials testing immune checkpoint inhibitors in combination with various chemotherapeutic agents across different cancer types.

In ovarian cancer, there are currently 5 randomized phase III trials adding PD-L1 blockade to chemotherapy: 2 are with avelumab and 3 are with atezolizumab. JAVELIN Ovarian 200 (NCT02580058) is the first one to compare avelumab alone or in combination with pegylated liposomal doxorubicin in patients with platinum-resistant/refractory recurrent ovarian, fallopian tube, or peritoneal cancer. The second trial is JAVELIN Ovarian 100 (NCT02718417), which will access the efficacy of avelumab in combination with conventional chemotherapy carboplatin and paclitaxel in patients with previously untreated ovarian cancer. The other 3 trials with atezolizumab involve adding both chemotherapy and bevacizumab (anti-VEGF) to atezolizumab. The NCT02891824 trial will assess the efficacy of atezolizumab in combination with bevacizumab plus platinum-based chemotherapy in patients with ovarian cancer who have platinum-sensitive relapse (platinum-free interval >6 months). The NCT03038100 trial will test the activity of atezolizumab in combination with bevacizumab paclitaxel and carboplatin in participants with newly diagnosed ovarian cancer. The NCT02839707 trial combines atezolizumab with bevacizumab and pegylated liposomal doxorubicin in platinum-resistant ovarian cancer.

Similarly, another PD-L1 inhibitor durvalumab and a PD-1 inhibitor in combination with chemotherapy are also being tested in several phase I/II clinical trials in ovarian cancer. These include durvalumab combined with PLD (NCT02431559) and pembrolizumab combined with paclitaxel and carboplatin (NCT02520154) or with dose-dense paclitaxel (NCT02440425).

Based on the published results and preliminary data, combinational therapy including PD-1/PD-L1 inhibitors and chemotherapy certainly has the potential to be superior to chemotherapy alone.[37,38] However, there are some ongoing challenges. Cytotoxic chemotherapy has historically been considered immunosuppressive because most chemotherapeutic agents indiscriminately impair cellular division and thus affect not only tumor cells but also effector lymphocytes and innate leukocytes.[39] Moreover, recent studies demonstrated that certain chemotherapy agents might attenuate the antitumor immune response.[40,41] Therefore, to thoroughly assess the combination with chemotherapy, selection of chemotherapy agents; optimization of the sequencing, timing, and dose; and management of concurrent toxicities will be required.

ADOPTIVE T-CELL THERAPY

ACT consists of the infusion of ex vivo–expanded tumor-specific T cells that can recognize and attack tumor cells, resulting in tumor regression.[12] There are currently 2 major forms of ACT being used for cancer treatment: isolating and expanding TIL or using genetically modified T cells that express a specific T-cell receptor (TCR) or a chimeric antigen receptor (CAR).[42] Both strategies have been tested in preclinical ovarian cancer models and currently being investigated in early phase trials.

Tumor-Infiltrating Lymphocyte Therapy

TIL therapy has been shown to induce long-lasting and complete regression of metastatic tumor in patients with melanoma.[43] Generally, ACT of TIL consists of several steps:

1. Isolation of TILs from fresh tumor biopsy;
2. Selection and expansion of tumor-specific T-cell population ex vivo;
3. Lymphodepletion of immunosuppressive components by chemotherapy or radiation; and
4. Infusion of expanded T cells to patients with interleukin 2 (IL-2) administration.

During this long-term procedure, both $CD4^+$ and $CD8^+$ T cells are expanded ex vivo and are subsequently infused back into the patient.[44]

TIL therapy produces melanoma response rates rangingfrom 47% to 72%.[45] The efficacy of TIL therapy in EOC has also been investigated in several early clinical studies (**Table 3**). The first trial of TIL therapy in EOC enrolled 17 patients with advanced or recurrent platinum-resistant disease. Among 7 patients who received TIL infusion, 1 CR and 4 PR were reported and tumor regression lasted for 3 to 5 months. Another group of 10 patients received TIL infusion combined with cisplatin-based chemotherapy. Seven patients had a CR, 2 had a PR, and 1 had an SD. The duration of response ranged from 13 to more than 26 months.[46] Later, a pilot study was conducted to determine the feasibility and clinical effects of TIL infusion plus low-dose IL-2 in patients with platinum-resistant ovarian cancer. Among 8 patients who received the treatment, 2 had reduction in ascites, 1 had reduction in tumor burden and CA-125, and 1 had surgically confirmed SD.[47] In 1995, Fujita and colleagues[48] tested the efficacy of maintenance therapy with TIL in patients with ovarian cancer with no evidence of disease after debulking surgery and adjuvant platinum-based chemotherapy. Thirteen patients received TIL and 11 additional patients (control group) received standard treatment. The TIL group had significantly improved 3-year overall survival (100% vs 65%, $P<.01$) and 3-year disease free survival (82.1% vs 54.5%, $P<.05$) compared with the control group. In summary, these early trials showed limited efficacy of TIL

Table 3
Completed clinical adoptive T-cell therapy trials in epithelial ovarian cancer

Agent	Target Antigens	Trial Identifier	Disease Status	Patients	Response
TIL	—	—	Advanced or recurrent EOC	17	CR 8, PR 6, SD 1
TIL	—	—	Recurrent EOC	8	CR 0, PR 0, SD 1
TIL	—	—	Advanced ovarian cancer after surgery and chemotherapy, 100% disease-free	13	Improved overall survival
CAR	Folate receptor α	NCT00019136	Recurrent FR^+ EOC	8	No clinical benefit
CAR	Mesothelin	NCT02159716	EOC	6	All patients showed stable disease at 1 month after treatment

Abbreviation: FR, folate receptor α.

therapy in EOC. However, it is notable that none of these trials used current chemotherapy regimens for lymphodepletion before TIL infusion, and the methods for ex-vivo TIL expansion have changed considerably. Therefore, there is still significant biological and clinical rationale to test TIL therapy in ovarian cancer (**Table 4**). An ongoing phase II trial is assessing the antitumor efficacy of TIL in metastatic digestive tract, urothelial, breast, or ovarian/endometrial cancer (NCT01174121). In this study, short-term cultured autologous TIL will be used after a lymphocyte depleting regimen, and checkpoint blockade pembrolizumab will be administered at time of progression. More recently, a phase I study focused on patients with platinum-resistant HGS ovarian, fallopian tube, or primary peritoneal cancer (NCT01883297) was opened. Patients will receive an infusion of autologous TIL, which will be stimulated ex vivo with autologous dendritic cells (DCs) and OKT3 (anti-CD3 antibody). This "restimulation" is believed to make autologous TIL work better.

T-cell Receptor–Engineered T Cells

Autologous T cells can be genetically modified to express a cloned TCR directed toward a specific antigen. T cells isolated from patient peripheral blood are used for transduction with a viral vector encoding TCR and then can rapidly be expanded to a great number for infusion within a short time. Similarl to the endogenous TCR-expressed T cells, TCR-engineered T cells recognize tumor-specific antigen in a major histocompatibility complex–dependent manner and its function can be negatively regulated by the immunosuppressive signals in the tumor microenvironment.[49]

The choice of antigen to be targeted determines the specificity of TCR-engineered T cells. To date, most of the studies have engineered TCRs to target TAAs, such as Melan-A/MART-1 and gp100, or cancer germline antigens, such as NY-ESO-1 and MAGE.[50,51] Although these TCR-engineered T cells have resulted in objective responses in most of the treated patients, especially in melanoma patients, they also caused "off-tumor-on-target" toxicity by reacting to healthy organs that expressed the targeted antigen.[52] In EOC, so far, there are no completed clinical trials using TCR-engineered T cells, and several phase I studies are ongoing (see **Table 4**). The study NCT02096614 evaluates the safety and effect of MAGE-A4–specific TCR gene transduced T cells in HLA-A*24:02 positive patients with refractory ovarian cancer that express the antigen MAGE-A4. Another 3 trials—NCT02366546, NCT01567891, and NCT02457650—all use T cells engineered with NY-ESO-1-specific TCR to treat patients with ovarian cancer with the HLA-A*02:01 or HLA-A*02:06 allele and whose tumor expresses the NY-ESO-1 antigen. NY-ESO-1 is highly expressed in various types of cancer, including EOC. Although in normal somatic tissues its expression is restricted to the germline cells, which lack human leukocyte antigen (HLA) molecules and cannot be recognized by T cells. Therefore, NY-ESO-1 has been selected as an attractive target for ACT in clinical trials. Most recently, efforts have been focused on the development of T cells engineered with TCRs specific to particular tumor neoantigens. A new pilot study has demonstrated the feasibility of the process from identification of neoantigen to production of the neoantigen-specific cytotoxic TCR-engineered T cells for ovarian cancer.[53]

Chimeric Antigen Receptor T Cells

CAR is another means for providing recognition specificity to engineered T cells. CAR molecule combines the antigen-binding domain of a single-chain variable fragment (scFv) derived from an antibody with cytoplasmic signaling motifs. The scFv fragment recognizes antigens that present on tumor cell surface. The cytoplasmic signaling motifs mediate T-cell activation, consisting of a CD3-zeta activation domain and 2

Table 4
Ongoing adoptive T-cell therapy clinical trials in epithelial ovarian cancer

Agent	Phase	Target Antigen	Infused Cells	Patients	Trial Identifier
TIL	II	—	Short-term cultured autologous TIL	Metastasis ovarian cancer	NCT01174121
TIL	I	—	Restimulated T cells	Platinum-resistant high-grade serous ovarian cancer	NCT01883297
TCR	I	MAGE-A4	MAGE-A4-specific TCR gene transferred T lymphocytes	HLA-A*24:02 positive MAGE-A4 expressing EOC	NCT02096614
TCR	I	NY-ESO-1	NY-ESO-1-specific TCR gene transduced T lymphocytes	HLA-A*02:01 or HLA-A*02:06 positive NY-ESO-1 expressing EOC	NCT02366546
TCR	I/II	NY-ESO-1	NY-ESO-1 (C259) transduced autologous T cells	Patients with HLA-A201, HLA-A205, and/or HLA-A206 allele and whose tumor expresses the NY-ESO-1	NCT01567891
TCR	I	NY-ESO-1	Anti-NY ESO-1 TCR-transduced T cells	Patients with HLA-A2+ NY-ESO-1 expressing tumor	NCT02457650
CAR	I/II	Mesothelin	Antimesothelin CAR transduced PBL	Metastatic or unresectable cancer that expresses mesothelin	NCT01583686
CAR	I	Mesothelin	Antimesothelin CAR transduced T cells	Refractory or relapsed mesothelin expressing tumor	NCT02580747
CAR	I	MUC16	4H11–28z/fIL-12/EGFRt + genetically modified T cells	EOC with MUC16 ecto antigen expression	NCT02498912
CAR	I/II	EGFR	Anti-EGFR-CAR transduced autologous T cells	Chemotherapy-resistant or relapsed EOC with EGFR expression	NCT01869166
CAR	I/II	ErbB2/Her2	Anti-HER-2-CAR transduced autologous T cells	Chemotherapy-resistant or relapsed EOC with Her2 expression	NCT01935843
CAR	I	CD133	Anti-CD133-CAR vector-transduced T cells	Chemotherapy refractory or relapsed CD133-positive EOC	NCT02541370

costimulatory domains, CD28 and CD137/4-1BB. On antigen encounter, intracellular domains of the CAR transduce the activation signals, leading to T-cell activation with cytotoxic function.[54,55] Recently, the first 2 CAR T-cell therapies (axicabtagene ciloleucel and tisagenlecleucel) have been approved for the treatment of refractory diffuse large B-cell lymphoma and refractory B-cell precursor acute lymphoblastic leukemia. They both use anti-CD19–redirected CAR T cells and have achieved impressive response rates. Thus, the field of CAR T-cell therapy is now booming and more than 200 CAR-T clinical trials are running.

In EOC, the first study of adoptive transfer of folate receptor α (FRα)-specific CAR T cells in patients with ovarian cancer showed no clinical benefit probably because of low expression of the CAR and poor persistence of the transferred T cells.[56] Another phase I trial (NCT02159716) tested the mesothelin-specific CAR T cells in 6 patients with recurrent serous ovarian cancer. The treatment was feasible and safe and trafficking of CAR T cells to the tumor site was observed. All 6 patients showed SD after 1-month treatment.[57] The effect of mesothelin-specific CAR T cells is promising and being tested in 2 more phase I/II clinical trials (NCT01583686, NCT02580747) in mesothelin-expressing cancers, including ovarian cancer. In addition to FRα and mesothelin, some other CAR T cells targeting TAAs are under investigation in clinical trials, including Mucin-16 (NCT02498912), epidermal growth factor receptor (NCT01869166), human epidermal growth factor receptor 2 (NCT01935843), CD133 (NCT02541370), and natural killer group 2D (NCT03018405). Identifying the tumor-specific surface antigens is the priority to manufacture effective CAR T cells against solid tumors. Moreover, the immunosuppressive environment within a solid tumor also inhibits the trafficking and effector function of CAR T cells. Therefore, various combinations of CAR T cells with other therapies would be expected to achieve greater persistence and response.

CANCER VACCINE

The biological principle of cancer vaccines is to provoke a tumor-specific immune response that involves both innate and adaptive immunity. Therapeutic cancer vaccine theoretically could increase TAA presentation by APCs and then generate TAA-specific CD8+ T cells to eradicate tumor cells. Moreover, vaccine-induced immune response has the ability of immunologic memory that can persist for long periods of time.[58] In EOC, many clinical studies have revealed induced antigen-specific T-cell response and improved survival in different degrees by using different vaccines, including recombinant protein or peptide vaccines and whole tumor lysate or DC-based autologous vaccines.

Protein-/Peptide-Based Vaccine

Protein-/peptide-based vaccines are usually based on the well-defined TAAs and administered together with an adjuvant to improve their presentation by endogenous DCs. The ideal TAA should be selective expression by tumor cells relative to normal tissue and high immunogenicity. Among antigens targeted for vaccination, NY-ESO-1 is one of the most spontaneously immunogenic tumor antigens that have been tested in clinical trials in various solid tumors, including ovarian cancer.[59] Vaccination of patients with HLA-A*0201-positive EOC with NY-ESO-1 peptide (NY-ESO-1 157-165) and Montanide, an incomplete Freund's adjuvant, induced specific T-cell immune response in patients with both NY-ESO-1-positive and NY-ESO-1-negative tumors.[60] Another study used the peptide NY-ESO-1 157-170 that contains both CD4+ and CD8+ T cell epitopes for vaccination in patients with advanced EOC. Long-lived and functional vaccine-elicited CD4+ and CD8+ T cells were detected in patients with no evidence of disease for greater than 6 months.[61] Overlapping long peptides (OLP) derived from NY-ESO-1 was also tested in various adjuvant combinations in patients with EOC. NY-ESO-1–specific antibody and CD8+ T-cell responses were detected in 6 of 13 (46%) and 8 of 13 (62%) patients after vaccination with OLP + Montanide, and both were detected in 10 of 11 (91%) patients receiving OLP + Montanide + poly-ICLC.[62] Recombinant poxviruses (vaccinia and fowlpox) expressing the whole protein of NY-ESO-1 was evaluated in a phase II clinical trials in 22 patients with ovarian cancer. Integrated NY-ESO-1–specific antibody and CD4+ and CD8+ T cells were induced in a high proportion of patients with EOC.[63] The expression of NY-ESO-1 is suppressed by DNA methylation and can be enhanced by the DNA methyltransferase (DNMT) inhibitor decitabine. A phase I trial combined the NY-ESO-1 peptide vaccine with escalating doses of decitabine and doxorubicin liposome chemotherapy in 12 patients with relapsed EOC. Increased NY-ESO-1–specific antibodies and CD8+ T cells were detected in most of the patients. Among 10 evaluable patients, 5 patients had SD and 1 had a PR.[64] Other antigens such as p53, Her2, and FRα have also been tested for vaccination in clinical studies of EOC. A p53 synthetic long peptide (p53-SLP) vaccine combined with low-dose cyclophosphamide was tested in a phase 2 single-arm trial in EOC. p53-specific effector T cells were observed in 90% of patients and SD was observed in 20% of patients.[65] Many different peptides derived from Her2 have also been tested in ovarian cancer. However, no immunogenicity was observed in most studies using single or mixed Her2 peptides and no clinical data were obtained.[66] FRα peptide vaccine was tested in a recent phase I clinical trial enrolling patients with EOC who showed no evidence of disease after conventional therapy. Vaccination was well tolerated in all patients and induced immune response in more than 90% of patients.[67]

Dendritic Cell–Based Vaccine

DC is the most potent APC population for activating antitumor T-cell response. Also because it rarely presents immune-related toxicities, DC has become the most frequently used cellular therapeutic in clinical trials. DC can be given alone after cytotoxic chemo- or radiotherapy or loaded ex vivo with various antigens, such as proteins, peptides, or the whole tumor lysate, before reinfusion into patients.[68]

Protein- or Peptide-Loaded Dendritic Cell

Similar with recombinant protein/peptide vaccine, this strategy is also based on well-defined TAAs. Autologous DCs are pulsed with recombinant protein or peptides before reinfusion. An early phase I study evaluated immunization with autologous DC pulsed with mannan-MUC1 fusion protein to treat patients with advanced cancer, including 2 patients with EOC. T-cell response was observed in all patients and 1 of 2 patients with EOC in progression at entry was stable after therapy for at least 3 years.[69] Later, lapuleucel-T, the Her-2-GM-CSF fusion protein–loaded DC vaccine was tested in 4 patients with Her2-positive ovarian cancer. Her-2–specific T-cell response was detected after vaccination and 2 patients had SD.[70] Peptide-loaded DC vaccines were also tested in ovarian cancer. A phase I trial enrolled 10 patients, including 3 patients with EOC, to receive immunization with DC pulsed with Her-2– or MUC-1–derived peptides. Antigen-specific T-cell responses were detected in 5 of 10 patients.[71] In another phase I trial, 11 patients with EOC were immunized with DC loaded with Her2, hTERT, and PADRE peptides with low-dose cyclophosphamide. Her2- and hTERT-specific T-cell responses were observed and the 3-year overall survival was 90%.[72]

Whole Tumor Lysate–Loaded Dendritic Cell

The advantage of whole tumor cells as a source of antigens for DC-based vaccine is that the entire repertoire of antigens associated with a particular tumor, including the specific neoantigens, may be processed and presented to the immune system. Therefore, this strategy is predicted to generate a better immune response and prevent tumor immune escape through antigen-loss variants or mutations. An earlier phase I study used DC loaded with crude whole tumor lysate to treat 8 patients, including 6 with recurrent EOC. Three patients showed SD lasting 25 to 45 weeks and tumor antigen–specific immunity was detected in 2 of 6 evaluable patients.[73] Later, oxidized whole tumor lysate with enhanced immunogenicity was used to load DC. A recent pilot trial tested the autologous oxidized lysate–loaded autologous DC in recurrent patients with ovarian cancer. DC vaccine was administered alone (cohort 1, n = 5), in combination with bevacizumab (cohort 2, n = 10), or bevacizumab plus low-dose cyclophosphamide (cohort 3, n = 10). Three patients had SD in cohort 1; 1 patient had PR and 4 patients had SD in cohort 2; and in cohort 3, 1 patient had PR and 6 patients had SD. Vaccination induced T-cell responses to tumor antigen, which were associated with significantly prolonged survival.[74]

The FANG vaccine is another whole tumor cell–based vaccine. Autologous tumor cells are electroporated with FANG vector, a plasmid expressing GM-CSF and a bifunctional short hairpin RNA against furin.[75] This vaccine has been tested in a phase I study recruiting 27 patients with advanced cancer, including 5 ovarian cancers.[75] Currently, this vaccine is being tested in a phase II study in patients with high-risk stage III/IV ovarian cancer (NCT02346747).

SUMMARY AND FUTURE DIRECTIONS
Checkpoint Blockade Combination Therapy

To date, checkpoint blockade is the most promising and studied immunotherapy in ovarian cancer. The combinations of PD(L)-1 antibodies with PARP inhibitors or conventional chemotherapy have achieved good response in clinical trials and demonstrate excellent clinical potential. Tumor cells create an immunosuppressive microenvironment through multiple mechanisms[10,76,77]; therefore combinatorial therapeutic strategies will be required to unleash the maximal antitumor immune response. Epigenetic modulators, including the inhibitors targeting HDAC, enhancer of zeste homolog 2 (EZH2), DNA methyltransferase 1 (DNMT1), and histone demethylase LSD1 are recently found to have the ability to regulate the antitumor immune response.[78–80] It has been showed that inhibitors of EZH2 and DNMT1 could induce chemokine expression in tumor cells, increase CD8+ T cell tumor infiltration and augment antitumor efficacy of PD-L1 blockade in an EOC preclinical model.[78] Two ongoing clinical trials in ovarian cancer are testing the combinations of PD-1 blockade pembrolizumab with epigenetic modulators: one is a DNMT1 inhibitor guadecitabine (NCT02901899) and another is a DNA methyltransferase inhibitor azacitidine (NCT02900560). Targeting tumor metabolism represents another promising strategy to combine with PD blockade. Growing evidence has shown that the tumor microenvironment supports metabolic reprogramming that dampens T-cell function. Indoleamine 2,3-dioxygenase (IDO)–mediated tryptophan catabolism has been recognized as a mechanism of immunosuppression in many types of cancer, including EOC. It has been well established that IDO inhibition could enhance antitumor immune response.[81] A current clinical trial involving patients with EOC is assessing the combination of IDO inhibitor epacadostat and PD-L1 blockade nivolumab.

In addition to the PD-L1/PD-1 axis, other immunosuppressive molecules, such as T-cell immunoglobulin mucin 3, lymphocyte activation gene 3 protein (LAG3), and T-cell immunoglobulin and ITIM domain (TIGIT), are all potential targets for developing immunotherapy.[19] The combinations of PD blockade with LAG3 blockade are under testing in clinical trials (NCT01968109).

Neoantigen Vaccine

Another promising approach is the development of EOC neoantigen vaccine. Cancer neoantigens are a class of HLA-bound peptides that are generated by tumor missense mutations. They are exclusively tumor specific and highly immunogenic, thus can be recognized by host immune system.[82] Neoantigen-derived vaccine has been recently tested in several clinical studies in patients with melanoma. The vaccine consisting of synthesized long peptides targeting up to 20 neoantigens per patient plus poly-ICLC (Hiltonol) was evaluated in a phase I study in patients with advanced cutaneous melanoma.[83] Vaccine-induced CD4[+] and CD8[+] T cells were detected against unique neoantigens. In 6 immunized patients, 4 had no recurrence at 25 months after vaccination. Two recurrent patients were further treated with PD1 blockade and experienced complete tumor regression. In another study, an RNA-based poly-neoepitope vaccine was tested in patients with advanced cutaneous melanoma.[84] Similarly, both CD4[+] and CD8[+] T-cell responses were detected against 66% and 25% of the candidate neoepitopes, respectively. These studies indicate that neoantigen vaccine can induce expansion of the repertoire of neoantigen-specific T cells and mediate tumor regression, which represents a novel strategy of personalized immunotherapy for patients with cancer, including EOC.

In summary, the tumor microenvironment is the main battleground between tumor cells and the host immune system. Major immunosuppressive networks have been identified in the human EOC microenvironment. Current checkpoint therapy targets the cancer immunosuppressive mechanisms and generates clinical therapeutic efficacy in a fraction of patients. However, it seems that patients with EOC are relatively insensitive to the single checkpoint therapy. Nonetheless, tumor-associated effector T cells are positively associated with ovarian cancer patient survival and response to chemotherapy.[3] As effector T-cell tumor trafficking is controlled by the cancer epigenetic pathway and T-cell effector function may be additionally affected by metabolic pathway, the combination therapy by targeting the immunosuppressive networks (eg, PD-L1/PD-1 pathway) and qualitatively supporting specific T cells may be a potential successful immunotherapy approach for patients with ovarian cancer.

REFERENCES

1. Jayson GC, Kohn EC, Kitchener HC, et al. Ovarian cancer. Lancet 2014; 384(9951):1376–88.
2. Ledermann JA, Raja FA, Fotopoulou C, et al. Newly diagnosed and relapsed epithelial ovarian carcinoma: ESMO Clinical Practice Guidelines for diagnosis, treatment and follow-up. Ann Oncol 2013;24(Suppl 6):vi24–32.
3. Wang W, Kryczek I, Dostal L, et al. Effector T cells abrogate stroma-mediated chemoresistance in ovarian cancer. Cell 2016;165(5):1092–105.
4. Lee N, Zakka LR, Mihm MC Jr, et al. Tumour-infiltrating lymphocytes in melanoma prognosis and cancer immunotherapy. Pathology 2016;48(2):177–87.
5. Zhang L, Conejo-Garcia JR, Katsaros D, et al. Intratumoral T cells, recurrence, and survival in epithelial ovarian cancer. N Engl J Med 2003;348(3): 203–13.

6. Curiel TJ, Coukos G, Zou L, et al. Specific recruitment of regulatory T cells in ovarian carcinoma fosters immune privilege and predicts reduced survival. Nat Med 2004;10(9):942–9.

7. Sato E, Olson SH, Ahn J, et al. Intraepithelial CD8+ tumor-infiltrating lymphocytes and a high CD8+/regulatory T cell ratio are associated with favorable prognosis in ovarian cancer. Proc Natl Acad Sci U S A 2005;102(51):18538–43.

8. Jackson SR, Yuan J, Teague RM. Targeting CD8+ T-cell tolerance for cancer immunotherapy. Immunotherapy 2014;6(7):833–52.

9. Lin H, Wei S, Hurt EM, et al. Host expression of PD-L1 determines efficacy of PD-L1 pathway blockade-mediated tumor regression. J Clin Invest 2018;128(2):805–15.

10. Zou W. Immunosuppressive networks in the tumour environment and their therapeutic relevance. Nat Rev Cancer 2005;5(4):263–74.

11. Postow MA, Callahan MK, Wolchok JD. Immune checkpoint blockade in cancer therapy. J Clin Oncol 2015;33(17):1974–82.

12. Restifo NP, Dudley ME, Rosenberg SA. Adoptive immunotherapy for cancer: harnessing the T cell response. Nat Rev Immunol 2012;12(4):269–81.

13. Hutchinson L. Immunotherapy: harmonizing the immune response with a cancer vaccine. Nat Rev Clin Oncol 2012;9(9):487.

14. Topalian SL, Taube JM, Anders RA, et al. Mechanism-driven biomarkers to guide immune checkpoint blockade in cancer therapy. Nat Rev Cancer 2016;16(5):275–87.

15. Qureshi OS, Zheng Y, Nakamura K, et al. Trans-endocytosis of CD80 and CD86: a molecular basis for the cell-extrinsic function of CTLA-4. Science 2011;332(6029):600–3.

16. Shrikant P, Khoruts A, Mescher MF. CTLA-4 blockade reverses CD8+ T cell tolerance to tumor by a CD4+ T cell- and IL-2-dependent mechanism. Immunity 1999;11(4):483–93.

17. Dong H, Strome SE, Salomao DR, et al. Tumor-associated B7-H1 promotes T-cell apoptosis: a potential mechanism of immune evasion. Nat Med 2002;8(8):793–800.

18. Hui E, Cheung J, Zhu J, et al. T cell costimulatory receptor CD28 is a primary target for PD-1-mediated inhibition. Science 2017;355(6332):1428–33.

19. Zou W, Wolchok JD, Chen L. PD-L1 (B7-H1) and PD-1 pathway blockade for cancer therapy: mechanisms, response biomarkers, and combinations. Sci Transl Med 2016;8(328):328rv324.

20. Ribas A, Shin DS, Zaretsky J, et al. PD-1 blockade expands intratumoral memory T cells. Cancer Immunol Res 2016;4(3):194–203.

21. Brahmer JR, Tykodi SS, Chow LQ, et al. Safety and activity of anti-PD-L1 antibody in patients with advanced cancer. N Engl J Med 2012;366(26):2455–65.

22. Hamanishi J, Mandai M, Ikeda T, et al. Safety and antitumor activity of anti-PD-1 antibody, nivolumab, in patients with platinum-resistant ovarian cancer. J Clin Oncol 2015;33(34):4015–22.

23. Varga A, Piha-Paul SA, Ott PA, et al. Antitumor activity and safety of pembrolizumab in patients (pts) with PD-L1 positive advanced ovarian cancer: Interim results from a phase Ib study. J Clin Oncol 2015;33(15_suppl):5510.

24. Infante JR, Braiteh F, Emens LA, et al. Safety, clinical activity and biomarkers of atezolizumab (atezo) in advanced ovarian cancer (OC). Ann Oncol 2016;27(suppl_6):871P.

25. Disis ML, Patel MR, Pant S, et al. Avelumab (MSB0010718C; anti-PD-L1) in patients with recurrent/refractory ovarian cancer from the JAVELIN Solid Tumor phase Ib trial: Safety and clinical activity. J Clin Oncol 2016;34(15_suppl):5533.

26. NCT01611558: phase II study of ipilimumab monotherapy in recurrent platinum-sensitive ovarian cancer - study results. 2016. Available at: https://clinicaltrials.gov/ct2/show/results/NCT01611558. Accessed May 24, 2016.

27. Wolchok JD, Chiarion-Sileni V, Gonzalez R, et al. Overall survival with combined nivolumab and ipilimumab in advanced melanoma. N Engl J Med 2017;377(14):1345–56.

28. Goodman AM, Kato S, Bazhenova L, et al. Tumor mutational burden as an independent predictor of response to immunotherapy in diverse cancers. Mol Cancer Ther 2017;16(11):2598–608.

29. Howitt BE, Shukla SA, Sholl LM, et al. Association of polymerase e-mutated and microsatellite-instable endometrial cancers with neoantigen load, number of tumor-infiltrating lymphocytes, and expression of PD-1 and PD-L1. JAMA Oncol 2015;1(9):1319–23.

30. Yarchoan M, Hopkins A, Jaffee EM. Tumor mutational burden and response rate to PD-1 inhibition. N Engl J Med 2017;377(25):2500–1.

31. Strickland KC, Howitt BE, Shukla SA, et al. Association and prognostic significance of BRCA1/2-mutation status with neoantigen load, number of tumor-infiltrating lymphocytes and expression of PD-1/PD-L1 in high grade serous ovarian cancer. Oncotarget 2016;7(12):13587–98.

32. Drew Y, de Jonge M, Hong S-H, et al. An open-label, phase II basket study of olaparib and durvalumab (MEDIOLA): results in germline BRCA-mutated (gBRCAm) platinum-sensitive relapsed (PSR) ovarian cancer (OC). Presented at: SGO Annual Meeting. New Orleans, LA, March 24–7, 2018. Late-breaking abstract.

33. Ott PA, Hodi FS, Buchbinder EI. Inhibition of immune checkpoints and vascular endothelial growth factor as combination therapy for metastatic melanoma: an overview of rationale, preclinical evidence, and initial clinical data. Front Oncol 2015;5:202.

34. Voron T, Colussi O, Marcheteau E, et al. VEGF-A modulates expression of inhibitory checkpoints on CD8+ T cells in tumors. J Exp Med 2015;212(2):139–48.

35. Bracci L, Schiavoni G, Sistigu A, et al. Immune-based mechanisms of cytotoxic chemotherapy: implications for the design of novel and rationale-based combined treatments against cancer. Cell Death Differ 2014;21(1):15–25.

36. Galluzzi L, Zitvogel L, Kroemer G. Immunological mechanisms underneath the efficacy of cancer therapy. Cancer Immunol Res 2016;4(11):895–902.

37. Mathios D, Kim JE, Mangraviti A, et al. Anti-PD-1 antitumor immunity is enhanced by local and abrogated by systemic chemotherapy in GBM. Sci Transl Med 2016;8(370):370ra180.

38. Langer CJ, Gadgeel SM, Borghaei H, et al. Carboplatin and pemetrexed with or without pembrolizumab for advanced, non-squamous non-small-cell lung cancer: a randomised, phase 2 cohort of the open-label KEYNOTE-021 study. Lancet Oncol 2016;17(11):1497–508.

39. Zitvogel L, Apetoh L, Ghiringhelli F, et al. Immunological aspects of cancer chemotherapy. Nat Rev Immunol 2008;8(1):59–73.

40. Emens LA, Middleton G. The interplay of immunotherapy and chemotherapy: harnessing potential synergies. Cancer Immunol Res 2015;3(5):436–43.

41. Galluzzi L, Buque A, Kepp O, et al. Immunological effects of conventional chemotherapy and targeted anticancer agents. Cancer Cell 2015;28(6):690–714.

42. Galluzzi L, Vacchelli E, Bravo-San Pedro JM, et al. Classification of current anti-cancer immunotherapies. Oncotarget 2014;5(24):12472–508.
43. Kelderman S, Heemskerk B, Fanchi L, et al. Antigen-specific TIL therapy for melanoma: a flexible platform for personalized cancer immunotherapy. Eur J Immunol 2016;46(6):1351–60.
44. Rosenberg SA, Restifo NP. Adoptive cell transfer as personalized immunotherapy for human cancer. Science 2015;348(6230):62–8.
45. Rosenberg SA, Yang JC, Sherry RM, et al. Durable complete responses in heavily pretreated patients with metastatic melanoma using T-cell transfer immunotherapy. Clin Cancer Res 2011;17(13):4550–7.
46. Aoki Y, Takakuwa K, Kodama S, et al. Use of adoptive transfer of tumor-infiltrating lymphocytes alone or in combination with cisplatin-containing chemotherapy in patients with epithelial ovarian cancer. Cancer Res 1991;51(7):1934–9.
47. Freedman RS, Edwards CL, Kavanagh JJ, et al. Intraperitoneal adoptive immunotherapy of ovarian carcinoma with tumor-infiltrating lymphocytes and low-dose recombinant interleukin-2: a pilot trial. J Immunother Emphasis Tumor Immunol 1994;16(3):198–210.
48. Fujita K, Ikarashi H, Takakuwa K, et al. Prolonged disease-free period in patients with advanced epithelial ovarian cancer after adoptive transfer of tumor-infiltrating lymphocytes. Clin Cancer Res 1995;1(5):501–7.
49. Abate-Daga D, Hanada K, Davis JL, et al. Expression profiling of TCR-engineered T cells demonstrates overexpression of multiple inhibitory receptors in persisting lymphocytes. Blood 2013;122(8):1399–410.
50. Rapoport AP, Stadtmauer EA, Binder-Scholl GK, et al. NY-ESO-1-specific TCR-engineered T cells mediate sustained antigen-specific antitumor effects in myeloma. Nat Med 2015;21(8):914–21.
51. Chapuis AG, Thompson JA, Margolin KA, et al. Transferred melanoma-specific CD8+ T cells persist, mediate tumor regression, and acquire central memory phenotype. Proc Natl Acad Sci U S A 2012;109(12):4592–7.
52. Fesnak AD, June CH, Levine BL. Engineered T cells: the promise and challenges of cancer immunotherapy. Nat Rev Cancer 2016;16(9):566–81.
53. Matsuda T, Leisegang M, Park JH, et al. Induction of neoantigen-specific cytotoxic T cells and construction of T-cell receptor-engineered T cells for ovarian cancer. Clin Cancer Res 2018;24(21):5357–67.
54. June CH, Sadelain M. Chimeric antigen receptor therapy. N Engl J Med 2018;379(1):64–73.
55. June CH, O'Connor RS, Kawalekar OU, et al. CAR T cell immunotherapy for human cancer. Science 2018;359(6382):1361–5.
56. Kershaw MH, Westwood JA, Parker LL, et al. A phase I study on adoptive immunotherapy using gene-modified T cells for ovarian cancer. Clin Cancer Res 2006;12(20 Pt 1):6106–15.
57. Tanyi JL, Haas AR, Beatty GL, et al. Anti-mesothelin chimeric antigen receptor T cells in patients with epithelial ovarian cancer. J Clin Oncol 2016;34(15_suppl):5511.
58. Guo C, Manjili MH, Subjeck JR, et al. Therapeutic cancer vaccines: past, present, and future. Adv Cancer Res 2013;119:421–75.
59. Thomas R, Al-Khadairi G, Roelands J, et al. NY-ESO-1 based immunotherapy of cancer: current perspectives. Front Immunol 2018;9:947.
60. Diefenbach CS, Gnjatic S, Sabbatini P, et al. Safety and immunogenicity study of NY-ESO-1b peptide and montanide ISA-51 vaccination of patients with epithelial ovarian cancer in high-risk first remission. Clin Cancer Res 2008;14(9):2740–8.

61. Odunsi K, Qian F, Matsuzaki J, et al. Vaccination with an NY-ESO-1 peptide of HLA class I/II specificities induces integrated humoral and T cell responses in ovarian cancer. Proc Natl Acad Sci U S A 2007;104(31):12837–42.

62. Sabbatini P, Tsuji T, Ferran L, et al. Phase I trial of overlapping long peptides from a tumor self-antigen and poly-ICLC shows rapid induction of integrated immune response in ovarian cancer patients. Clin Cancer Res 2012;18(23):6497–508.

63. Odunsi K, Matsuzaki J, Karbach J, et al. Efficacy of vaccination with recombinant vaccinia and fowlpox vectors expressing NY-ESO-1 antigen in ovarian cancer and melanoma patients. Proc Natl Acad Sci U S A 2012;109(15):5797–802.

64. Odunsi K, Matsuzaki J, James SR, et al. Epigenetic potentiation of NY-ESO-1 vaccine therapy in human ovarian cancer. Cancer Immunol Res 2014;2(1):37–49.

65. Vermeij R, Leffers N, Hoogeboom BN, et al. Potentiation of a p53-SLP vaccine by cyclophosphamide in ovarian cancer: a single-arm phase II study. Int J Cancer 2012;131(5):E670–80.

66. Martin Lluesma S, Wolfer A, Harari A, et al. Cancer vaccines in ovarian cancer: how can we improve? Biomedicines 2016;4(2) [pii:E10].

67. Kalli KR, Block MS, Kasi PM, et al. Folate receptor alpha peptide vaccine generates immunity in breast and ovarian cancer patients. Clin Cancer Res 2018; 24(13):3014–25.

68. Jung NC, Lee JH, Chung KH, et al. Dendritic cell-based immunotherapy for solid tumors. Transl Oncol 2018;11(3):686–90.

69. Loveland BE, Zhao A, White S, et al. Mannan-MUC1-pulsed dendritic cell immunotherapy: a phase I trial in patients with adenocarcinoma. Clin Cancer Res 2006; 12(3 Pt 1):869–77.

70. Peethambaram PP, Melisko ME, Rinn KJ, et al. A phase I trial of immunotherapy with lapuleucel-T (APC8024) in patients with refractory metastatic tumors that express HER-2/neu. Clin Cancer Res 2009;15(18):5937–44.

71. Brossart P, Wirths S, Stuhler G, et al. Induction of cytotoxic T-lymphocyte responses in vivo after vaccinations with peptide-pulsed dendritic cells. Blood 2000;96(9):3102–8.

72. Chu CS, Boyer J, Schullery DS, et al. Phase I/II randomized trial of dendritic cell vaccination with or without cyclophosphamide for consolidation therapy of advanced ovarian cancer in first or second remission. Cancer Immunol Immunother 2012;61(5):629–41.

73. Hernando JJ, Park TW, Kubler K, et al. Vaccination with autologous tumour antigen-pulsed dendritic cells in advanced gynaecological malignancies: clinical and immunological evaluation of a phase I trial. Cancer Immunol Immunother 2002;51(1):45–52.

74. Tanyi JL, Bobisse S, Ophir E, et al. Personalized cancer vaccine effectively mobilizes antitumor T cell immunity in ovarian cancer. Sci Transl Med 2018;10(436) [pii:eaao5931].

75. Senzer N, Barve M, Kuhn J, et al. Phase I trial of "bi-shRNAi(furin)/GMCSF DNA/ autologous tumor cell" vaccine (FANG) in advanced cancer. Mol Ther 2012;20(3): 679–86.

76. Li W, Tanikawa T, Kryczek I, et al. Aerobic glycolysis controls myeloid-derived suppressor cells and tumor immunity via a specific CEBPB isoform in triple-negative breast cancer. Cell Metab 2018;28(1):87–103.e6.

77. Cui TX, Kryczek I, Zhao L, et al. Myeloid-derived suppressor cells enhance stemness of cancer cells by inducing microRNA101 and suppressing the corepressor CtBP2. Immunity 2013;39(3):611–21.

78. Peng D, Kryczek I, Nagarsheth N, et al. Epigenetic silencing of TH1-type chemo-kines shapes tumour immunity and immunotherapy. Nature 2015;527(7577): 249–53.

79. Guerriero JL, Sotayo A, Ponichtera HE, et al. Class IIa HDAC inhibition reduces breast tumours and metastases through anti-tumour macrophages. Nature 2017;543(7645):428–32.

80. Sheng W, LaFleur MW, Nguyen TH, et al. LSD1 ablation stimulates anti-tumor im-munity and enables checkpoint blockade. Cell 2018;174(3):549–63.e19.

81. Zhai L, Spranger S, Binder DC, et al. Molecular pathways: targeting IDO1 and other tryptophan dioxygenases for cancer immunotherapy. Clin Cancer Res 2015;21(24):5427–33.

82. Katsnelson A. Mutations as munitions: neoantigen vaccines get a closer look as cancer treatment. Nat Med 2016;22(2):122–4.

83. Ott PA, Hu Z, Keskin DB, et al. An immunogenic personal neoantigen vaccine for patients with melanoma. Nature 2017;547(7662):217–21.

84. Sahin U, Derhovanessian E, Miller M, et al. Personalized RNA mutanome vac-cines mobilize poly-specific therapeutic immunity against cancer. Nature 2017; 547(7662):222–6.

Adoptive T-Cell Therapy for Solid Malignancies

Mohammad S. Jafferji, MD*, James C. Yang, MD

KEYWORDS

- Adoptive T-cell transfer • Tumor-infiltrating lymphocytes • Neoantigens
- Gene engineered T-cell receptor • Chimeric antigen receptor T cell

KEY POINTS

- Adoptive transfer involves the harvesting of autologous T lymphocytes, in vitro expansion and/or manipulation, and infusion of the expanded cell product.
- Lymphodepletion before adoptive cell transfer is critical to improve clinical response.
- Adoptive T-cell therapy of autologous TIL can cause durable regression of metastatic melanoma.
- Chimeric antigen receptor T cells (CAR-T) have shown significant therapeutic value in hematologic malignancies but limited benefit in solid cancers because of the limited tumor-specific surface antigens.
- Adoptive transfer of neoantigen-specific T cells from TIL can cause significant regression of common epithelial malignancies.

INTRODUCTION: ADOPTIVE CELL TRANSFER

The use of immunotherapies for solid and hematologic malignancies has demonstrated durable antitumor effects.[1,2] The use of checkpoint inhibitors allows for immunologic reactivation of the adaptive immune system against tumor-specific neoantigens and effective rejection. Similarly, recent developments in adoptive transfer of T cells has shown effective immune rejection of solid malignancies and durable regression. Adoptive cell transfer involves the extraction of in vivo T lymphocytes, selection for or introduction of tumor reactive cells, in vitro expansion, and delivery of the T-cell product back to the patient. This article discusses the different approaches, challenges, and further directions of adoptive T-cell transfer in solid malignancies.

Disclosure Statement: The authors have nothing to disclose.
Surgery Branch, National Cancer Institute, National Institutes of Health, 10 Center Drive, CRC Building 10, Room: 3-3832, Bethesda, MD 20892, USA
* Corresponding author.
E-mail address: Mohammad.Jafferji@nih.gov

THE TUMOR MICROENVIRONMENT AND TUMOR-INFILTRATING LYMPHOCYTES

One of the insights that has been observed for decades is the presence of CD4[+] and CD8[+] lymphocytes within primary and metastatic lesions. They are found in virtually all solid malignancies. Early murine work on allograft rejection in the 1960s demonstrated that T cells played a critical role in mediating rejection. Attempts at treating transplanted murine models were met with difficulty in in vitro expansion and cell culture. Additionally, further investigation revealed that host immune inhibitory mechanisms limited any observed response to adoptive transferred cells.[3–5] A major advancement in the development of adoptive cell transfer was the demonstration of interleukin (IL)-2 as a potent growth factor for T cells in vitro.[6] This allowed for the opportunity for not only expansion but also selection and manipulation of T cells. Treatment with checkpoint inhibitors alone can induce robust responses in some tumors but not against most human cancers. The efficacy of immune checkpoint inhibitors in smoking-induced non–small cell lung cancer versus nonsmokers, microsatellite unstable colorectal cancers versus microsatellite stable colorectal cancers, and solar-induced cutaneous versus mucosal melanomas indicates that the abundance of mutated neoantigens seems to drive the immunologic repertoire in those cancers that respond to immunotherapies.[7,8] The lack of antigenic targets and the poor antitumor T-cell repertoire in most patients are major factors limiting cancer immunotherapies. Tumor vaccines by and large have not improved the immunologic antitumor repertoire or resulted in clinically significant responses. Adoptive T-cell therapy may represent the best means of overcoming these limitations. Yet the immunologically hostile tumor microenvironment represents a major obstacle to tumor rejection. A critical asset of adoptive T-cell therapy is that the antitumor immune response is removed from this environment and manipulated independently in vivo, whereas the host and the tumor microenvironment are simultaneously prepared to receive and nurture infused immune cells. The clinical responses seen with early efforts at adoptive therapy show that the concept can work, and a better understanding of the factors at work in this complex set of interactions will allow the modality to be effectively applied to a wider array of cancers in the future.

ADOPTIVE T-CELL THERAPY IN METASTATIC MELANOMA

Adoptive transfer of cultured autologous tumor infiltrating lymphocytes (TIL) was first shown to cause durable regression in patients with metastatic melanoma.[1] Melanoma in many ways has become the clinical model for cancer immunotherapy and adoptive T-cell transfer. Immunotherapies including IL-2, checkpoint inhibitors against CTLA-4 and PD-1, and adoptive T-cell transfer have revolutionized the care and improved the durable regression of this malignancy. The first studies using high-dose systemic IL-2 monotherapy for metastatic melanoma demonstrated that IL-2, a potent activator of multiple arms of the immune system including cytotoxic T cells, could cause tumor regression.[9] Overall response rates achieved with this strategy were 16% with a complete response achieved in 6% of patients. Importantly, most of those who achieved a complete response remained disease free for years after treatment, some now with 30 years of follow-up. IL-2 also allowed for stable ex vivo culture of T cells from patients with cancer.[6] Furthermore, the unique property of melanoma to grow in vitro and establish long-lived autologous tumor lines allowed precise immunologic studies of tumor recognition by these T cells. Initial studies with expanded autologous TIL in combination with high-dose systemic IL-2 provided a majority of short responses and response rates were similar to high-dose systemic IL-2 alone.[10] A major insight into improving response rates and duration was the addition of pretransfer nonmyeloablative chemotherapy (cyclophosphamide and fludarabine) to induce host lymphodepletion, which encouraged the growth and persistence of transferred T cells.[11] This regimen results in complete depletion of lymphocytes and neutrophils for about 7 to 10 days. This induces the lymphotrophic cytokines IL-7 and IL-15 and depletes T-regulatory cells and myeloid suppressor cells immediately before adoptive transfer.[12] Analysis of patients who received the conditioning regimen in these studies showed persistence of transferred cells in the circulation by detection of immunologic reactivity and the presence of the T-cell receptors (TCR) from transferred TIL as demonstrated by TCR DNA sequencing. In some patients up to 80% of circulating T lymphocytes months after adoptive transfer were those from the infused cultured T cells. Although enhanced host lymphodepletion using such modalities as total body irradiation were investigated, these did not demonstrate clear benefit compared with basich cyclophosphamide and fludarabine.[13] The important finding from these studies was that durable complete responses could be achieved using a strategy of preparative lymphodepletion and transfer of a large dose of effector T cells with many patient disease free 5 and even 10 years after a single treatment. A major effort to identify the tumor-associated rejection antigens recognized by effective TIL followed. Melanoma TIL were found to often contain reactivity against proteins involved in melanin synthesis.[14] In addition, reactivity against tumor-specific mutated proteins was occasionally seen as were T cells recognizing a family of proteins termed tumor-germline antigens. The efforts to clone tumor-reactive receptors from these T cells and engineer them into the T cells of any patient is discussed later. Investigations into on-target, off-tumor normal tissue recognition revealed that some TIL recognized shared normal antigens, such as melanoma antigen recognized by T cell 1 (MART-1), which is expressed by normal melanocytes and malignant melanoma. Protocols focusing on attacking these tissue differentiation antigens were necessary to determine whether they could induce tumor regressions and whether they were safe.

The studies with expanded endogenous melanoma TIL established that effective adoptive transfer against solid cancers could be consistently achieved with three main components: (1) a preparative regimen of lymphodepleting chemotherapy, (2) expansion and transfer of large numbers of autologous T cells and (3) systemic administration of high-dose IL-2. Most patients tolerate the entirety of the treatment with minimal to no lasting adverse events. Nausea, vomiting, and fatigue related to the lymphodepletion regimen is common. The infusion of the expanded TIL is usually well tolerated with minimal side effects most commonly transient rigors; however, shortness of breath and transient hypoxia can occur.[13] High-dose IL-2 has a narrow therapeutic window and most patient develop symptoms that limit dosing. Generalized symptoms, such as malaise, fevers, and anorexia, are common.[14] High-dose IL-2 can affect multiple organ systems and can cause generalized rash, mucositis, diarrhea, acute kidney injury, total body fluid overload, pulmonary edema, delirium, and hypotension. Timely discontinuation of IL-2 and supportive care typically resolves these symptoms.

Melanoma contains a high nonsynonymous mutational frequency that is highest among solid malignancies.[15] A high frequency of mutations has been thought to allow more unique mutation-specific epitopes for immune recognition and thus a larger repertoire of mutation-specific TCR that can recognize the malignancy and mediate rejection. This is one factor thought to contribute to the success of melanoma TIL therapy. The role of mutation frequency is also supported by multiple studies where higher response rates are seen with checkpoint inhibition for melanoma and microsatellite unstable gastrointestinal cancers. Nevertheless, these associations are typically seen in large studies and a review of TIL from patients with metastatic melanoma found that somatic mutation frequencies ranged from 200 to more than 3000 with no significant correlation seen with response when studying small numbers of patients.[16] Another consideration arises with the Food and Drug Administration approval of anti-PD-1 and anti-CTLA-1 monoclonal antibodies (checkpoint inhibitors) for treatment of several different tumor types. The widespread use of these agents may change the landscape of patients presenting for treatment with adoptive transfer of TIL. Those patients most likely to respond to checkpoint inhibitors may also have the best chance of responding to TIL, but may delay or not receive TIL at all because of a preemptive response to checkpoint inhibitors. The most telling arenas in which to evaluate TIL may be as salvage therapy after checkpoint failure, or against cancers with very low response rates to checkpoint inhibition. Several interesting trials are in progress looking at melanoma patients who progress on checkpoint inhibitors and using TIL against epithelial gastrointestinal cancers with extremely low response rates to checkpoint inhibition. These represent the greatest need in oncology, because most cancer deaths are caused by such cancers and most patients with these tumors show little or no long-term benefit from checkpoint blockade.

GENE-ENGINEERED T-CELL THERAPIES

The demonstration that adoptive transfer of autologous TIL could cause durable regression in patients with metastatic melanoma along with advancements in high-efficiency transduction methods of T cells and identification of cancer-specific antigens led to investigation of genetically modified T cells targeting specific antigens.[17] Understanding what antigens were being recognized by successful TIL populations and if shared between patients, having the ability to create such cells from Peripheral Blood Lymphocytes (PBL) might allow other patients with metastatic melanoma to receive effective T cells. The two main strategies developed are cloning genes encoding tumor-reactive TCR or construction of hybrid receptors fusing antibody-binding domains with TCR activating components in what is called a chimeric antigen receptor (CAR) (**Table 1**). The latter is further discussed later. Either of these can be introduced into a lymphocyte and confer the reactivity of that receptor.

The ideal genetically modified T cells expresses a TCR against a tumor-specific antigen and is Major Histocompatibility Complex (MHC) dependent without off-target or on-target, off-tumor effects. The first type of antigens recognized by TIL were tissue differentiation antigens, such as proteins involved in melanin production. MHC class A02:01 restricted TCRs against the melanocyte differentiation antigens MART-1 and gp100 were isolated (using TIL or PBL from patients) and retrovirally introduced into autologous T cells.[18] MART-1 and gp100 are also expressed on normal melanocytes within the ear, skin, and eyes.[19] Clinical trials in HLA-A0201 patients with metastatic melanoma using these receptors were conducted. Objective clinical responses

Table 1	
Key differences between TCR and CAR gene-engineered T cells in cancer immunotherapy	
TCR Modified T Cell	**CAR Modified T Cell**
Target antigen is processed and presented by MHC	Target antigen is recognized intact
Any protein made in the cytoplasm could be recognized	Only proteins on the external cell surface are recognized
Requires patient have correct HLA allele	No HLA restriction

Abbreviation: MHC, major histocompatibility complex.

were seen with a 30% odds ratio using the high-affinity MART-1 TCR and 19% in those receiving the gp100 TCR. However, on-target, off-tumor toxicities in tissue resident melanocytes in the skin, eye, and inner ear were common. Those affected experienced skin rash, uveitis, and/or hearing loss, many requiring local steroid therapy. Additionally, the objective response with this approach was lower than what was seen with adoptive transfer of unselected TIL in patients with metastatic melanoma (30% vs 51%) with a higher toxicity profile. Although regression is seen with the use of a single high-affinity TCR, the presence of the antigen in normal tissues, with resultant toxicities, limited the use of these TCRs in melanoma. The difference in on-target toxicity compared with TIL also provided a clue that perhaps these antigenic targets did not play a major role in TIL responses. A similar approach targeting a carcinoembryonic antigen (CEA) epitope overexpressed in colon cancer was also tried in human clinical trials.[20] A TCR reactive to a human CEA epitope was isolated after vaccination of transgenic mice. The A02:01 restricted murine TCRs were then retrovirally transduced into a patient's autologous PBL and adoptively transferred. Three patients with the required HLA A02:01 allele and overexpressing CEA on their metastatic colon cancer were treated with this anti-CEA TCR. One of three patients had an objective partial response lasting 6 months before tumor progression. Serum CEA levels dropped in all three patients by 74% to 99% but this was transient and rose from their nadir 3 to 4 months following treatment. Most importantly, all three patients developed severe life-threating inflammatory colitis seen at around 7 days after treatment. Pretreatment colonic mucosal biopsies revealed weak staining of CEA and post-treatment biopsies showed severe colitis with denudation of the colonic epithelium and infiltration of CD3[+] cells. Given this experience, the study was halted and demonstrates the limited clinical benefit of targeting CEA especially because of its on-target, off-tumor toxicity.

Cancer germline antigens, such as NY-ESO-1 and MAGE (melanoma-associated antigen), are a class of nonmutated, tumor-associated antigens that are often not expressed in normal adult tissues but present on germline tissues and some cancers.[21] However, because germline tissues are somewhat immunologically privileged and may lack expression of MHC, there has been interest in TCR-directed therapies against this class of antigens (**Table 2**). These antigens are expressed in varying frequencies among different tumor histologies. NY-ESO-1 is expressed in 13% of metastatic melanomas but in only 1% of the most common epithelial cancers, such colon, pancreatic, prostate, and ovarian cancers.[22–25] It is highly expressed in synovial sarcoma with upward of 80% expressing this antigen.[26] MAGE is expressed in multiple tumor histologies, most frequently in melanoma, where it is found in up to 32% of metastatic melanoma samples. Although found less frequently, this antigen has been shown to be expressed in up to 10% of common epithelial cancers. MHC class A02:01-restricted TCRs against NY-ESO-1 were identified and retrovirally cloned

Table 2
Key differences between unmutated self-antigens, such as germline antigens, and mutated non-self-antigens, such as neoantigens commonly found in TIL

Unmutated Self-Antigens	Mutated Non-Self-Antigens
Constant between patients (off-the-shelf reagents)	Totally patient specific
Potential for autoimmune toxicity	Very low potential for autoimmunity
T-cell repertoire may be limited by thymic editing	No central thymic tolerance (neoantigens)

into CD8$^+$ enriched peripheral blood lymphocytes of patients with heavily treated metastatic melanoma and synovial sarcoma and positive expression on tumor biopsies. Eighteen patients with synovial sarcoma and 20 with metastatic melanoma were treated at the National Cancer Institute (NCI) using this strategy.[27] The objective response rate for those with synovial sarcoma and melanoma was 61% (n = 11) and 55% (n = 11), respectively. Two patients with synovial sarcoma had durable complete regression of multiple metastatic sites that are ongoing. Four patients with metastatic melanoma had a complete response, three of which were durable. Unlike those treated with the anti-MART, gp100, or CEA TCR transduced cells, no on-target, off-tumor toxicities were seen. Only the expected adverse events related to lymphodepletion and IL-2 were seen. These trials demonstrated that a high-efficiency TCR clone against a single antigen present on a tumor, but not present on normal adult tissue, can mediate durable complete regression in solid tumors. Other trials have focused on virally induced cancer, such as cervical, anal, and head/neck cancers from human papilloma virus (HPV)-16. HPV integrates and constitutively expresses oncoproteins, chiefly E6 and E7.[28] TCRs against naturally processed E6 and E7 epitopes were developed and similarly cloned into peripheral blood lymphocytes. In vitro assays with the E6 TCR clone showed tumor cell line killing and a clinical trial conducted in 12 patients with either HPV-16-related cervical, anal, oropharyngeal, or vaginal cancer was performed.[29] Two partial responses were seen with the longest lasting 6 months. Again, there were no associated on-target, off-tumor toxicities reported. A clinical trial using an A02:01-restricted TCR generated against an E7 epitope is ongoing in high-risk HPV-associated cancers. Other trials using PBL engineered with off-the-shelf TCRs recognizing the most frequent shared mutations in the common KRAS oncogene are ongoing. KRAS point mutations are found in 70% of pancreatic cancers, 30% to 50% of colorectal cancers, and 30% of non–small cell lung cancers.[30–32] KRAS mutations in codon 12, pG12D, and pG12V account for the most KRAS mutations in pancreatic and colon cancers. It is an important driver mutation of oncogenesis and is found expressed only in tumor cells and thus is an attractive immunologic target. At the NCI, murine TCR reactive to KRAS G12D and G12V were generated after vaccination of transgenic mice and cloned into human T cells. Treatment in an HLA A11:01-restricted pancreatic cancer cell line xenograft model showed significant reduction in tumor burden in NSG mice.[33] Phase I/II human trials using both G12V and G12D are ongoing in patients with these point mutations and express the HLA A11 allele.

Given the paucity of shared expressed tumor antigens, such as germline antigens in solid cancers, a focus on generation of tumor-derived, neoantigen-specific high-affinity TCRs is currently under investigation and its results will be important in determining the efficacy and toxicities of a personalized high-efficiency, highly clonal T-cell treatment.

CHIMERIC ANTIGEN RECEPTORS T-CELL THERAPY IN SOLID MALIGNANCIES

CAR T cells (CAR-T) have become an important treatment option for relapsed hematologic malignancies, such as acute lymphoblastic leukemia and non-Hodgkin lymphoma.[34] As reported elsewhere in this issue, its recent success in treating these malignancies and Food and Drug Administration approval has led to an interest in treating solid cancers. Unfortunately, attempts at applying this strategy has been met with only anecdotal success. CAR-T are autologous T cells obtained from the peripheral blood and transduced with a chimera of the TCR transmembrane domain, intracellular costimulatory domain (eg, CD28 or 4-1BB), and a signaling domain (eg, CD3 zeta) and fused with the extracellular domain of an antibody, usually the single-chain variable region.[35] This allows specific antibody antigen recognition of a surface or soluble molecule and direct activation of the T cell and killing of the tumor cells. The most clinically successful CAR-T uses the cell surface antigen CD19, which is expressed in B-cell lymphomas and leukemias but also on normal B cells. This CD19 CAR-T allows recognition, activation, and killing of any cell expressing CD19 including normal B cells.[36] B-cell aplasia is almost always seen after treatment and represents on-target off-tumor effect of this therapy but has minimal impact because B-cell aplasia is well tolerated.

There has been a large effort to identify surface molecules in solid cancers that can be recognized by a CAR and mediated tumor destruction. Preclinical murine models showed that this strategy could elicit tumor regression. Unfortunately, despite exhaustive searches for safe tumor-associated cell surface antigens, there have been few that have been found on solid cancers and not on normal cells. Use of an antibody-derived CAR binding domain means the antigen must not only be widely shared but be displayed on the surface of the tumor cell membrane. There about 30 unique antigens that are currently being investigated for clinical efficacy and toxicity using this strategy in solid cancers.[37] Unfortunately, there are few mutated cell surface antigens that would allow for recognition by a CAR. Multiple clinical trials have evaluated some of the few overexpressed surface molecules, such as HER2, EGFRvIII, CEA, and mesothelin, to assess safety and efficacy in multiple solid cancers.[38] However, all of these surface molecules are also expressed in varying levels in normal tissue, or are inconsistently expressed by tumor cells. Treatment using these CAR-T has been met with either limited efficacy or high on-target, off-tumor toxicity related to the antigens being present in the normal tissues.

For example, HER2 (ERBB2) is a cell surface tyrosine kinase commonly overexpressed in multiple cancers, such as breast, ovarian, gastric, and sometimes colon cancer. Monoclonal antibodies against Her2/neu (trastuzumab) are a standard option and have been shown to improve disease-free and overall survival in patients with Her2/neu amplification and have an acceptable toxicity profile.[39] Our group constructed a CAR using the monoclonal antibody against HER2; 10^{10} cells were adoptively transferred after lymphodepletion in a patient with metastatic colon cancer.[40] Unfortunately, the patient developed a severe cytokine storm with respiratory failure within 15 minutes of cell infusion. This was followed by severe hypotension, arrhythmia, multiple cardiac arrests, and gastrointestinal bleeding, and the patient died despite maximal intensive care 5 days after infusion. Postmortem examination revealed that the patient had systemic ischemia and widespread microangiopathic injury. Acute respiratory distress syndrome, rhabdomyolysis, and diffuse intestinal hemorrhage was seen. Serum samples obtained following adoptive transfer revealed a rapid and marked increase of cytokines. Deep sequencing of the vector-specific DNA was also performed and found high levels of CAR infiltration in lung and mediastinal lymph nodes without preferential infiltration into tumors. Overall, it is hypothesized that the HER2 CAR also recognized lower levels of expressed ERBB2 on normal tissues and led to widespread activation and destruction of these normal tissues leading to multiorgan failure and death.

One of the unique mutations expressed on the surface of about 30% of glioblastoma is EGFR variant III (EFGRvIII).[41] This mutation of the EGFR is expressed on the surface and represents a unique and rare antigen that can be targeted by a CAR because it is mutated in tumor cells but not in normal tissues. Thus, multiple human clinical studies have sought to treat glioblastoma expressing EGFRvIII mutation with a CAR specific to this surface molecule. At the NCI, the Surgery Branch conducted a phase I/II dose escalation trial using the EGFRvIII CAR using single-chain variable region from an antibody clone (mAb139) and intracellular signaling domain from CD28, 4-1BB, and CD3ζ.

Preclinical mouse glioma models treated EGFRvIII CAR-T infused demonstrated long-term persistence in vivo and observed responses were seen.[42] Unfortunately, no objective responses have been seen in human trials ongoing at the NCI. Novel delivery methods, such as epidural infusion of EGFRvIII-specific CAR-T, have also been anecdotally performed with evidence of only short-term partial regression.[43] Overall, despite the unique surface expression of mutated EGFRvIII in this population, clinical response has been poor. Although it is unclear as to the mechanism for lack of response, antigen expression may be inconsistent and the blood-brain barrier may play a limiting role in some patients.

Pediatric neuroblastomas uniformly overexpress GD2, a disialoganglioside antigen on the cell surface, which is also expressed in melanoma and at lower levels on normal neurons, melanocytes, and peripheral nerve fibers. CAR-T were generated against GD2 and a phase I clinical trial with 11 pediatric patients with high-risk disease were treated with the anti-GD2 CAR.[44] There was one complete response that was durable and three others had short partial responses. No off-tumor toxicities were reported. That this tumor can show spontaneous regression in some patients may mean that this experience may not be generalizable to other cancers.

To date, there have been no data demonstrating consistent clinical effect of CAR-T on solid malignancies. Further elucidation of novel cancer surface antigens is needed to allow tumor specific CAR-T targeting. An example of a novel target under clinical investigation is CD70, a member of the tumor necrosis factor superfamily and a type II integral membrane glycoprotein, which is normally restricted to activated T and B lymphocytes but is overexpressed on most clear cell renal cell cancers.[45] CD70 binds to its ligand CD27 and this interaction plays a role in proliferation and differentiation of T and B lymphocytes. CD70 antibody drug conjugates have shown antitumor activity in renal cell carcinoma and Hodgkin lymphoma. Preclinical mouse models treated with a CAR constructed from human CD27 binding moieties combined with CD3-zeta demonstrated renal cell carcinoma tumor shrinkage and no apparent effect on the host adaptive immune system.[46,47] At the NCI, a phase I/II study is currently treating patients with CD70-positive renal cell cancer with adoptive transfer of anti-CD70 CAR-T after nonmyeloablative chemotherapy.

Despite the success of CAR-T in lymphoma and leukemias, the role of CAR-T as an effective targeted therapy is limited in solid malignancies. This limitation is mainly caused by the current paucity of cancer-specific cell surface molecules available for antibody recognition. In contrast, TCR recognition of cancer-specific mutated or overexpressed antigens in the context of MHC may be a better alternative because every protein made in the cytoplasm of a cancer cell can potentially be processed and presented on MHC to T cells.

ADOPTIVE T-CELL TRANSFER IN COMMON EPITHELIAL MALIGNANCIES

Most cancer deaths in the United States are from epithelial cancers, such as lung, colon, breast, and pancreatic cancers. Despite modern multimodal therapies including surgery, chemotherapy, and radiotherapy, which have modestly improved survival, metastatic epithelial cancers are largely lethal and durable regression is rare. The demonstration that adoptive transfer of TIL could mediate durable complete regression in metastatic melanoma has led to an interest in this approach in these common epithelial cancers. Initial studies using the same methods used to treat melanoma (discussed previously) with unselected in vitro expanded TIL showed no significant response in those with epithelial cancers. In light of the recent appreciation of the key role of neoantigens in T-cell-dependent immunotherapy, efforts to develop tumor-reactive T cells has focused on this class of antigens. The development of rapid whole exome sequencing allows all nonsynonymous mutations of a tumor to be rapidly identified. Unlike melanoma, most epithelial cancers do not harbor a large burden of mutations with most ranging from 30 to 80 mutations in the cancer exome.[48] Metastatic epithelial cancer TIL were again selected as a source of T cells and processed into 24 tumor fragments, from which separate TIL cultures were grown (**Fig. 1**). Representative tumor samples are sequenced and compared with the normal patient tissue genome. Because autologous epithelial tumor lines can seldom be established in vitro, an alternate method of displaying mutated epitopes in the context of all MHC alleles was needed. Autologous antigen-presenting cells were either pulsed with peptide containing all nonsynonymous tumor-specific mutations, or they were electroporated with synthetic minigenes encoding all candidate mutated epitopes. Cultured TIL from the individual fragment cultures are then cocultured overnight with these antigen-presenting cells "mutation displays" to assess immune recognition. Those fragments that show immunologic reactivity are then expanded in vitro then infused into the patient after lymphodepletion. Approximately 80% of epithelial tumor TIL contain mutation reactive T cells against one to five neoantigens and most are unique to that patient's tumor. Reactive TIL tend to be more frequently CD4$^+$, whereas melanoma-reactive TIL are predominately CD8$^+$. As a proof of principle, adoptive transfer using this approach has shown dramatic regression in a few heavily pretreated patients with multiple epithelial tumor histologies including metastatic cholangiocarcinoma, colorectal cancer, and breast cancer. However, in its current form, the overall response remains low in patients treated and most have no response.

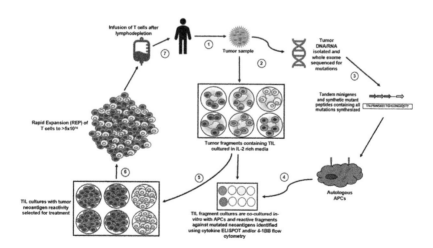

Fig. 1. Adoptive TIL transfer strategy in epithelial cancers. (1) Tumor is resected from patient with metastatic cancer. (2) Tumor is dissected into 24 fragments. Tumor tissue exome is sequenced to identify all somatic mutations. Fragments are cultured in IL-2-rich media to allow TIL growth. (3) Mutations identified by sequencing are then coded into tandem minigenes and synthetic mutated peptides. These are then electroporated and pulsed on autologous antigen-presenting cells (APCs), respectively. (4) APCs are then cocultured with all 24 TIL cultures. Cytokine and 4-1BB activity are used to identify neoantigen reactive TIL fragments. (5) Neoantigen reactive TIL cultures are then selected and cultured for treatment. (6) Selected TIL cultures are then expanded in vitro often achieving T-cell counts >5 × 10^{10}. (7) Expanded TIL product is infused back into patient after lymphodepletion chemotherapy.

At the NCI, a heavily pretreated patient with cholangiocarcinoma with metastasis to the lungs and liver underwent adoptive transfer of 4.2×10^{10} initially unselected TIL cells from a resected lung metastasis after lymphodepletion and followed with 4 doses of IL-2.[49] The patient had only a minor response to this treatment with progression at 7 months. The lung metastasis was sequenced and 26 nonsynonymous mutations were found. Reactivity was detected against mutated erbb2 interacting protein (ERB-B2IP). The patient received a second TIL infusion this time with the selected reactive fragments containing approximately 95% of CD4+ cells recognizing ERBB2IP. The patient had a near complete regression of the liver lesions and significant shrinkage of the lung lesions lasting 3 years before showing signs of progression in the lungs. A biopsy of these lesions showed that the transferred T cells were still persisting but expressed the inhibitory PD-1 receptor. Six doses of pembrolizumab were then administered resulting in an additional partial response now ongoing nearly 2 years later with no additional therapy.

Another patient with metastatic colon cancer to the lungs who had progression after multiple standard treatments was treated with 1.48×10^{11} selected TIL cultured from three resected pulmonary metastases.[50] CD8+ reactivity against KRAS G12D mutation was found and comprised 45% of the T cells received. The patient had significant regression of all seven lung tumors for 9 months until one lesion began to progress and sequencing analysis found loss of the HLA B08:02 allele presenting the mutated KRAS

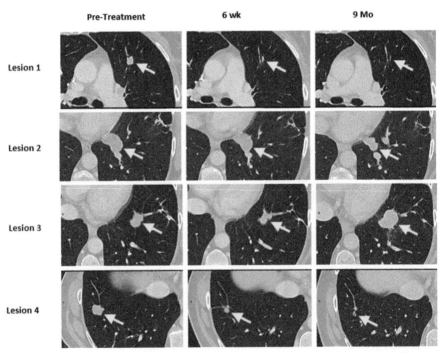

Fig. 2. Contrast-enhanced computed tomography scan of a 54-year-old woman with metastatic colon cancer before and approximately 6 weeks and 9 months after infusion with TIL of which 45% comprised KRAS G12D specific T cells. *Arrows* highlight lung lesions before and after therapy. Shown are four of seven lesions; the remaining three lesions (not shown) completely regressed by 9 months. Lesion 3 progressed and was resected and the patient remains without evidence of disease.

epitope after resection of that lesion (**Fig. 2**). Currently, the patient remains without evidence of disease 2 years following that surgery.

A heavily pretreated patient with ER + HER2-metastatic breast cancer to the chest wall and liver treated by Surgery Branch at NCI underwent treatment with selected TIL therapy from a resected breast mass.[51] Reactivity to two mutated neoantigens, SLC3A2 and KIAA0368, was found and the patient received a single dose of 1.32×10^{11} cells. Interestingly, sampling of peripheral lymphocytes after treatment detected two new neoantigen reactivities against a CTSB CADPS2 epitope that were not detected in the initial screening. By 6 weeks after cell transfer, the patient had achieved a 51% reduction in target lesions and ultimately reached complete regression that continues 22 months after treatment (**Fig. 3**).

Despite these striking examples that selected TIL therapy can induce durable responses in epithelial cancers, most of the greater than 30 patients treated with this strategy at the NCI had either no response or short-term partial responses with the overall response remaining low. In addition, the creation of these cell products can take several months. Investigations as to reasons for poor response are ongoing. First, relying on the endogenous starting population for TIL expansion often results in very low frequencies of tumor neoantigen reactivity in the final cell infusion after expansion. Additionally, T cells harvested from TIL typically have effector memory and effector phenotypes to start and after expansion, may be exhausted and unable to expand and persist in vivo. It is clear that epithelial malignancies in general have much lower numbers of tumor-mutation-reactive TIL than melanoma and selection methods to enrich for these cells are needed to get responses. However, another approach that may help improve responses is the cloning of neoantigen-specific TCR and retroviral introduction into less exhausted peripheral blood lymphocytes to achieve the populations desired. Retroviral transduction of TCR is achieved with high efficiency. Instead

Pre-Treatment   **22 Mo**

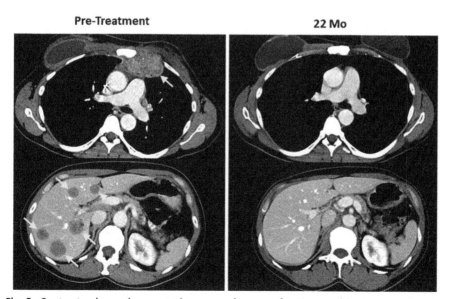

Fig. 3. Contrast-enhanced computed tomography scan of a 49-year-old woman with metastatic ER + Her2-breast cancer to the chest wall (*arrow*) and liver (*arrows*) before (*left*) and after (*right*) adoptive transfer of selected TIL. At 22 months the patient had a complete response that is ongoing.

of reactive fragments being rapidly expanded and infused, reactive TCR clones generated and expanded leading to a higher percentage of reactive T cells administered to the patient. This "re-engineering" of the infused product can also be extended to modifications in T-cell function to resist inhibitory pathways and improve survival. Enrollment of patients at the NCI using this strategy is beginning and will be important in improving efficacy and applicability of adoptive transfer in the treatment of common epithelial malignancies.

FUTURE DIRECTIONS OF ADOPTIVE T-CELL THERAPIES

Immunotherapies for cancer have had an important impact on the treatment of multiple cancers. Additionally, the understanding of cancer biology and its interaction with the host immune system has played an important role in developing novel personalized treatments. Adoptive T-cell transfer affords the advantage of in vitro manipulation; expansion; and with the advent of gene editing tools, such as CRISPR-Cas9, potentially enhancing T-cell function to overcome in vivo and tumor intrinsic immunosuppression. Other obstacles, such as tumor heterogeneity and antigen loss, are areas that need to be further investigated to enhance responses to this strategy. Better detection of neoantigens either from the peripheral blood or from tumor biopsies is needed to increase identification of the available neoantigen repertoire. Further research is also needed to identify unique surface antigens in common solid malignancies in order for CAR-directed therapies to be feasible in these cancers. Finally, T-cell therapies are labor intensive and require large amounts of resources and time. Interest from the government, academic, and private sectors is crucial in improving the delivery of these treatments in a modern health care system.

REFERENCES

1. Rosenberg SA, Yang JC, Sherry RM, et al. Durable complete responses in heavily pretreated patients with metastatic melanoma using T-cell transfer immunotherapy. Clin Cancer Res 2011;17(13):4550–7.
2. Kochenderfer JN, Dudley ME, Kassim SH, et al. Chemotherapy-refractory diffuse large B-cell lymphoma and indolent B-cell malignancies can be effectively treated with autologous T cells expressing an anti-CD19 chimeric antigen receptor. J Clin Oncol 2015;33(6):540–9.
3. Delorme EJ, Alexander P. Treatment of primary fibrosarcoma in the rat with immune lymphocytes. Lancet 1964;2(7351):117–20.
4. Fefer A. Immunotherapy and chemotherapy of Moloney sarcoma virus-induced tumors in mice. Cancer Res 1969;29(12):2177–83.
5. Fernandez-Cruz E, Woda BA, Feldman JD. Elimination of syngeneic sarcomas in rats by a subset of T lymphocytes. J Exp Med 1980;152(4):823–41.
6. Morgan D, Ruscetti F, Gallo R. Selective in vitro growth of T lymphocytes from normal human bone marrows. Science 1976;193(4257):1007–8.
7. Rizvi NA, Hellmann MD, Snyder A, et al. Mutational landscape determines sensitivity to PD-1 blockade in non–small cell lung cancer. Science 2015;348(6230): 124–8.
8. Le DT, Durham JN, Smith KN, et al. Mismatch-repair deficiency predicts response of solid tumors to PD-1 blockade. Science 2017;357(6349):409–13.
9. Rosenberg SA, Mulé JJ, Spiess PJ, et al. Regression of established pulmonary metastases and subcutaneous tumor mediated by the systemic administration of high-dose recombinant interleukin 2. J Exp Med 1985;161(5):1169–88.

10. Rosenberg SA, Lotze MT, Muul LM, et al. Observations on the systemic administration of autologous lymphokine-activated killer cells and recombinant interleukin-2 to patients with metastatic cancer. N Engl J Med 1985;313(23): 1485–92.

11. Dudley ME, Wunderlich JR, Robbins PF, et al. Cancer regression and autoimmunity in patients after clonal repopulation with antitumor lymphocytes. Science 2002;298(5594):850–4.

12. Gattinoni L, Finkelstein SE, Klebanoff CA, et al. Removal of homeostatic cytokine sinks by lymphodepletion enhances the efficacy of adoptively transferred tumor-specific CD8+ T cells. J Exp Med 2005;202(7):907–12.

13. Goff SL, Dudley ME, Citrin DE, et al. Randomized, prospective evaluation comparing intensity of lymphodepletion before adoptive transfer of tumor-infiltrating lymphocytes for patients with metastatic melanoma. J Clin Oncol 2016;34(20):2389–97.

14. Shaker MA, Younes HM. Interleukin-2: evaluation of routes of administration and current delivery systems in cancer therapy. J Pharm Sci 2009;98(7):2268–98.

15. Alexandrov LB, Nik-Zainal S, Wedge DC, et al. Signatures of mutational processes in human cancer. Nature 2013;500(7463):415–21.

16. Crystal JS, et al. Diversity of mutated antigen recognition by tumor infiltrating lymphocytes from patients with metastatic melanoma. J Immunother Cancer 2015; 3(2):P9.

17. Dembić Z, Haas W, Zamoyska R, et al. Transfection of the CD8 gene enhances T-cell recognition. Nature 1987;326:510.

18. Morgan RA, Dudley ME, Wunderlich JR, et al. Cancer regression in patients after transfer of genetically engineered lymphocytes. Science 2006;314(5796):126–9.

19. Johnson LA, Morgan RA, Dudley ME, et al. Gene therapy with human and mouse T-cell receptors mediates cancer regression and targets normal tissues expressing cognate antigen. Blood 2009;114(3):535–46.

20. Parkhurst MR, Yang JC, Langan RC, et al. T cells targeting carcinoembryonic antigen can mediate regression of metastatic colorectal cancer but induce severe transient colitis. Mol Ther 2011;19(3):620–6.

21. Caballero OL, Chen YT. Cancer/testis (CT) antigens: potential targets for immunotherapy. Cancer Sci 2009;100(11):2014–21.

22. Chen YT, Scanlan MJ, Sahin U, et al. A testicular antigen aberrantly expressed in human cancers detected by autologous antibody screening. Proc Natl Acad Sci U S A 1997;94(5):1914–8.

23. Barrow C, Browning J, MacGregor D, et al. Tumor antigen expression in melanoma varies according to antigen and stage. Clin Cancer Res 2006;12(3 Pt 1): 764–71.

24. Gure AO, Chua R, Williamson B, et al. Cancer-testis genes are coordinately expressed and are markers of poor outcome in non-small cell lung cancer. Clin Cancer Res 2005;11(22):8055–62.

25. Kerkar SP, Wang ZF, Lasota J, et al. MAGE-A is more highly expressed than NY-ESO-1 in a systematic immunohistochemical analysis of 3668 cases. J Immunother 2016;39(4):181–7.

26. Jungbluth AA, Antonescu CR, Busam KJ, et al. Monophasic and biphasic synovial sarcomas abundantly express cancer/testis antigen NY-ESO-1 but not MAGE-A1 or CT7. Int J Cancer 2001;94(2):252–6.

27. Robbins PF, Kassim SH, Tran TL, et al. A pilot trial using lymphocytes genetically engineered with an NY-ESO-1-reactive T cell receptor: long term follow up and correlates with response. Clin Cancer Res 2015;21(5):1019–27.

28. Hinrichs CS, Rosenberg SA. Exploiting the curative potential of adoptive T-cell therapy for cancer. Immunol Rev 2014;257(1):56–71.
29. Draper LM, Kwong ML, Gros A, et al. Targeting of HPV-16+ epithelial cancer cells by TCR gene engineered T cells directed against E6. Clin Cancer Res 2015; 21(19):4431–9.
30. Hruban RH, van Mansfeld AD, Offerhaus GJ, et al. K-ras oncogene activation in adenocarcinoma of the human pancreas. A study of 82 carcinomas using a combination of mutant-enriched polymerase chain reaction analysis and allele-specific oligonucleotide hybridization. Am J Pathol 1993;143(2):545–54.
31. Laghi L, Orbetegli O, Bianchi P, et al. Common occurrence of multiple K-RAS mutations in pancreatic cancers with associated precursor lesions and in biliary cancers. Oncogene 2002;21(27):4301–6.
32. Karapetis CS, Khambata-Ford S, Jonker DJ, et al. K-ras mutations and benefit from cetuximab in advanced colorectal cancer. N Engl J Med 2008;359(17): 1757–65.
33. Wang QJ, Yu Z, Griffith K, et al. Identification of T-cell receptors targeting KRAS-mutated human tumors. Cancer Immunol Res 2016;4(3):204–14.
34. June CH, Sadelain M. Chimeric antigen receptor therapy. N Engl J Med 2018; 379(1):64–73.
35. Kochenderfer J, Feldman SA, Zhao Y, et al. Construction and pre-clinical evaluation of an anti-CD19 chimeric antigen receptor. Blood 2008;112(11):4623.
36. Kochenderfer JN, et al. Anti-CD19 CAR T cells administered after low-dose chemotherapy can induce remissions of chemotherapy-refractory diffuse large B-cell lymphoma. Blood 2014;124(21):550.
37. D'Aloia MM, Zizzari IG, Sacchetti B, et al. CAR-T cells: the long and winding road to solid tumors. Cell Death Dis 2018;9(3):282.
38. Tanyi JL, Stashwick C, Plesa G, et al. Possible compartmental cytokine release syndrome in a patient with recurrent ovarian cancer after treatment with mesothelin-targeted CAR-T cells. J Immunother 2017;40(3):104–7.
39. Carter P, Presta L, Gorman CM, et al. Humanization of an anti-p185HER2 antibody for human cancer therapy. Proc Natl Acad Sci U S A 1992;89(10):4285–9.
40. Morgan RA, Yang JC, Kitano M, et al. Case report of a serious adverse event following the administration of T cells transduced with a chimeric antigen receptor recognizing ERBB2. Mol Ther 2010;18(4):843–51.
41. Padfield E, Ellis HP, Kurian KM. Current therapeutic advances targeting EGFR and EGFRvIII in glioblastoma. Front Oncol 2015;5:5.
42. Bullain SS, Sahin A, Szentirmai O, et al. Genetically engineered T cells to target EGFRvIII expressing glioblastoma. J Neurooncol 2009;94(3):373–82.
43. Brown CE, Alizadeh D, Starr R, et al. Regression of glioblastoma after chimeric antigen receptor T-cell therapy. N Engl J Med 2016;375(26):2561–9.
44. Pule MA, Savoldo B, Myers GD, et al. Virus-specific T cells engineered to coexpress tumor-specific receptors: persistence and antitumor activity in individuals with neuroblastoma. Nat Med 2008;14(11):1264–70.
45. Diegmann J, Junker K, Gerstmayer B, et al. Identification of CD70 as a diagnostic biomarker for clear cell renal cell carcinoma by gene expression profiling, real-time RT-PCR and immunohistochemistry. Eur J Cancer 2005;41(12):1794–801.
46. Wang QJ, Yu Z, Hanada KI, et al. Preclinical evaluation of chimeric antigen receptors targeting CD70-expressing cancers. Clin Cancer Res 2017;23(9):2267–76.
47. Shaffer DR, Savoldo B, Yi Z, et al. T cells redirected against CD70 for the immunotherapy of CD70-positive malignancies. Blood 2011;117(16):4304–14.

48. Tran E, Ahmadzadeh M, Lu YC, et al. Immunogenicity of somatic mutations in human gastrointestinal cancers. Science 2015;350(6266):1387–90.
49. Tran E, Turcotte S, Gros A, et al. Cancer immunotherapy based on mutation-specific CD4+ T cells in a patient with epithelial cancer. Science 2014;344(6184):641–5.
50. Tran E, Robbins PF, Lu YC, et al. T-cell transfer therapy targeting mutant KRAS in cancer. N Engl J Med 2016;375(23):2255–62.
51. Zacharakis N, Chinnasamy H, Black M, et al. Immune recognition of somatic mutations leading to complete durable regression in metastatic breast cancer. Nat Med 2018;24(6):724–30.

Role of Surgery in Combination with Immunotherapy

Nicholas D. Klemen, MD[a], Mackenzie L. Shindorf, MD[b],
Richard M. Sherry, MD[c],*

KEYWORDS

- Metastatic melanoma • Surgery • Metastasectomy • Oligometastatic
- Immunotherapy • Checkpoint inhibitors • Solid tumors

KEY POINTS

- The treatment landscape for patients with advanced melanoma has dramatically changed and there are few data on how to best sequence therapy.
- Metastasectomy in selected patients with isolated immunorefractory disease can be followed by long progression-free survival (PFS).
- In the current era of effective cancer immunotherapy, there are limited data pertaining to patient selection for metastasectomy and evolving indications for palliative procedures.

INTRODUCTION: THE RAPIDLY CHANGING LANDSCAPE OF TREATMENT FOR MELANOMA

The development of highly effective immunotherapies therapies over the last decade has dramatically altered the therapeutic landscape for patients with advanced melanoma and several other types of solid tumors. The first Food and Drug Administration–approved immunotherapy was high-dose interleukin-2 (IL-2) for advanced renal cell cancer (RCC) in 1992 and for metastatic melanoma in 1998. The 7% to 8% of patients that achieved a complete and durable cancer regression of their disease after IL-2 demonstrated the potential and promise of cancer immunotherapy.[1,2] Subsequent studies of adoptive cell transfer (ACT) of autologous tumor-infiltrating lymphocytes (TIL) and gene-modified peripheral blood lymphocytes provided important insights into the mechanisms of immunotherapy and demonstrated

Disclosure Statement: The authors have nothing to disclose.
[a] Department of Surgery, Yale University School of Medicine, Yale School of Medicine, 333 Cedar Street, New Haven, CT 06511, USA; [b] Surgery Branch, National Cancer Institute, National Institutes of Health, CRC Room 3-3888, 9000 Rockville Pike, Bethesda, MD 20892, USA; [c] Surgery Branch, National Cancer Institute, National Institutes of Health, CRC Room 3-5942, 9000 Rockville Pike, Bethesda, MD 20892, USA
* Corresponding author.
E-mail address: sherryr@mail.nih.gov

that selected patients could achieve overall response rates exceeding 50%.[3–5] The checkpoint inhibitor (CPI) revolution began in earnest in 2011 with the Food and Drug Administration approval of anti-CTLA-4 antibodies[6] and was bolstered by the approval of anti-PD-1[7] and anti-PD-L1 antibodies.[8] The combination therapy of anti-CTLA-4 and anti-PD-1 antibodies can mediate objective response rates in excess of 60% and complete response rates of 20%.[9] Together, these advances have shifted the treatment landscape so rapidly that the median survival of patients with advanced melanoma, a dismal 6 to 10 months only a decade ago, has yet to be re-established.

Immunotherapy treatments have unique patterns of response compared with other systemic therapies. Patients who achieve a complete response to immunotherapy, whether by IL-2, ACT, or CPI, are usually disease-free for years or even decades.[10] Moreover, some patients achieve durable partial tumor regression, which suggests the immune system is capable of sterilizing or permanently suppressing a patient's metastatic disease burden. The potential durability of immunotherapy responses stands in stark contrast to responses typically seen after systemic cytotoxic or targeted therapies, which can cause dramatic regressions but which are almost inevitably followed by relapse.

Unfortunately, it remains true that most patients treated with immunotherapy do not respond, or develop progressive disease after a partial response. For some of these patients, surgical resection of isolated immunorefractory lesions is followed by long progression-free survival (PFS). A new challenge for surgeons is to define patient selection criteria, indications, timing, and the potential impact of metastasectomy in the era of effective systemic immunotherapies. Although this article focuses on the role of surgery in combination with immunotherapy, the principles and clinical issues discussed herein may also apply to the application of surgery in combination with new and effective targeted therapies.

THE TRADITIONAL ROLE OF METASTASECTOMY FOR PATIENTS WITH ADVANCED MELANOMA

Long-standing principles of metastasectomy for advanced melanoma, and for many other types of solid tumors, have been derived from retrospective data that predate the CPI era. For selected patients with metastatic melanoma, metastasectomy is an excellent treatment option. Retrospective data indicate that surgery in highly selected patients is safe, associated with long PFS in 20% to 40% of patients, and can even be curative.[11,12] Clinical factors associated with favorable outcomes after metastasectomy are well established and include a long disease-free interval, the number of metastatic lesions, and M-stage. In addition, failure to achieve R0 resection is a prognostic marker (because it indicates aggressive biology) and is thought to directly contribute to recurrence risk.

THE ROLE OF METASTASECTOMY IN THE ERA OF EFFECTIVE IMMUNOTHERAPY

Despite recent advances in immunotherapy, many patients with advanced melanoma develop immunorefractory progressive disease. Some of these patients may be excellent candidates for surgical metastasectomy; the challenge for surgeons is to identify characteristics that can reliably select those patients most likely to benefit from surgery following immunotherapy.

The Biology of Response and Resistance to Cancer Immunotherapy

Although the cellular mechanisms of cancer immunotherapy are incompletely understood, emerging data have provided some crucial insights. These mechanisms provide biologic rationale for performing metastasectomy following immune manipulation. Increasing evidence supports the hypothesis that the final common pathway for immunotherapy treatments can be understood as stimulation or creation of autologous lymphocytes that recognize and react to the gene products of cancer-specific mutations (neoantigens). This mechanism likely explains the clinical impact of IL-2; CPIs, such as anti-CTLA-4 and anti-PD-1 antibodies; and ACT of autologous lymphocytes.[13] Several lines of evidence have supported this hypothesis: cancer mutational burden correlates with T-cell infiltration of tumors and clinical response to CPI; T cells recognizing neoantigens have been isolated from a variety of solid tumors; and in some patients, lymphocytes transduced with specific T-cell receptors or chimeric antibody receptors can mediate complete and durable regression of metastatic disease.[3,7,14,15]

Although this hypothesis is oversimplified, it provides a general insight into the complex and numerous potential mechanisms that can generate immune resistance. These include, but are not limited to, a lack of neoantigens in tumors with a low burden of somatic mutations, defects in pathways that involve antigen presentation by tumors, intrinsic declines in T-cell physiology (ie, terminal differentiation and exhaustion), suppressive mechanisms in the tumor microenvironment (eg, T regulatory cells, myeloid derived suppressors), and cancer antigen loss. Despite this complexity, and perhaps because of it, it is possible that effective immunotherapy alters tumor biology and as a result may alter the indications for metastasectomy.

A highly illustrative example of the phenomena of oncologic immune resistance is the report of a patient with advanced refractory colon cancer with a 9-month partial response to ACT using TIL that included a CD8$^+$ T-cell response against a KRAS G12D mutation presented on HLA B08:02.[16] This patient had regression of multiple lesions but progressed at a single pulmonary site that was ultimately resected. Molecular analysis of this immunorefractory lesion demonstrated loss of the HLA B08:02 locus and thus explained the isolated tumor progression. This patient has remained disease free following metastasectomy for more than 2 years and has not required further treatment.

Metastasectomy Following Immunotherapy

The reported clinical experience of metastasectomy following immunotherapy has been limited to case reports and small single institutional series. Metastasectomy after IL-2 was first reported in patients with advanced RCC and metastatic melanoma.[17] After experiencing a partial response, many patients developed progressive disease and a selected group were salvaged by surgical resection. With long follow-up, it was shown that 20% of patients with melanoma and 33% of patients with RCC had PFS more than 5 years after surgical resection of immunorefractory disease. Other reports of metastasectomy for RCC and/or melanoma have also shown some patients can achieve prolonged PFS after resection.[18,19]

The experience with metastasectomy following immunotherapy using checkpoint blockade thus far has been limited to reports from Memorial Sloan Kettering Cancer Institute. In 2013 Gyorki and colleagues[20] reported on 23 patients with metastatic melanoma treated with surgery during or after CTLA-4 blockade with ipilimumab. Surgery was safe and well tolerated, and a few patients had long survival after resection. An update of the Memorial Sloan Kettering Cancer Institute experience was recently presented at the Society of Surgical Oncology Annual Symposium, and included 237 patients with advanced melanoma who were treated with CPI and then surgery.[21] Although the patient selection criteria and the indications for surgery were not detailed in the abstract, the authors reported that favorable outcomes were associated with complete resection and a response to immunotherapy.

The National Cancer Institute Surgery Branch reported a series of patients with advanced melanoma who underwent metastasectomy following ACT treatment with autologous lymphocytes.[22] There were 115 patients that had an objective cancer regression (by RECIST) or stable disease at least 6 months before documented tumor progression (excluding central nervous system sites), and 26 of these 115 patients (23%) underwent metastasectomy as the next treatment strategy. Before immunotherapy there were a median of five metastases per patient (including one patient with more than 20 metastases) but after ACT the 26 patients selected for surgery had disease progression in one or two sites. The 5-year survival after surgery was 57%, and 42% enjoyed PFS longer than 1 year. Most patients had a complete resection, but some patients had selected surgical resection of sites of progressive disease while stable or regressing tumors were left in situ because of the potential morbidity of resecting all disease. This approach may be reasonable for patients who exhibit signs of a mixed response to immunotherapy.

Patient Selection for Metastasectomy in the Era of Effective Immunotherapy

The challenge for surgeons is to identify patients who may benefit from metastasectomy in the era of immunotherapy. Historically, a patient with an initial diagnosis of metastatic melanoma, with a solitary metastasis or other favorable prognostic markers, might be considered an excellent surgical candidate. Although this is still a reasonable strategy, the therapeutic options are now more complex and the optimal treatment sequence less clear. Should such a patient receive upfront systemic therapy with CPI? Should surgery be reserved for patients with nonresponding tumors? Because such a patient is likely to receive postoperative adjuvant therapy, should CPI be offered in the neoadjuvant setting? These management decisions are also complicated by the potential for major side effects from CPI therapy including pneumonitis, colitis, and permanent endocrine dysfunction.[9]

The role of metastasectomy for patients that have documented melanoma progression following CPI has yet to be precisely defined. Selected patients with isolated progression of immunorefractory disease might achieve prolonged PFS and overall survival following surgical resection. Because immunotherapy can mediate prolonged disease stabilization, the traditional goal and prognostic significance of an R0 resection may ultimately be challenged. Ultimately it may not be necessary to resect lesions that seem to be responding to immunotherapy or that have been stable for some defined interval and it is possible that only progressing lesions need to be removed (ie, selective surgical resection). The concept of limited progression following immunotherapy because of immune escape likely will lead to expanded indications for metastasectomy.

The Role of Palliative Surgery in the Context of Immunotherapy

As systemic therapies have improved, indications for palliative surgeries have also changed. Without effective systemic therapies, patients with major complications from advanced cancer might appropriately be referred to hospice. Given the potential effectiveness of CPI, targeted therapies, and ACT, appropriate patients should be managed with the goal of palliation as a bridge to effective systemic treatment. On occasion, palliative surgery may be required during immunotherapy.[20]

NEOADJUVANT IMMUNOTHERAPY

The recognition that immunotherapy is effective for patients with a wide variety of metastatic cancers combined with the convincing evidence that CPI is effective in the adjuvant setting for high-risk patients with melanoma has fueled interest in exploring the use of CPIs in the neoadjuvant setting.[23,24] Tarhini and colleagues[25] evaluated neoadjuvant ipilimumab for patients with melanoma, which resulted in increased lymphocyte infiltration and memory generation. These findings suggested an immuno-modulating impact of neoadjuvant ipilimumab therapy. Huang and colleagues[26] from the University of Pennsylvania evaluated 27 patients with melanoma who received one dose of neoadjuvant pembrolizumab followed by resection 3 weeks later. Eight of these patients were found to have a complete or near complete pathologic response. Not surprisingly, these investigators found that TIL infiltration correlated with patho-logic response. Early data reported from the Netherlands Cancer Institute on the impact of two courses of neoadjuvant ipilimumab and nivolumab in 10 patients with locally advanced melanoma. This group noted seven patients with complete or near complete pathologic responses and one patient with a 75% reduction in tumor burden. Two patients had stable or progressive disease (Rozeman and colleagues 2017 ESMO Congress).[27]

Forde and colleagues[28] recently published data on the safety and feasibility of neo-adjuvant nivolumab for patients with resectable non–small cell lung cancer. These au-thors confirmed this strategy was safe and documented 9 of 20 of these patients generated a complete pathologic response. In addition, they found that the neoadju-vant nivolumab induced expansion of circulating tumor-reactive T cells.

The clinical impact of neoadjuvant immunotherapy is under intense investigation in patients with multiple different tumors. For example, there are four ongoing studies evaluating neoadjuvant immunotherapy in melanoma and two recently completed studies that have yet to publish the data (NCT02519322 and NCT01608594). Because most of these patients receive continued CPI therapy in the adjuvant setting, it will be difficult if not impossible to confirm any clinical impact of this strategy. What is clear from current reports is that neoadjuvant immunotherapy with CPI can alter the tumor microenvironment. Whether those changes have a meaningful clinical impact needs to be established by randomized trials. Nonetheless, these neoadjuvant strategies are certain to identify insights and clinical correlates that may serve to elucidate the role of the immune system in eliminating or controlling cancer.

IMMUNOTHERAPY FOR OTHER SOLID TUMORS

Cutaneous melanoma is the most immune-responsive tumor and therefore it is no sur-prise that the principles and practices of cancer immunotherapy have largely been established treating these patients. For patients with other advanced solid tumors, the extent to which immunotherapy can alter tumor biology and clinical outcomes needs to be more clearly elucidated. Potential changes in the role for metastasectomy, palliative surgery, and neoadjuvant therapy in patients with other advanced solid tu-mors will no doubt be a function of the therapeutic effectiveness of the treatment, and a basic understanding of immune response and resistance mechanisms. It will be interesting to determine if the evolving principles of surgery for patients with met-astatic melanoma apply to other solid tumors.

CONCLUSIONS AND FUTURE DIRECTIONS

Effective cancer immunotherapy has improved overall survival for many patients with advanced cancer and is associated with unique patterns of cancer regression. The observation that these therapies can mediate durable complete and partial responses suggests that immunotherapy may alter tumor biology, and as a result may expand the indication for potentially curative metastasectomy or palliative surgery. The widespread use of CPI therapy, and the rapid development of ACT and other investigational immunotherapies has produced a clear need to define if and how surgery can best complement these novel treatments. The opportunities for surgeons to participate in this clinical research effort are abundant and might at a minimum include a prospective multi-institutional database. For patients with advanced melanoma and multifocal relapse following immunotherapy, clinicians are often forced to choose between bad options that include continued treatment with ineffective systemic therapies, investigational therapies, or morbid and aggressive surgery. In that situation, a randomized clinical trial would be ethical and might provide valuable insights into how these complex patients are best managed.

REFERENCES

1. Rosenberg SA. IL-2: the first effective immunotherapy for human cancer. J Immunol 2014;192(12):5451–8.
2. Rosenberg SA, Packard BS, Aebersold PM. Use of tumor-infiltrating lymphocytes and interleukin-2 in the immunotherapy of patients with metastatic melanoma. A preliminary report. N Engl J Med 1988;319(25):1676–80.
3. Morgan RA, Dudley ME, Wunderlich JR, et al. Cancer regression in patients after transfer of genetically engineered lymphocytes. Science 2006;314(5796):126–9.
4. Rosenberg SA, Yang JC, Sherry RM, et al. Durable complete responses in heavily pretreated patients with metastatic melanoma using T-cell transfer immunotherapy. Clin Cancer Res 2011;17(13):4550–7.
5. Goff SL, Dudley ME, Citrin DE, et al. Randomized, prospective evaluation comparing intensity of lymphodepletion before adoptive transfer of tumor-infiltrating lymphocytes for patients with metastatic melanoma. J Clin Oncol 2016;JCO667220. https://doi.org/10.1200/JCO.2016.66.7220.
6. Hodi FS, O'Day SJ, McDermott DF, et al. Improved survival with ipilimumab in patients with metastatic melanoma. N Engl J Med 2010;363(8):711–23.
7. Topalian SL, Hodi FS, Brahmer JR, et al. Safety, activity, and immune correlates of anti-PD-1 antibody in cancer. N Engl J Med 2012;366(26):2443–54.
8. Brahmer JR, Tykodi SS, Chow LQM, et al. Safety and activity of anti-PD-L1 antibody in patients with advanced cancer. N Engl J Med 2012;366(26):2455–65.
9. Larkin J, Chiarion-Sileni V, Gonzalez R, et al. Combined nivolumab and ipilimumab or monotherapy in untreated melanoma. N Engl J Med 2015;373(1):23–34.
10. Prieto PA, Yang JC, Sherry RM, et al. CTLA-4 blockade with ipilimumab: long-term follow-up of 177 patients with metastatic melanoma. Clin Cancer Res 2012;18(7):2039–47.
11. Howard JH, Thompson JF, Mozzillo N, et al. Metastasectomy for distant metastatic melanoma: analysis of data from the first Multicenter Selective Lymphadenectomy Trial (MSLT-I). Ann Surg Oncol 2012;19(8):2547–55.
12. Faries MB, Thompson JF, DeConti RC, et al. Long-term survival after complete surgical resection and adjuvant immunotherapy for distant melanoma metastases. Ann Surg Oncol 2017;24(13):3991–4000.
13. Tran E, Robbins PF, Rosenberg SA. "Final common pathway" of human cancer immunotherapy: targeting random somatic mutations. Nat Immunol 2017;18(3):255–62.
14. Lawrence MS, Stojanov P, Polak P, et al. Mutational heterogeneity in cancer and the search for new cancer-associated genes. Nature 2013;499(7457):214–8.

15. Tran E, Turcotte S, Gros A, et al. Cancer immunotherapy based on mutation-specific CD4+ T cells in a patient with epithelial cancer. Science 2014; 344(6184):641–5.
16. Tran E, Robbins PF, Lu Y-C, et al. T-cell transfer therapy targeting mutant KRAS in cancer. N Engl J Med 2016;375(23):2255–62.
17. Yang JC, Abad J, Sherry R. Treatment of oligometastases after successful immunotherapy. Semin Radiat Oncol 2006;16(2):131–5.
18. Daliani DD, Tannir NM, Papandreou CN, et al. Prospective assessment of systemic therapy followed by surgical removal of metastases in selected patients with renal cell carcinoma. BJU Int 2009;104(4):456–60.
19. Hughes T, Broucek J, Iodice G, et al. Metastasectomy following incomplete response to high-dose interleukin-2. J Surg Oncol 2017;117(4):572–8.
20. Gyorki DE, Yuan J, Mu Z, et al. Immunological insights from patients undergoing surgery on ipilimumab for metastatic melanoma. Ann Surg Oncol 2013;20(9): 3106–11.
21. Bello DM, Panageas KS, Hollmann TJ, et al. Outcomes of patients with metastatic melanoma selected for surgery after immunotherapy. Society of Surgical Oncology Annual Cancer Symposium, Abstract 5. Presented Chicago, March 23, 2018.
22. Klemen ND, Feingold PL, Goff SL, et al. Metastasectomy following immunotherapy with adoptive cell transfer for patients with advanced melanoma. Ann Surg Oncol 2017;24(1):135–41.
23. Eggermont AMM, Chiarion-Sileni V, Grob J-J, et al. Prolonged survival in stage III melanoma with ipilimumab adjuvant therapy. N Engl J Med 2016;375(19): 1845–55.
24. Weber J, Mandalà M, Del Vecchio M, et al. Adjuvant nivolumab versus ipilimumab in resected stage III or IV melanoma. N Engl J Med 2017;377(19):1824–35.
25. Tarhini AA, Edington H, Butterfield LH, et al. Immune monitoring of the circulation and the tumor microenvironment in patients with regionally advanced melanoma receiving neoadjuvant ipilimumab. PLoS One 2014;9(2):e87705.
26. Huang A. Abstract CT181: Safety, activity, and biomarkers for neoadjuvant anti-PD-1 therapy in melanoma. Cancer Res. 2018;78(Suppl 13):CT181.
27. Rozeman E.A. Abstract (Neo-)adjuvant ipilimumab + nivolumab (IPI+ NIVO) in palpable stage 3 melanoma – updated relapse free survival (RFS) data from the OpACIN trial and first biomarker analyses. ESMO Annals of Oncology Abstract Book of 42nd ESMO Congress; 2017.
28. Forde PM, Chaft JE, Smith KN, et al. Neoadjuvant PD-1 blockade in resectable lung cancer. N Engl J Med 2018;378(21):1976–86.

Induced Pluripotent Stem Cell-Derived T Cells for Cancer Immunotherapy

Sunny J. Patel, BS[a,b], Takayoshi Yamauchi, PhD[a,c,d], Fumito Ito, MD, PhD[a,e,f],*

KEYWORDS

- Reprogramming • Induced pluripotent stem cells • T cells • Adoptive T cell therapy
- Immunotherapy • Stem cells

KEY POINTS

- Despite full effector function, differentiated T cells currently available for adoptive cell therapy exhibit less expansion, persistence, and antitumor efficacy in vivo against solid malignancies compared with less-differentiated T cells.
- Induced pluripotent stem cells (iPSCs) can self-renew and provide an unlimited number of autologous less-differentiated antigen-specific T cells that can mediate effective regression of established tumor and establish antigen-specific immunologic memory in vivo.
- Development of highly reproducible and robust differentiation protocols for clinically applicable large-scale production of tumor-specific iPSC-derived T cells is needed.

BACKGROUND

T Cells for Cancer Immunotherapy

$CD8^+$ T cells play a critical role in adaptive immunity by virtue of their ability to initiate killing following receptor-mediated engagement by antigens expressed on the surface of tumor cells.[1] $CD8^+$ T cell-mediated cytotoxicity requires direct contact with target cells, thereby limiting damage to bystander cells. The attractiveness of target-specific

Disclosure Statement: The authors have nothing to disclose.

[a] Center for Immunotherapy, Roswell Park Comprehensive Cancer Center, Buffalo, NY, USA; [b] Medical College of Georgia, Augusta University, 1120 Fifteen Street, Augusta, GA 30912-3600, USA; [c] Department of Molecular Enzymology, Faculty of Life Sciences, Kumamoto University, Kumamoto, 860-8556, Japan; [d] Center for Metabolic Regulation of Healthy Aging, Faculty of Life Sciences, Kumamoto University, Kumamoto, 860-8556, Japan; [e] Department of Surgical Oncology, Roswell Park Comprehensive Cancer Center, Elm and Carlton Streets, CCC-539, Buffalo, NY 14263, USA; [f] Department of Surgery, Jacobs School of Medicine and Biomedical Sciences, State University of New York at Buffalo, Buffalo, NY, USA

* Corresponding author. Department of Surgical Oncology, Roswell Park Comprehensive Cancer Center, Elm and Carlton Streets, CCC-539, Buffalo, NY 14263.

E-mail address: fumito.ito@roswellpark.org

approaches lies in avoidance of the serious side effects of other conventional treatments such as chemotherapy and radiation, which have relatively nonspecific mechanisms of action. A unique feature of the immune response, unlike conventional cancer therapies, is that it can elicit long-term protection from recurring disease (immunologic memory).[2] Another significant advantage of T cell-based immunotherapies is that T cells can search out and traffic to widely disseminated heterogeneous tumor cell targets by using chemokine-chemokine receptor interaction and generalized Lévy walks.[3,4]

Current Status of Adoptive T Cell Therapy

Significant advances have been made in the development of adoptive cell therapy (ACT) aiming to boost the immune response directed against chronic viral infections and various cancers.[5–14] ACT using autologous tumor-infiltrating lymphocytes (TILs) has been used clinically for several decades, and was found to mediate objective tumor regression in 50% to 70% of patients with interleukin-2 (IL-2)-refractory metastatic melanoma in combination with lymphodepleting chemotherapy and systemic high-dose IL-2 administration.[14,15] In addition, ACT using genetic modification of peripheral blood lymphocytes with a T cell receptor (TCR)- or a chimeric antigen receptor (CAR)-specific for tumor-specific antigen can mediate regression in multiple cancer histologies.[5–12] Both technologies can augment T cell function by altering receptor specificity and signaling functions that control proliferative capacity and other cellular functions.[5–12] In the former approach, T cells with enhanced affinity or novel specificity are created by expression of TCR α/β heterodimers in peripheral blood T cells.[10–13] The endogenous repertoire for TCRs is generally of low affinity when targeting shared tumor-associated antigen because of the impact of central tolerance; however, TCRs targeting neoantigens, in which mutations in the cancer genome create neo-epitopes, have high affinity.[16,17] Furthermore, the affinity and functional avidity of tumor antigen-specific TCRs can be enhanced by high-throughput genetic approaches.[18–20] NY-ESO-1 is expressed in a variety of cancers, but not in normal adult tissues, except for germ cells of the testis, making it an ideal target for immunotherapy.[21,22] NY-ESO-1-specific TCR-engineered T cells have generated clinical responses in patients with advanced multiple myeloma, melanoma, and synovial cell sarcoma.[11–13] TCR-based targeting approaches are, however, often susceptible to the common tumor escape mechanisms of major histocompatibility complex (MHC) down-modulation and altered peptide processing.[23]

The concept of CAR technology dates to the 1980s when Gross and colleagues[24] engineered and expressed chimeric TCR genes comprising antigen-binding domains fused to T cell signaling domains. Because the target-binding moiety is derived from antibodies with higher affinity than TCRα/β, CARs enable highly specific targeting of antigen in an MHC-independent fashion.[5–9] Adoptive transfer of CD19-directed CAR-T cells has generated complete and durable remissions in patients with refractory and relapsed B cell malignancies, such as acute lymphoblastic leukemia, chronic lymphocytic leukemia, and non-Hodgkin lymphoma.[6–9] There is growing optimism as we develop a better understanding of these technologies, which continue to reveal the potential in adoptive T cell therapy.

Limitations to Adoptive T Cell Therapy for Solid Malignancies

Whereas adoptive T cell therapy demonstrated impressive clinical response with long-term remission for hematological malignancies, this success has not yet been concluded in solid malignancies.[25] Despite encouraging results in preclinical models and in patients, poor survival of infused T cells and the existence of immune suppressive pathways seem to restrict the full potential of ACT for solid tumors. Current clinical ACT protocols require extensive ex vivo manipulation of autologous T cells to obtain large numbers, resulting in the generation of fully differentiated effector T cells. Whereas these differentiated T cells are equipped with full effector function, they are severely impaired in their proliferative capacity (**Fig. 1**).[26–28] Trafficking of infused T cells to the tumor is a critical step for successful immunotherapy that correlates with clinical responses in patients.[29] However, the tumor microenvironment (TME) characterized by abnormal tumor vessels and interstitium limits lymphocyte adhesion, extravasation, and infiltration.[30] As a result, only a fraction of ex vivo expanded T cells can infiltrate into the tumor tissue.[29]

Cancer cells reprogram their metabolism to meet the rapid energy requirements for proliferation, survival, and metastasis.[31] Glycolytic metabolism of glucose results in lactic acid, which can acidify the TME.[32] Acidosis and hypoxia are considered biochemical hallmarks of the TME[33,34] that not only modulate cancer cell metabolism but also influence T cell proliferation and effector function.[35] Hypoxia induces FoxP3, a key transcriptional regulator for regulatory T cells (Tregs),[36] and polarizes CD4$^+$ T cells toward a Th2 phenotype,[37] allowing the resultant IL-4 and IL-13 to induce macrophage M2 polarization.[38]

Tumor-associated macrophages (TAMs) are the major immunoregulatory cells in tumors, considered to have an M2 phenotype and secrete an array of cytokines, chemokines, and enzymes, which can suppress T cell effector function.[39] TAMs secrete chemokines, CCL5, CCL20, and CCL22 that recruit natural Treg cells (nTreg) and arginase I, which inhibit TCR ζ chain re-expression in activated T cells by the depletion of L-arginine.[40] IL-10 and transforming growth factor β produced by TAMs can induce regulatory functions by the upregulation of the Foxp3 and cytotoxic T lymphocyte antigen 4 (CTLA-4) in CD4$^+$ T cells, and the expression of the programmed death-ligand 1 (PD-L1) in monocytes—a coinhibitory molecule that can inhibit CD8$^+$ T cell functions.[40–44] Through hypoxia-inducible factor 1α signaling, myeloid-derived suppressor cells and TAMs in the hypoxic TME upregulate PD-L1 on macrophages.[45] Continuous exposure to chronically expressed tumor antigens drives T cells into senescence and exhaustion, characterized by expression of coinhibitory molecules such as T cell immunoglobulin, mucin domain-containing protein 3, lymphocyte activation gene 3 protein, PD-1, and CTLA-4 with impaired effector functions and proliferative capacity.[27,46–48]

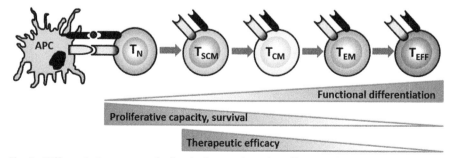

Fig. 1. Differentiation status of adoptively transferred T cells inversely correlates with therapeutic efficacy. APC, antigen-presenting cell; T_{CM}, central memory T cells; T_{EFF}, effector T cells; T_{EM}, effector memory T cells; T_N, naive T cells; T_{SCM}, stem cell memory T cells. (*Data from* Sallusto F, Lanzavecchia A. Memory in disguise. Nat Med 2011;17(10):1182–3.)

Ideal T Cell Subsets for Adoptive T Cell Therapy

These limitations signify the necessity of identifying T cell subsets that maintain the ability to proliferate, effectively traffic to the TME, exhibit robust effector function, and mediate regression of tumors for ACT. Accumulating evidence from preclinical and clinical studies has shown that less-differentiated "younger" T cells with longer telomere persist longer and exhibit more potent antitumor efficacy than differentiated T cells after adoptive transfer.[26,27,49–54] Using murine B16 melanoma model with Pmel-1 TCR transgenic mice specific for the gp100 antigen expressed on B16 tumors, adoptive transfer of central memory T cells (T_{CM}: CD62L^{hi} CD44^{hi}) exhibited superior expansion, persistence, and antitumor efficacy in vivo compared with effector memory T cells (T_{EM}: CD62L^{lo} CD44^{hi} KLRG-1^{lo}) or terminally differentiated effector T cells (T_{EFF}: CD62L^{lo} CD44^{hi} KLRG-1^{hi}).[26,27,49] Even more resounding was the result that stem cell memory T cells (T_{SCM}: CD62L^{hi} CD44^{lo} stem cell antigen-1^{hi} CD122^{hi}) were even more potent than T_{CM} on a per-cell basis.[52–55] Preclinical and clinical studies found a significant correlation between T cell differentiation status and antitumor efficacy, indicating the superiority of T_{SCM} cells over other memory CD8$^+$ T cell subsets.[52–54] Finally, in addition to evaluating memory and effector subsets individually, the ability of natural Ag-specific T_{EFF} derived from different CD8$^+$ T cell subsets, specifically naive T cells (T_N) and T_{CM}, has also been assessed in mice and humans.[56,57] Compared with T_{EFF} derived from T_{CM}, naive-derived T_{EFF} retained the ability to release IL-2 while withholding the acquisition of the senesce marker, KLRG-1.[56,57] When adoptively transferred into tumor-bearing mice, T_N-derived T_{EFF} demonstrated superior in vivo expansion, persistence, and antitumor efficacy relative to T_{CM}-derived T_{EFF}.[57] In humans, these cells also maintained significantly higher CD27 and longer telomere lengths after ex vivo expansion, suggesting greater proliferative potential.[56] These results suggest that the ability of T cells to mediate tumor regression decreases with differentiation. Overall, the increased potential to self-proliferate and differentiate into memory and effector T cell subsets allows less-differentiated forms, such as T_{SCM} and T_N, to regulate and sustain effective tumor regression and foster superior antitumor efficacy relative to differentiated effector cells.

An array of possible approaches has been proposed to enhance the efficacy of ACT. Initial antigen signal strength,[58] quality of costimulation,[59] and the presence of cytokines, such as IL-2, IL-7, and IL-15,[49,60] may influence the relative ratio of T_{CM} to T_{EM} and T_{EFF} generated in response to antigen. Therefore, modulating immunomodulatory cytokines used in ACT along with adapting the duration and nature of T cell ex vivo culture conditions can enhance the in vivo function of tumor-specific CD8$^+$ T cells by selecting and generating optimal memory T cells in patients with cancer. Another strategy involves altering metabolism within T cells, primarily inhibiting glycolytic pathways noted to be drivers of terminal effector differentiation. This may promote long-lived CD8$^+$ T cell immunity and enhanced tumor destruction.[61] In vitro culturing of T cells in the presence of small molecules provides cell products with superior engraftment, expansion, and antitumor immunity after adoptive transfer. Inhibition of GSK3, a vital component of the oncogenic WNT signaling pathway, maintains stemness in mature memory CD8$^+$ T cells providing self-renewal capability and multipotency superior to central memory T cells.[54] Collectively, less-differentiated tumor antigen-specific T cells are ideal T cell subsets for ACT; however, generating large numbers of these "younger" T cells is problematic.

Classification of Stem Cells Based on Differentiation Potential

Stem cells are defined by dual hallmark features of self-renewal and differentiation potential.[62–64] These cells are classified into several types according to their capacity to differentiate into specialized cells. A totipotent cell such as a zygote (a fertilized egg) and blastomeres during early cleavage of the embryo can give rise to a new organism given appropriate maternal support. They can also differentiate into embryonic and extra-embryonic cell types such as the fetal membranes and placenta.[65]

Pluripotent stem cells (PSCs) can self-renew and have the ability to form all 3 embryonic germ layers (ie, ectoderm, endoderm, and mesoderm). Embryonic stem cells (ESCs) epitomize quintessential PSCs that can be isolated from the inner cell mass of blastocysts and cultured as immortal cell lines.[66,67] Multipotent stem cells can self-renew, but differentiate into all cell types within one particular lineage.[64] These include neural stem cells that are derived from neural tissues and can give rise to all cell types (neurons, astrocytes, and oligodendrocytes) of the nervous system.[68] Mesenchymal stem cells are also multipotent stromal cells that can be isolated from the bone marrow.[69] They are nonhematopoietic, multipotent stem cells with the capacity to differentiate into mesodermal lineage such as bone cells, cartilage cells, muscle cells, and fat cells.

The Rise of Induced Pluripotency

The understanding of induced pluripotency has developed over the last 6 decades with the aid of advancing discoveries and technologies. The first PSCs cultured in vitro were derived from a type of germ line tumor called teratocarcinoma.[70] The breakthrough came when researchers showed that PSCs can be isolated from mouse blastocysts and propagated in vitro as immortalized, nontransformed cell lines.[66,67] Later, Thomson and colleagues[71] showed that PSCs can be derived from human embryos. However, ethical concerns using human zygotes and immune rejection of grafted stem cells limit the use of human ESCs.

In 2006 Takahashi and Yamanaka demonstrated that the transient expression of only 4 transcription factors (Oct4, Sox2, Klf4, and c-Myc) was sufficient to convert murine fibroblasts into induced PSCs (iPSCs), which are embryonic stemlike cells that demonstrate the same pluripotency and self-renewal properties.[72] Only a year later, the successful derivation of human iPSCs from fibroblasts was reported.[73,74] Human iPSCs circumvent the ethical controversies and rejection problem associated with using autologous stem cells; they provide a valuable source of patient-specific cells for the study and potential treatment of human diseases. Remarkable progress made in reprogramming technology over the past decade has also facilitated the generation of human iPSCs with a minimally invasive approach from several human cell types such as keratinocytes, dental stem cells, oral gingival, oral mucosa fibroblasts, and cord blood cells.[75–80]

In 2010, 3 groups reported the generation of human iPSCs from peripheral blood T cells.[81–83] The use of peripheral blood cells as a source for iPSCs is a less invasive procedure compared with having patients undergo skin biopsy for obtaining fibroblasts. Although all 3 groups used the same 4 transcription factors (Oct4, Sox2, Klf4, and c-Myc) to generate T cell-derived human iPSCs (T-iPSCs), reprogramming efficiency was different. Seki and colleagues[81] introduced the 4 factors with Sendai virus vectors and found that only 1 mL of whole blood was sufficient to generate human iPSCs. In addition to higher induction efficiency, Sendai virus vectors have some advantages for the generation of human iPSCs. Unlike integrating viral (eg, retroviral or lentiviral) vectors, Sendai virus vectors only replicate in the cytoplasm of infected cells and do not integrate into the host genome.[84] Moreover, temperature-sensitive mutations in the viral genome allow for rapid removal of residual viral genomic RNA from reprogrammed cells.[85] Generation of transgene-free iPSCs by nonintegrating Sendai virus vectors minimizes the risk of tumor formation associated with random oncogene activation or tumor supressor inactivation.

During normal αβ T cell development, *TCRA* and *TCRB* genes are rearranged in the thymus. Detection of TCR gene arrangement in iPSCs indicates derivation from cells of the T lineage.[81–83] Using Sendai virus vectors, we have also found efficient generation of human iPSCs from peripheral blood T cells (**Fig. 2**). Furthermore, we have shown successful derivation of human iPSCs from melanoma TILs expressing high levels of PD-1.[86] A wide variety of TCR gene rearrangement patterns in TIL-derived iPSCs confirmed the heterogeneity of T cells infiltrating melanomas.[86] These findings also suggest the feasibility of rejuvenating fully differentiated and exhausted antigen-specific T cells by reprogramming and redifferentiation techniques for adoptive T cell therapy.

Potential of iPSCs to Generate T Cells for Adoptive Cell Therapy

Subsequently, a series of studies have provided insights into the function of rejuvenated antigen-specific T-iPSC-derived T cells. The tumor specificity of T-iPSC-derived T cells can be conferred by way of 2 approaches. One is to reprogram tumor antigen-specific T cells and redifferentiate T-iPSCs for the generation of T cells carrying the TCR recognizing the same tumor antigen (**Fig. 3**A). Vizcardo and colleagues[87] established T-iPSCs from a CD8$^+$ T cell clone specific for the melanoma antigen MART-1 using the Sendai virus reprogramming system. All regenerated CD8$^+$ T cells from T-iPSCs were found to express TCR specific for MART-1 antigen and produce interferon-γ (IFN-γ) in vitro.[87] Nishimura and colleagues[88] rejuvenated a HIV-1-specific CD8$^+$ T cell clone and demonstrated that regenerated iPSC-derived T cells have high proliferative capacity, antigen-specific killing activity, and elongated telomeres. Wakao and colleagues[89] generated T-iPSCs from human cord blood mucosal-associated invariant T (MAIT) cells, innate-like T cells that recognize derivatives of

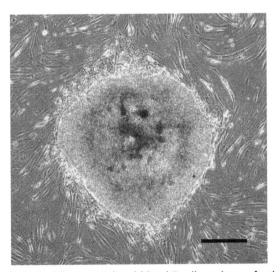

Fig. 2. Human iPSCs derived from peripheral blood T cells under on-feeder conditions. Peripheral blood T cells were reprogrammed by viral transduction of a Sendai virus vector carrying a cassette of the OCT3/4, SOX2, KLF4, and c-MYC. One day after reprogramming, cells were replated on to feeder cells. A human iPSC on feeder cells on day 19 is shown. Scale bar, 500 μm.

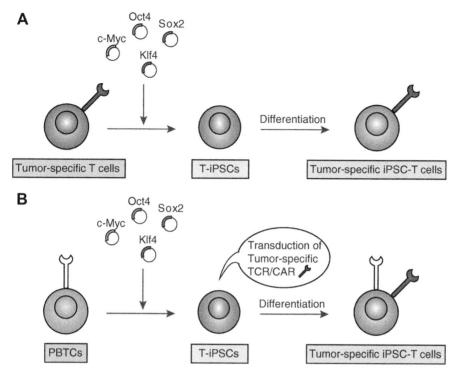

Fig. 3. Two approaches of generating tumor-specific T cells using autologous induced pluripotent stem cells (iPSCs) and reprogramming technology. (*A*) Reprogramming of tumor-specific T cells to generate T cell-derived human iPSCs (T-iPSCs) followed by redifferentiation to naive tumor-specific iPSC-derived T cells. (*B*) Reprogramming of peripheral blood T cells followed by transduction of TCR or CAR recognizing tumor antigen to T-iPSCs. Genetically engineered T-iPSCs differentiated to naive tumor-specific TCR/CAR-transduced iPSC-derived T cells.

precursors of bacterial riboflavin presented by the MHC class I-related molecule MR1. Regenerated MAIT cells possessed the ability to produce a wide variety of cytokines and chemokines in the presence of bacteria-fed monocytes.[89]

Whereas these studies use a strategy of reprogramming T cells with known antigen specificity and redifferentiating T-iPSCs for the generation of rejuvenated antigen-specific T cells, another approach is to genetically transfer a receptor with known specificity for an antigen into established iPSCs (**Fig. 3**B). Themeli and colleagues[90] have shown that T-iPSCs transduced with CAR specific for CD19 antigen can generate T cells that display antitumor immunity in a xenograft model of lymphoma. These studies suggest that iPSCs with CAR genetic modification have the potential to generate functional and expandable T cells specialized for tumor eradication.

In vivo Antitumor Efficacy of iPSC-Derived T Cells Against Solid Malignancies

Although these studies suggest in vivo antitumor efficacy of T-iPSC-derived T cells, it remains uncertain whether iPSC-derived T cells escape immune rejection (immunogenicity) and mediate effective regression of established tumor following adoptive transfer in an immunocompetent host. Some studies have shown that certain iPSC-derived cells, such as smooth muscle cells and cardiomyocytes, are immunogenic, whereas other cell types, such as retinal pigment epithelial, hepatocytes, and neuronal cells, exhibit little to no immunogenicity.[91–94]

To this end, we have recently established a preclinical murine model in which Pmel-1 TCR transgenic CD8$^+$ T cells able to recognize gp100 antigen were rejuvenated to iPSC-derived T cells using the Sendai virus reprogramming system (**Fig. 4**).[95] This novel preclinical model has provided us with a variety of new findings and insights into not only the reprogramming process of iPSC technology but also its therapeutic potential through in vitro and in vivo analysis in an immunocompetent mouse model. We demonstrated for the first time that murine T cells, like human T cells, can be reprogrammed into iPSCs with the Sendai virus reprogramming system without the use of gene knockout mice or drug-inducible gene expression systems.[96,97] Of equal importance was our finding that dual inhibition (2i) of both prodifferentiation MEK and GSK-3 pathways, which was shown to support the establishment of mouse iPSCs from partially reprogrammed cells,[98] was required for reprogramming of Pmel-1 T cells. Rejuvenated iPSC-derived T cells were less-differentiated phenotypes that expressed memory T cell markers and acquired effector functions producing IFN-γ and tumor necrosis factor alpha after stimulation with the cognate antigen, gp100.[95] Furthermore, adoptive transfer of iPSC-derived regenerated T cells significantly delayed B16 tumor growth and improved overall survival in a lethal murine model of melanoma (**Fig. 5A, B**).[95] Importantly, an establishment of antigen-specific immunologic memory provides insight into immunogenicity of iPSC-derived T cells, and reveals the feasibility of generating long-lived tumor-specific T cells by way of reprogramming to pluripotency and redifferentiation (**Fig. 5C**).[95]

CHALLENGES/FUTURE DIRECTIONS

ESCs and iPSCs are tumorigenic cells that can cause teratoma on transplantation.[99] For clinical translation of iPSC-derived T cell therapies, the tumorigenic potential of contaminated iPSCs and the malignant transformation of differentiated iPSCs (tumorigenicity) are major safety concerns.[100,101] Whereas the tumorigenic risks of iPSC-derived products can be reduced by several methods,[102–105] these methods may not be satisfactory because tumorigenic risk arises not only from contamination with undifferentiated iPSCs, but also from intermediate products having altered proliferation potential and/or with tumorigenic transformed cells.[100]

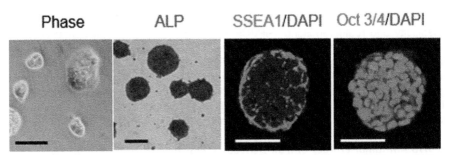

Fig. 4. Generation of iPSCs from Pmel-1 TCR transgenic CD8$^+$ T cells. Morphology, alkaline phosphatase (ALP) activity, and expression of pluripotency and surface markers (SSEA1 and Oct3/4) in Pmel-1 iPSCs. Scale bars, 200 μm. (*From* Saito H, Okita K, Chang AE, et al. Adoptive transfer of CD8+ T cells generated from induced pluripotent stem cells triggers regressions of large tumors along with immunologic memory. Cancer Res 2016;76(12):3473–83; with permission.)

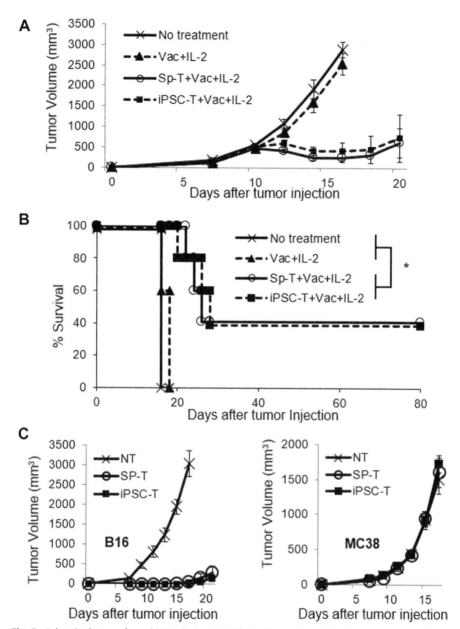

Fig. 5. Adoptively transferred iPSC-derived CD8$^+$ T cells mediate effective regression of large tumors and establish immunologic memory. (*A, B*) Tumor growth curves (*A*) and survival curves (*B*) in C57BL/6 mice bearing B16 melanomas established for 11 days in different treatment groups. Vac, vaccination with the gp100 antigen, anti-CD40 mAb, poly(I:C), and imiquimod cream. Tumor volume results are the mean of measurements from 5 mice per group (*$P<.0001$ using log-rank [Mantel-Cox] test). (*C*) Surviving mice (n = 4) after adoptive transfer of Pmel-1 iPSC-derived or splenic T cells, vaccination, and IL-2 were rechallenged with B16 cells into the contralateral flank and MC38 cells on the back on day 80. Tumor growth curves are depicted in which $T = 0$ corresponds to the time of injection of secondary tumors. As a control, tumor growth was monitored following inoculation of the same tumor cell dose into nontumor (NT) experienced naive C57BL/6 mice (n = 5). (*From* Saito H, Okita K, Chang AE, et al. Adoptive transfer of CD8+ T cells generated from induced pluripotent stem cells triggers regressions of large tumors along with immunological memory. Cancer Res 2016;76(12):3473–83; with permission.)

Current methods of in vitro differentiation of T lymphocytes from human iPSCs use coculture with murine OP9 bone marrow stromal cells expressing the Notch ligand delta-like 1 (OP9-DL1).[106] To translate this strategy into routine clinical practice, it will be essential to find a way to differentiate iPSCs under xeno-free conditions. Furthermore, regenerated human iPSC-derived T cells express CD3, TCRαβ, and CD8α, but not CD8β. Therefore, these regenerated iPSC-derived T cells possess CD8αα homodimers but not CD8αβ heterodimers.[107] CD8αα homodimer has been found only on a small portion of developing thymocytes, gut intraepithelial lymphocytes, and a subset of NK cells and dendritic cells.[108] Although both forms of the CD8 molecule bind to MHC class I with similar affinity, studies have shown that the CD8αα homodimer is a functionally weaker coreceptor than CD8αβ for TCR-based activation.[109,110] Moreover, Themeli and colleagues[90] have shown that CAR-iPSC-derived T cells possess an innate γδ T cell-like profile. In contrast, we have found that regenerated murine iPSC-derived T cells express both CD8α and CD8β (CD8αβ heterodimer), which might be because of the use of the sorting procedure performed before activation with the cognate antigen.[95] In line with our study, Maeda and colleagues[107] have recently shown that isolating CD4+CD8+ double-positive (DP) T cells before activation with anti-CD3 antibody can generate human CD8αβ iPSC-derived T cells. Nevertheless, development of feeder-free and xeno-free culture procedures for the generation of CD8αβ T cells will be ideal for clinical use of iPSC-derived T cells. Of note, Vizcardo and colleagues[111] recently developed a 3D thymic culture system in a preclinical model and showed successful generation of murine CD8αβ iPSC-derived T cells without the use of OP9-DL1 feeder cells.

Lastly, TCRα gene rearrangement takes place when T cells are at the CD4+CD8+ DP stage in the thymus.[112,113] Additional rearrangement of TCR α chain may occur when iPSC-derived T cells become CD4+CD8+ DP T cells. This may produce T cells with unpredictable antigen specificity, and adoptive transfer of these T cells may cause unpredictable autoimmune reactions because they do not go through thymic positive and negative selection. A possible solution would be to downregulate the expression of the recombination activating genes 1 and 2 to stop further endogenous TCRα gene rearrangement by CRISPR/Cas9 genome editing.[114–116]

SUMMARY

ACT with antigen-specific T cells is a promising approach for treating patients with a variety of malignancies. Despite remarkable success seen in the treatment of hematological malignancies, the difficulty with generating sufficient numbers of tumor-specific T cells harboring characteristics necessary for in vivo effectiveness remains a major obstacle to ACT for solid malignancies. Use of iPSCs to provide an unlimited number of autologous less-differentiated antigen-specific T cells can theoretically overcome these limitations, and holds great promise for adoptive T cell therapy. Whereas autologous iPSC-derived T cells provide a bright future for personalized cancer treatment, many challenges still remain before these cells can be used clinically in patients. Safety and therapeutic efficacy of iPSC-derived T cells need to be further evaluated in preclinical models before they are translated into clinic.

ACKNOWLEDGMENTS

We would like to acknowledge funding support from the Roswell Park Alliance Foundation, the Melanoma Research Alliance, the Sarcoma Foundation of America, and the National Cancer Institute (NCI) grant, K08CA197966 (F. Ito).

REFERENCES

1. Zhang N, Bevan MJ. CD8(+) T cells: foot soldiers of the immune system. Immunity 2011;35(2):161–8.
2. Williams MA, Bevan MJ. Effector and memory CTL differentiation. Annu Rev Immunol 2007;25:171–92.
3. Harris TH, Banigan EJ, Christian DA, et al. Generalized Levy walks and the role of chemokines in migration of effector CD8+ T cells. Nature 2012;486(7404): 545–8.
4. Nagarsheth N, Wicha MS, Zou W. Chemokines in the cancer microenvironment and their relevance in cancer immunotherapy. Nat Rev Immunol 2017;17(9): 559–72.
5. Kochenderfer JN, Wilson WH, Janik JE, et al. Eradication of B-lineage cells and regression of lymphoma in a patient treated with autologous T cells genetically engineered to recognize CD19. Blood 2010;116(20):4099–102.
6. Maus MV, Fraietta JA, Levine BL, et al. Adoptive immunotherapy for cancer or viruses. Annu Rev Immunol 2014;32:189–225.
7. Porter DL, Levine BL, Kalos M, et al. Chimeric antigen receptor-modified T cells in chronic lymphoid leukemia. N Engl J Med 2011;365(8):725–33.
8. Grupp SA, Kalos M, Barrett D, et al. Chimeric antigen receptor-modified T cells for acute lymphoid leukemia. N Engl J Med 2013;368(16):1509–18.
9. Maude SL, Frey N, Shaw PA, et al. Chimeric antigen receptor T cells for sustained remissions in leukemia. N Engl J Med 2014;371(16):1507–17.
10. Morgan RA, Dudley ME, Wunderlich JR, et al. Cancer regression in patients after transfer of genetically engineered lymphocytes. Science 2006;314(5796): 126–9.
11. Rapoport AP, Stadtmauer EA, Binder-Scholl GK, et al. NY-ESO-1-specific TCR-engineered T cells mediate sustained antigen-specific antitumor effects in myeloma. Nat Med 2015;21(8):914–21.
12. Robbins PF, Morgan RA, Feldman SA, et al. Tumor regression in patients with metastatic synovial cell sarcoma and melanoma using genetically engineered lymphocytes reactive with NY-ESO-1. J Clin Oncol 2011;29(7):917–24.
13. Robbins PF, Kassim SH, Tran TL, et al. A pilot trial using lymphocytes genetically engineered with an NY-ESO-1-reactive T-cell receptor: long-term follow-up and correlates with response. Clin Cancer Res 2015;21(5):1019–27.
14. Rosenberg SA, Yang JC, Sherry RM, et al. Durable complete responses in heavily pretreated patients with metastatic melanoma using T-cell transfer immunotherapy. Clin Cancer Res 2011;17(13):4550–7.
15. Rosenberg SA, Packard BS, Aebersold PM, et al. Use of tumor-infiltrating lymphocytes and interleukin-2 in the immunotherapy of patients with metastatic melanoma. A preliminary report. N Engl J Med 1988;319(25):1676–80.
16. Tran E, Robbins PF, Lu YC, et al. T-cell transfer therapy targeting mutant KRAS in cancer. N Engl J Med 2016;375(23):2255–62.
17. Tran E, Ahmadzadeh M, Lu YC, et al. Immunogenicity of somatic mutations in human gastrointestinal cancers. Science 2015;350(6266):1387–90.
18. Chervin AS, Aggen DH, Raseman JM, et al. Engineering higher affinity T cell receptors using a T cell display system. J Immunol Methods 2008;339(2):175–84.
19. Li Y, Moysey R, Molloy PE, et al. Directed evolution of human T-cell receptors with picomolar affinities by phage display. Nat Biotechnol 2005;23(3):349–54.

20. Kuball J, Hauptrock B, Malina V, et al. Increasing functional avidity of TCR-redirected T cells by removing defined N-glycosylation sites in the TCR constant domain. J Exp Med 2009;206(2):463–75.

21. Chen YT, Scanlan MJ, Sahin U, et al. A testicular antigen aberrantly expressed in human cancers detected by autologous antibody screening. Proc Natl Acad Sci U S A 1997;94(5):1914–8.

22. Odunsi K, Jungbluth AA, Stockert E, et al. NY-ESO-1 and LAGE-1 cancer-testis antigens are potential targets for immunotherapy in epithelial ovarian cancer. Cancer Res 2003;63(18):6076–83.

23. Itoh Y, Hemmer B, Martin R, et al. Serial TCR engagement and down-modulation by peptide:MHC molecule ligands: relationship to the quality of individual TCR signaling events. J Immunol 1999;162(4):2073–80.

24. Gross G, Waks T, Eshhar Z. Expression of immunoglobulin-T-cell receptor chimeric molecules as functional receptors with antibody-type specificity. Proc Natl Acad Sci U S A 1989;86(24):10024–8.

25. Klebanoff CA, Rosenberg SA, Restifo NP. Prospects for gene-engineered T cell immunotherapy for solid cancers. Nat Med 2016;22(1):26–36.

26. Gattinoni L, Klebanoff CA, Palmer DC, et al. Acquisition of full effector function in vitro paradoxically impairs the in vivo antitumor efficacy of adoptively transferred CD8+ T cells. J Clin Invest 2005;115(6):1616–26.

27. Restifo NP, Dudley ME, Rosenberg SA. Adoptive immunotherapy for cancer: harnessing the T cell response. Nat Rev Immunol 2012;12(4):269–81.

28. Sallusto F, Lanzavecchia A. Memory in disguise. Nat Med 2011;17:1182.

29. Pockaj BA, Sherry RM, Wei JP, et al. Localization of 111indium-labeled tumor infiltrating lymphocytes to tumor in patients receiving adoptive immunotherapy. Augmentation with cyclophosphamide and correlation with response. Cancer 1994;73(6):1731–7.

30. Chung AS, Lee J, Ferrara N. Targeting the tumour vasculature: insights from physiological angiogenesis. Nat Rev Cancer 2010;10(7):505–14.

31. Hanahan D, Weinberg RA. Hallmarks of cancer: the next generation. Cell 2011; 144(5):646–74.

32. Gatenby RA, Gillies RJ. Why do cancers have high aerobic glycolysis? Nat Rev Cancer 2004;4(11):891–9.

33. Gatenby RA, Gillies RJ. A microenvironmental model of carcinogenesis. Nat Rev Cancer 2008;8(1):56–61.

34. Brahimi-Horn MC, Bellot G, Pouyssegur J. Hypoxia and energetic tumour metabolism. Curr Opin Genet Dev 2011;21(1):67–72.

35. Mellor AL, Munn DH. Creating immune privilege: active local suppression that benefits friends, but protects foes. Nat Rev Immunol 2008;8(1):74–80.

36. Clambey ET, McNamee EN, Westrich JA, et al. Hypoxia-inducible factor-1 alpha-dependent induction of FoxP3 drives regulatory T-cell abundance and function during inflammatory hypoxia of the mucosa. Proc Natl Acad Sci U S A 2012;109(41):E2784–93.

37. Yang M, Ma C, Liu S, et al. Hypoxia skews dendritic cells to a T helper type 2-stimulating phenotype and promotes tumour cell migration by dendritic cell-derived osteopontin. Immunology 2009;128(1 Suppl):e237–49.

38. Murray PJ, Allen JE, Biswas SK, et al. Macrophage activation and polarization: nomenclature and experimental guidelines. Immunity 2014;41(1):14–20.

39. Grivennikov SI, Greten FR, Karin M. Immunity, inflammation, and cancer. Cell 2010;140(6):883–99.

40. Adeegbe DO, Nishikawa H. Natural and induced T regulatory cells in cancer. Front Immunol 2013;4:190.
41. Daurkin I, Eruslanov E, Stoffs T, et al. Tumor-associated macrophages mediate immunosuppression in the renal cancer microenvironment by activating the 15-lipoxygenase-2 pathway. Cancer Res 2011;71(20):6400–9.
42. Ng TH, Britton GJ, Hill EV, et al. Regulation of adaptive immunity; the role of inter-leukin-10. Front Immunol 2013;4:129.
43. Oh SA, Li MO. TGF-beta: guardian of T cell function. J Immunol 2013;191(8):3973–9.
44. Kuang DM, Zhao Q, Peng C, et al. Activated monocytes in peritumoral stroma of hepatocellular carcinoma foster immune privilege and disease progression through PD-L1. J Exp Med 2009;206(6):1327–37.
45. Henze AT, Mazzone M. The impact of hypoxia on tumor-associated macrophages. J Clin Invest 2016;126(10):3672–9.
46. Baitsch L, Baumgaertner P, Devevre E, et al. Exhaustion of tumor-specific CD8(+) T cells in metastases from melanoma patients. J Clin Invest 2011;121(6):2350–60.
47. Ahmadzadeh M, Johnson LA, Heemskerk B, et al. Tumor antigen-specific CD8 T cells infiltrating the tumor express high levels of PD-1 and are functionally impaired. Blood 2009;114(8):1537–44.
48. Wherry EJ. T cell exhaustion. Nat Immunol 2011;12(6):492–9.
49. Klebanoff CA, Gattinoni L, Torabi-Parizi P, et al. Central memory self/tumor-reactive CD8+ T cells confer superior antitumor immunity compared with effector memory T cells. Proc Natl Acad Sci U S A 2005;102(27):9571–6.
50. Dudley ME, Gross CA, Langhan MM, et al. CD8+ enriched "young" tumor infil-trating lymphocytes can mediate regression of metastatic melanoma. Clin Cancer Res 2010;16(24):6122–31.
51. Zhou J, Shen X, Huang J, et al. Telomere length of transferred lymphocytes cor-relates with in vivo persistence and tumor regression in melanoma patients receiving cell transfer therapy. J Immunol 2005;175(10):7046–52.
52. Gattinoni L, Klebanoff CA, Restifo NP. Paths to stemness: building the ultimate antitumour T cell. Nat Rev Cancer 2012;12(10):671–84.
53. Gattinoni L, Lugli E, Ji Y, et al. A human memory T cell subset with stem cell-like properties. Nat Med 2011;17(10):1290–7.
54. Gattinoni L, Zhong X-S, Palmer DC, et al. Wnt signaling arrests effector T cell dif-ferentiation and generates CD8+ memory stem cells. Nat Med 2009;15(7):808–13.
55. Lugli E, Dominguez MH, Gattinoni L, et al. Superior T memory stem cell persis-tence supports long-lived T cell memory. J Clin Invest 2013;123(2):594–9.
56. Hinrichs CS, Borman ZA, Gattinoni L, et al. Human effector CD8+ T cells derived from naive rather than memory subsets possess superior traits for adoptive immunotherapy. Blood 2011;117(3):808–14.
57. Hinrichs CS, Borman ZA, Cassard L, et al. Adoptively transferred effector cells derived from naive rather than central memory CD8+ T cells mediate superior antitumor immunity. Proc Natl Acad Sci U S A 2009;106(41):17469–74.
58. van Faassen H, Saldanha M, Gilbertson D, et al. Reducing the stimulation of CD8+ T cells during infection with intracellular bacteria promotes differentiation primarily into a central (CD62LhighCD44high) subset. J Immunol 2005;174(9):5341–50.
59. Gett AV, Sallusto F, Lanzavecchia A, et al. T cell fitness determined by signal strength. Nat Immunol 2003;4(4):355–60.

60. Klebanoff CA, Finkelstein SE, Surman DR, et al. IL-15 enhances the in vivo anti-tumor activity of tumor-reactive CD8+ T cells. Proc Natl Acad Sci U S A 2004; 101(7):1969–74.

61. Sukumar M, Liu J, Ji Y, et al. Inhibiting glycolytic metabolism enhances CD8+ T cell memory and antitumor function. J Clin Invest 2013;123(10):4479–88.

62. De Los Angeles A, Ferrari F, Xi R, et al. Hallmarks of pluripotency. Nature 2015; 525(7570):469–78.

63. Hanna JH, Saha K, Jaenisch R. Pluripotency and cellular reprogramming: facts, hypotheses, unresolved issues. Cell 2010;143(4):508–25.

64. Daley GQ. Stem cells and the evolving notion of cellular identity. Philos Trans R Soc Lond B Biol Sci 2015;370(1680):20140376.

65. Condic ML. Totipotency: what it is and what it is not. Stem Cells Dev 2014;23(8): 796–812.

66. Evans MJ, Kaufman MH. Establishment in culture of pluripotential cells from mouse embryos. Nature 1981;292(5819):154–6.

67. Martin GR. Isolation of a pluripotent cell line from early mouse embryos cultured in medium conditioned by teratocarcinoma stem cells. Proc Natl Acad Sci U S A 1981;78(12):7634–8.

68. Conti L, Cattaneo E. Neural stem cell systems: physiological players or in vitro entities? Nat Rev Neurosci 2010;11(3):176–87.

69. Joyce N, Annett G, Wirthlin L, et al. Mesenchymal stem cells for the treatment of neurodegenerative disease. Regen Med 2010;5(6):933–46.

70. Hogan BL. Changes in the behaviour of teratocarcinoma cells cultivated in vitro. Nature 1976;263(5573):136–7.

71. Thomson JA, Itskovitz-Eldor J, Shapiro SS, et al. Embryonic stem cell lines derived from human blastocysts. Science 1998;282(5391):1145–7.

72. Takahashi K, Yamanaka S. Induction of pluripotent stem cells from mouse embryonic and adult fibroblast cultures by defined factors. Cell 2006;126(4): 663–76.

73. Takahashi K, Tanabe K, Ohnuki M, et al. Induction of pluripotent stem cells from adult human fibroblasts by defined factors. Cell 2007;131(5):861–72.

74. Yu J, Vodyanik MA, Smuga-Otto K, et al. Induced pluripotent stem cell lines derived from human somatic cells. Science 2007;318(5858):1917–20.

75. Aasen T, Raya A, Barrero MJ, et al. Efficient and rapid generation of induced pluripotent stem cells from human keratinocytes. Nat Biotechnol 2008;26(11): 1276–84.

76. Yan X, Qin H, Qu C, et al. iPS cells reprogrammed from human mesenchymal-like stem/progenitor cells of dental tissue origin. Stem Cells Dev 2010;19(4): 469–80.

77. Egusa H, Okita K, Kayashima H, et al. Gingival fibroblasts as a promising source of induced pluripotent stem cells. PLoS One 2010;5(9):e12743.

78. Miyoshi K, Tsuji D, Kudoh K, et al. Generation of human induced pluripotent stem cells from oral mucosa. J Biosci Bioeng 2010;110(3):345–50.

79. Haase A, Olmer R, Schwanke K, et al. Generation of induced pluripotent stem cells from human cord blood. Cell Stem Cell 2009;5(4):434–41.

80. Giorgetti A, Montserrat N, Aasen T, et al. Generation of induced pluripotent stem cells from human cord blood using OCT4 and SOX2. Cell Stem Cell 2009;5(4): 353–7.

81. Seki T, Yuasa S, Oda M, et al. Generation of induced pluripotent stem cells from human terminally differentiated circulating T cells. Cell Stem Cell 2010;7(1): 11–4.

82. Loh YH, Hartung O, Li H, et al. Reprogramming of T cells from human peripheral blood. Cell Stem Cell 2010;7(1):15–9.
83. Staerk J, Dawlaty MM, Gao Q, et al. Reprogramming of human peripheral blood cells to induced pluripotent stem cells. Cell Stem Cell 2010;7(1):20–4.
84. Li HO, Zhu YF, Asakawa M, et al. A cytoplasmic RNA vector derived from non-transmissible Sendai virus with efficient gene transfer and expression. J Virol 2000;74(14):6564–9.
85. Fusaki N, Ban H, Nishiyama A, et al. Efficient induction of transgene-free human pluripotent stem cells using a vector based on Sendai virus, an RNA virus that does not integrate into the host genome. Proc Jpn Acad Ser B Phys Biol Sci 2009;85(8):348–62.
86. Saito H, Okita K, Fusaki N, et al. Reprogramming of melanoma tumor-infiltrating lymphocytes to induced pluripotent stem cells. Stem Cells Int 2016; 2016(8394960):11.
87. Vizcardo R, Masuda K, Yamada D, et al. Regeneration of human tumor antigen-specific T cells from iPSCs derived from mature CD8(+) T cells. Cell Stem Cell 2013;12(1):31–6.
88. Nishimura T, Kaneko S, Kawana-Tachikawa A, et al. Generation of rejuvenated antigen-specific T cells by reprogramming to pluripotency and redifferentiation. Cell Stem Cell 2013;12(1):114–26.
89. Wakao H, Yoshikiyo K, Koshimizu U, et al. Expansion of functional human mucosal-associated invariant T cells via reprogramming to pluripotency and re-differentiation. Cell Stem Cell 2013;12(5):546–58.
90. Themeli M, Kloss CC, Ciriello G, et al. Generation of tumor-targeted human T lymphocytes from induced pluripotent stem cells for cancer therapy. Nat Biotechnol 2013;31(10):928–33.
91. Zhao T, Zhang ZN, Westenskow PD, et al. Humanized mice reveal differential immunogenicity of cells derived from autologous induced pluripotent stem cells. Cell Stem Cell 2015;17(3):353–9.
92. de Almeida PE, Meyer EH, Kooreman NG, et al. Transplanted terminally differentiated induced pluripotent stem cells are accepted by immune mechanisms similar to self-tolerance. Nat Commun 2014;5:3903.
93. Araki R, Uda M, Hoki Y, et al. Negligible immunogenicity of terminally differentiated cells derived from induced pluripotent or embryonic stem cells. Nature 2013;494(7435):100–4.
94. Guha P, Morgan JW, Mostoslavsky G, et al. Lack of immune response to differentiated cells derived from syngeneic induced pluripotent stem cells. Cell Stem Cell 2013;12(4):407–12.
95. Saito H, Okita K, Chang AE, et al. Adoptive transfer of CD8+ T cells generated from induced pluripotent stem cells triggers regressions of large tumors along with immunological memory. Cancer Res 2016;76(12):3473–83.
96. Hong H, Takahashi K, Ichisaka T, et al. Suppression of induced pluripotent stem cell generation by the p53-p21 pathway. Nature 2009;460(7259):1132–5.
97. Eminli S, Foudi A, Stadtfeld M, et al. Differentiation stage determines potential of hematopoietic cells for reprogramming into induced pluripotent stem cells. Nat Genet 2009;41(9):968–76.
98. Silva J, Barrandon O, Nichols J, et al. Promotion of reprogramming to ground state pluripotency by signal inhibition. PLoS Biol 2008;6(10):e253.
99. Ben-David U, Benvenisty N. The tumorigenicity of human embryonic and induced pluripotent stem cells. Nat Rev Cancer 2011;11(4):268–77.

100. Lee AS, Tang C, Rao MS, et al. Tumorigenicity as a clinical hurdle for pluripotent stem cell therapies. Nat Med 2013;19(8):998–1004.
101. Nori S, Okada Y, Nishimura S, et al. Long-term safety issues of iPSC-based cell therapy in a spinal cord injury model: oncogenic transformation with epithelial-mesenchymal transition. Stem Cell Reports 2015;4(3):360–73.
102. Tang C, Lee AS, Volkmer JP, et al. An antibody against SSEA-5 glycan on human pluripotent stem cells enables removal of teratoma-forming cells. Nat Biotechnol 2011;29(9):829–34.
103. Ben-David U, Gan QF, Golan-Lev T, et al. Selective elimination of human pluripotent stem cells by an oleate synthesis inhibitor discovered in a high-throughput screen. Cell Stem Cell 2013;12(2):167–79.
104. Lee MO, Moon SH, Jeong HC, et al. Inhibition of pluripotent stem cell-derived teratoma formation by small molecules. Proc Natl Acad Sci U S A 2013; 110(35):E3281–90.
105. Tateno H, Onuma Y, Ito Y, et al. Elimination of tumorigenic human pluripotent stem cells by a recombinant lectin-toxin fusion protein. Stem Cell Reports 2015;4(5):811–20.
106. Schmitt TM, de Pooter RF, Gronski MA, et al. Induction of T cell development and establishment of T cell competence from embryonic stem cells differentiated in vitro. Nat Immunol 2004;5(4):410–7.
107. Maeda T, Nagano S, Ichise H, et al. Regeneration of CD8alphabeta T cells from T-cell-derived iPSC imparts potent tumor antigen-specific cytotoxicity. Cancer Res 2016;76(23):6839–50.
108. Hayday A, Theodoridis E, Ramsburg E, et al. Intraepithelial lymphocytes: exploring the Third Way in immunology. Nat Immunol 2001;2(11):997–1003.
109. Renard V, Romero P, Vivier E, et al. CD8 beta increases CD8 coreceptor function and participation in TCR-ligand binding. J Exp Med 1996;184(6):2439–44.
110. Witte T, Spoerl R, Chang HC. The CD8beta ectodomain contributes to the augmented coreceptor function of CD8alphabeta heterodimers relative to CD8alphaalpha homodimers. Cell Immunol 1999;191(2):90–6.
111. Vizcardo R, Klemen ND, Islam SMR, et al. Generation of tumor antigen-specific iPSC-derived thymic emigrants using a 3D thymic culture system. Cell Rep 2018;22(12):3175–90.
112. Krangel MS. Mechanics of T cell receptor gene rearrangement. Curr Opin Immunol 2009;21(2):133–9.
113. von Boehmer H. Selection of the T-cell repertoire: receptor-controlled checkpoints in T-cell development. Adv Immunol 2004;84:201–38.
114. Cho SW, Kim S, Kim JM, et al. Targeted genome engineering in human cells with the Cas9 RNA-guided endonuclease. Nat Biotechnol 2013;31(3):230–2.
115. Cong L, Ran FA, Cox D, et al. Multiplex genome engineering using CRISPR/Cas systems. Science 2013;339(6121):819–23.
116. Mali P, Yang L, Esvelt KM, et al. RNA-guided human genome engineering via Cas9. Science 2013;339(6121):823–6.

Future Research Goals in Immunotherapy

Tyler W. Hulett, PhD[a,1], Bernard A. Fox, PhD[a,b,c,*,1], David J. Messenheimer, PhD[d], Sebastian Marwitz, PhD[a], Tarsem Moudgil, MS[a], Michael E. Afentoulis, MS[a], Keith W. Wegman, PhD[a], Carmen Ballesteros-Merino, PhD[a], Shawn M. Jensen, PhD[a]

KEYWORDS

- Biomarkers • Immunoprofiling • Combination immunotherapy • Seromics
- T-cell agonists • Cancer vaccines

KEY POINTS

- There is a need to improve the ability to characterize and monitor anticancer immunity. Multiplex immunohistochemistry and liquid tumor biopsies are rapidly evolving to provide improved biomarkers and insights.
- Seromics is providing evidence of coordinated B- and CD8 T-cell responses to nonmutated cancer antigens in mice and patients with NSCLC. This provides evidence of immunosurveillance in humans.
- Broadening the repertoire of approved immunotherapies requires combination immunotherapy trials that evaluate and optimize the impact of individual agents on the development, expansion, and persistence of anticancer immunity.
- Clinical development of T-cell agonists alone or combined with checkpoint blockade has been disappointing. Trials combining vaccines that upregulate agonist receptors with agonists are needed.

Disclosure Statement: D.J. Messenheimer is an employee of Boehringer Ingelheim. S.M. Jensen, C. Ballesteros-Merino, and B.A. Fox have research support from Bristol-Myers Squibb, PerkinElmer, Macrogenics, Definiens/AstraZeneca, OncoSec, Macrogenics, NanoString, and Viralytics. S.M. Jensen and B.A. Fox have research support from Janssen/Johnson and Johnson. B. A. Fox has research support from Quanterix and Shimadzu, is cofounder and CEO of and has equity in UbiVac, and has served as consultant or on advisory boards for Argos, AstraZeneca, Bayer, Bristol-Myers Squibb, CellDex therapeutics, Definiens, Janssen/Johnson and Johnson, Macrogenics, PerkinElmer, and PrimeVax. T.W. Hulett, T. Moudgil, M.S. Afentoulis, K.W. Wegman, and S. Marwitz have nothing to disclose.
Funding for S. Marwitz has been provided by Deutsche Forschungsgemeinschaft (MA 7800/1-1).
[a] Laboratory of Molecular and Tumor Immunology, Robert W. Franz Cancer Center, Earle A. Chiles Research Institute, Providence Cancer Institute, Providence Portland Medical Center, Portland, OR, USA; [b] Oregon Health & Science University, Portland, OR, USA; [c] UbiVac, Portland, OR, USA; [d] Boehringer Ingelheim Pharmaceuticals, Inc., 900 Ridgebury Road, Ridgefield, CT 06877-0368, USA
[1] Contributed equally to this work as co-first authors.
* Corresponding author. Earle A. Chiles Research Institute, 2N56 North Pavilion, 4805 Northeast Glisan Street, Portland, OR 97213.
E-mail addresses: Bernard.Fox@Providence.org; foxb@foxlab.org
; @BernardAFox (B.A.F.)

INTRODUCTION

Although few oncologists today would doubt that the immune system can mediate regression of cancer, this is a recent development. Less than a decade ago, little clinical evidence existed to suggest that an anticancer immune response might be therapeutic for solid tumors beyond malignant melanoma. In the case of melanoma, it was already established that adoptive immunotherapy patients receiving nonmyeloablative chemotherapy had response rates of about 50% in patients for whom tumor-infiltrating lymphocytes (TIL) could be generated and expanded.[1] In addition to these TIL data, treatment of melanoma and renal cancer with high-dose systemic interleukin (IL)-2 remained a bright spot. Not because the response rates were so great, but because patients who obtained a complete response had a 90% chance of surviving more than 20 years without a recurrence, suggestive of curative therapy.[2] Now, checkpoint blockade has transformed much of oncology by allowing oncologists to take the brakes off pre-existing anticancer immunity, resulting in objective clinical responses or durable stable disease in patients with a wide spectrum of cancers.[3–6] Although it will take another 20 years to appreciate whether these responses duplicate the success of IL-2 and result in possible cures, the scope and breadth of the clinical responses to checkpoint blockade immunotherapy has provided oncology with a paradigm shift.

These findings are occurring in a wider context where biomarkers linking antitumor immunity to patient outcomes are rapidly evolving,[6,7] demonstrating that the outcomes of traditional cancer treatments, including surgery, benefit from increased antitumor immunity.[8,9] However, for patients with most cancers, even those patients on the latest combination immunotherapy trials, many develop secondary immune resistance mechanisms that cause therapies to fail.[10] This article outlines the research objectives most critical for achieving these goals.

GOAL 1: IMPROVE THE ABILITY TO CHARACTERIZE AND MONITOR ANTICANCER IMMUNITY

For more than 100 years associations between brisk infiltrates of mononuclear cells into an individual patient's cancer and improved outcomes have been recognized for most cancers.[11] In 2006, the application of digital imaging and computer assessment provided a more objective approach to assess infiltrates of $CD3^+$ and $CD8^+$ T cells in resected colon cancer samples with striking results.[9] This prognostic biomarker was recently validated in an international study assessing colon cancers from 13 countries[8] and we expect similar immunoscore tests will prove useful for a variety of diverse cancer types and potentially guide personalized treatment administration. However, these digital pathology tools and manual observations only establish the presence of T cells within a tumor microenvironment; they leave oncologists blind to whether a tumor has evolved escape mechanisms that are preventing immune-mediated destruction. Detection of PD-L1 expression before checkpoint blockade is being used and enriches for objective responders, but patients lacking PD-L1 expression in their biopsy still respond to checkpoint blockade, albeit at a lower frequency.[12,13] To understand a more complete picture of a patient's endogenous battle with cancer, we posit that it is necessary to measure both number and interactions of T cells in relationship to other immune cell types and checkpoint molecules within the microenvironment, and to identify whether antigen presentation defects exist.

Methods for Defining Anticancer Immunity with Biopsy

Multiplex immunohistochemistry

Multiplex immunohistochemistry (IHC) with four to nine fluorescent markers assessed on a single 4-μm section of formalin-fixed paraffin embedded tissue[14] generates more information from a single section than conventional IHC and allows an evaluation of relationships of cells that express specific markers to one another. Using this approach to evaluate the CD8+/FoxP3+ and CD8+/PD-L1+ cell ratio of infiltrating lymphocytes in formalin-fixed paraffin-embedded melanoma tissue identified a correlation with the ability to isolate tumor-reactive T cells from that tumor.[15] Such an evaluation was also shown to play a critical role as a prognostic biomarker for human papilloma virus negative head and neck squamous cell carcinoma.[16] Furthermore, assessments of density and spatial colocalization were recently reported to be associated with improved prognostic[17] and predictive power for non–small cell lung cancer (NSCLC) receiving immunotherapy.[18] Considering that the "approved" IHC for PD-L1 expression informs on a single parameter, the integration of additional markers in and around the tumor and immune infiltrates will provide a substantially improved predictive biomarker over PD-L1 alone.

mRNA expression profiling

Although mRNA profiling of the tumor microenvironment can enrich for patients likely to respond to checkpoint blockade, it has not yet provided a means to identify all patients who will fail to respond to anti-PD-1.[19] One recent advance in mRNA data filtering, coined CIBERSORT, has been shown to approximately elucidate immune population numbers.[20] Therefore, CIBERSORT presents an alternative to multiplex IHC but sacrifices important information about context and cell-to-cell interactions. Attempts are being made to overcome this barrier via spatial transcriptomics[21] and the Digital Spatial Profiler (NanoString). The Digital Spatial Profiler is directed by multiplex IHC to evaluate tissue sections for spatially resolved gene expression in micronscale areas of interest. The depth and detail provided by such new methods seemed unimaginable only a few years ago and we believe that information garnered using these methods will ultimately allow development of effective therapies for the toughest to treat cancers.

Tumor mutational burden and neoantigen profiling

Rizvi and colleagues[22] were first to report that patients with high tumor mutational burden (TMB) have an increased response to anti-PD-1, yet 50% of the responders with the most highly mutated cancers experienced progression by 16 months. Progression in the face of an anticancer immune response may be secondary to many mechanisms.[23] One of those mechanisms is immunoediting where the cancer cells expressing the neoantigen are eliminated by the immune system, leaving behind cancer cells that do not express that mutation. Evidence for this mechanism in patients receiving anti-PD-1 was recently presented.[24] If one accepts that a preexisting anticancer immune response is required for patients to respond to checkpoint blockade, a possible explanation for the lack of response may be that some highly mutated tumors still fail to induce or maintain anticancer immunity. As reported by Spranger and colleagues,[25] a tumor "inflamed" signature is distributed across the spectrum of TMB and perhaps a better measure of immunity than TMB itself. In support of this observation is a study where severely mutated mismatch repair deficient tumors that lacked or had low T cell infiltrates fared as poorly as mismatch repair sufficient cancers with absent or low levels of T-cell infiltrates.[26] One explanation for this observation is that severe copy number and epigenetic dysregulation often accompanies high TMB, meaning that although high TMB tumors may have more neoantigens and abnormally expressed self-antigens, such tumors simultaneously have a high evolutionary diversity that allows for more complex forms of growth, metastasis, and immune evasion.

Biopsy-Free Methods for Defining Antitumor Immunity

Liquid tumor biopsies

Given the caveats associated with repeated biopsy, a great deal of interest has focused on evaluating whether serum proteins, cell-free DNA, or tumor-derived extracellular vesicles found in the plasma provide an approach to assess the tumor and/or immune cells. Both mass spectroscopic evaluation of serum proteins and cell-free DNA have provided biomarkers that enrich for responders to checkpoint blockade[27,28] and cell-free DNA is being explored as an alternative to biopsy for the identification of neoantigenic epitopes for cancer vaccine manufacture.[29]

Analysis of extracellular vesicles has also provided a window into in vivo processes. The ability to identify vesicles derived from tumor or immune cells provides opportunities to overlay these studies with other strategies outlined previously.[30] Such extracellular vesicles are directly immunosuppressive, and recent work demonstrated this suppressive capability is correlated to vesicle PD-L1 expression.[30] Overall, there are advantages, theoretic and practical, for each of the liquid biomarker assessments discussed.

Lymphocyte receptor sequencing

The availability of T-cell receptor (TCR) and B-cell receptor sequencing has made it possible to track clonal lymphocyte populations across time.[31] One future research goal is to develop a high-throughput monitoring method that uses TCR or B-cell receptor sequencing, to pair identification of the receptor with antigen and a proof-of-concept of this strategy has been reported.[32] Another possibility is to reverse the process and stain lymphocyte populations of interest with fluorescent tetramer libraries that have unique barcodes, sequence the TCR of those cells, and link the TCR with the antigen it bound. These types of methods are evolving rapidly and hold promise to not just characterize anticancer immunity but potentially identify TCRs that have therapeutic activity.

Antibody seromics

Evidence is growing that some features of antigen-specific immune surveillance are observed in the antibody repertoire. Currently, there are several nearly proteome-wide methods available for analyzing human autoantibodies,[33–37] and upcoming technologies, such as phage display immunoprecipitation sequencing (PhIP Seq), should allow for massive single-well screens targeted to smaller epitopes.[35] Indeed, PhIP Seq was recently used to survey antibody recognition of all known human viruses in the Immune Epitope Database,[34] and we envision this same technology might eventually be applied to survey the entire universe of known cancer neoantigens and overexpressed proteins identified by The Cancer Genome Atlas.

Recently, Tripathi and colleagues[38] characterized the HLA-presented peptidome of a panel of NSCLC cell lines, identifying a large number of common nonmutated epitopes presented by NSCLC. Simultaneously, they were collecting serum on a large cohort of normal donors. Twenty-five of these normal donors eventually developed NSCLC, and their pretreatment sera were found to have IgG antibodies to dozens of proteins related to peptides that were presented on HLA by the NSCLC tumor cells. They went on to show that patients could mount a cytotoxic lymphocyte (CTL) response to nonmutated peptides from those same proteins that were the target of IgG responses, and that these CTL could lyse an HLA-matched allogeneic NSCLC cell line that naturally presented that peptide. Although it is well known in the viral immunology literature that B-cell responses often correlate with T-cell responses to the same protein, it has been less well studied in cancer. Vaccination with cancer testis antigens has been reported to result in coordinated antibody and T-cell responses to epitopes of the same protein,[39] but to our knowledge, it was Kwek and colleagues[36] who first identified an immunotherapy induced T-cell response to a new shared cancer antigen, PAK6, via a surrogate IgG antibody response to the same. Recently, Hulett and colleagues[40] studying the immune response to a cancer vaccine containing proteins overexpressed by 4T1 mammary carcinoma identified a coordinated IgG antibody and CD8$^+$ T-cell response to short peptide antigens. Focusing on proteins that contained neoantigen mutations, they identified a correlation between IgG responses to long peptides containing the mutated or wild-type sequence and CD8$^+$ T-cell responses to the minimal H2 binding epitope of the same. For most antigens the CD8$^+$ T-cell response could be detected against the neoantigen and wild-type epitopes. These reports are provocative because they suggest (1) that observable antibody immunosurveillance is occurring in these patients before the time of their diagnosis, (2) that IgG antibody responses can be used to identify proteins that are targeted by T-cell responses, and (3) that T-cell responses in untreated patients might be directed against mutated and nonmutated shared cancer antigens.

Summary

The challenge for personalized cancer immunotherapy is to assemble, in a short period of time following diagnosis or time of progression, a spectrum of robust assessments, obtained from validated platforms, that can be rapidly and accurately applied to influence clinical decision-making. This includes stratification for clinical trials, evaluation of immunologic response, and ultimately the true personalization of immunotherapy based on an assessment of the patient's anticancer immune response and the tumor's ability to counter that response.

GOAL 2: BROADEN THE REPERTOIRE OF APPROVED IMMUNOTHERAPIES AND IMMUNE-MODULATING COMBINATION TREATMENTS
Tools to Improve the Efficacy of Extant Anticancer Immunity

Checkpoint blockers
The vast and rapidly growing list of cancer immunotherapy clinical trials is heavily focused on combining checkpoint blockade with conventional therapies. In our opinion, the greatest potential for increasing durable responses and potential cures remains with combinations of immunotherapeutic agents that build on the current understanding of how the immune system works. Specifically, strategies that amplify the immune response and broaden the number of cancer targets recognized and the types of immune effector mechanisms brought to bear on the cancer.

T-cell agonists
Agonists are agents that provide a positive or costimulatory signal to cells of the immune system. Agents with anticancer activity include agonists that boost T-cell, natural killer cell, or APC function. In the case of T-cell agonists, expression of the agonist receptor is typically upregulated as a consequence of T-cell activation. Examples of T-cell agonist receptors are CD27, CD28, CD40, CD137 (4-1BB), GITR, ICOS, and OX40.[41] Unfortunately, most of the clinical trials evaluating T-cell agonists have not provided the signals required to support their development as single agents.[41–44] Although the number of clinical objective responses may be limited, the administration of T-cell agonists to patients has demonstrated some cases with striking immunologic

effects.[45] This includes a recent report that approximately a quarter of patients receiving neoadjuvant anti-OX40 experienced increased infiltration of CD8 T cells into head and neck cancers.[46]

Clinical trials of T-cell agonists in combination with checkpoint blockade are also in the early phase, but the lack of substantial clinical responses to the concurrent administration of anti-OX40 and anti-PD-L1[47] as well as concurrent combinations of anti-OX40, or other T cell agonists, with anti-PD-1, are stifling the development of this class of immune modulators. Our own work using the pymt/MMTV spontaneous mammary cancer model found that the combination of anti-OX40 and anti-PD-1 or anti-PD-L1 was significantly less therapeutic than anti-OX40 alone while the sequential administration provided significantly improved survival and apparent cure.[48] These data first presented at the American Association of Cancer annual meeting in 2016, before the first report of the combination in clinical trials,[47] and shared prepublication with interested pharmaceutical companies, provided a hint into the complexities around developing combination immunotherapy.[49] Working with a different model, Shrimali and colleagues[50] reported a similar negative effect when anti-OX40 was administered concurrently with anti-PD-1. Although at this point a sequenced combination anti-OX40 with checkpoint blockade has not been initiated, to these authors it seems an important trial to perform. We also believe that it is critical to incorporate appropriate monitoring to interpret the clinical observations.

Cytokine therapies: systemic

Strategies using T-cell growth factors, such as IL-2, IL-7, IL-15, and IL-21, have shown potent immune cell proliferation leading to increased numbers of immune cells in tumors,[51,52] and for IL-2 therapeutic and potentially curative effects.[2,53] Consequently, extensive efforts are being made by multiple groups to engineer cytokines that reduce their toxicity and/or increase their half-life.[54] One example is an IL-2 conjugated to releasable polyethylene glycol chains (NKTR-214), increasing the in vivo half-life of IL-2 and improving tolerability.[55] Current results from a phase 1/2 dose escalation trial where NKTR-214 was combined with anti-PD-1 are promising; additionally only 10.5% grade 3 or 4 treatment-related adverse events have been observed.[56]

IL-15 is a key cytokine regulating lymphocyte homeostasis, particularly CD8[+] memory T cells and natural killer cells. The first in human clinical trial of intravenous rIL-15 showed increased frequencies of effector memory CD8+ T cells, effector memory CD4+ T cells, and natural killer cells.[57] Naturally occurring IL-15 in vivo exists as a heterodimer composed of IL-15 with IL-15 receptor α.[58] Systemic administration of hetIL-15 in preclinical tumor models augmented the frequency of tumor-specific T cells within the tumor. These tumor-infiltrating T cells displayed a "nonexhausted" phenotype characterized by interferon-γ secretion, proliferation, cytotoxic potential, and low levels of PD-1.[59] Presently, clinical trials examining human hetIL-15 alone and in combination with anti-PD-1 are underway.

Cytokine therapies: intratumoral

An alternative to systemic administration of cytokines that result in toxicities is targeted local administration of cytokines or plasmids encoding the cytokine within the tumor microenvironment.[60] Preclinical studies examining electroporation of plasmid IL-12 DNA into tumors has demonstrated interferon-γ-mediated tumor cell killing, immune cell recruitment, and tumor regressions in animal models including regression of untreated lesions.[61–63] Clinical studies of this approach have demonstrated local expression of IL-12 within the injected tumor, recruitment of T cells, and enhanced Th1 immune responses with minimal systemic toxicity.[64] A clinical trial is evaluating the efficacy of this approach in combination with anti-PD-1 in patients with advanced metastatic melanoma that are progressing on anti-PD-1 alone.

Modifiers of transforming growth factor-β pathway

Transforming growth factor (TGF)-β is a growth factor long known to limit the proliferative capacity and effector function of T cells,[65] but can also impact cancer biology.[66] Therefore, interfering with this pathway may dampen the malignant capacity of cancer,[67] impact the tumor microenvironment, and improve the anticancer immune response. Mariathasan and colleagues[68] analyzed patients with metastatic urothelial cancer who were treated with atezolizumab to inhibit PD1/PD-L1 interaction. A TGF-β signaling signature in stromal fibroblasts (F-TBRS) was associated with lack of response. Several TGF-β "traps" are currently in testing, including a bifunctional fusion protein that targets PD-L1 and the extracellular domain of the TGF-β receptor II.[69] Efficacy was shown to be increased in multiple mouse models and seemed to be mediated by innate and adaptive immune responses.

Tools to Broaden Antigenic Diversity

Cancer vaccines: neoantigens

An active area of cancer vaccine development is the identification of immunogenic neoantigens and transforming them into personalized cancer vaccines. Most vaccine strategies have focused on single-nucleotide variant targets, most of which are private to the individual.[70] Future research goals include improvements to the efficacy of HLA peptide-binding algorithms for the spectrum of human HLA molecules and determination of which neoantigens are actually naturally presented on the membrane of tumor cells.

Cancer vaccines: overexpressed or ectopically expressed self

The potential for shared antigen cancer vaccines has been appreciated for a long time, but disappointing results from almost every clinical trial of vaccines as a single agent has significantly tempered enthusiasm for this approach. In retrospect, the results of clinical trials closely mirror the preclinical data, where vaccines as single agents universally failed to provide significant therapeutic effects against tumors that had been established for as little as 7 days.[71] Although objective clinical response data have been lacking, evidence for induction or boosting of an anticancer immune response provided encouragement and has kept alive investigations in this area.[72–76] Other studies have provided evidence for native T-cell responses to shared antigens in the absence of vaccination, buttressing the concept that induction and/or boosting of these responses by vaccination, in combination with other immune intervention, might improve therapeutic efficacy.[36,38,77] Our own experience with complex tumor-derived autophagosome vaccines suggest that vaccines based on shared antigenic targets are protective and therapeutic against unrelated tumors.[78–80]

Cancer vaccines: combination immunotherapy

In 1999, Allison and colleagues[81] combined a granulocyte-macrophage colony–stimulating factor producing tumor cell vaccine with anti-CTLA-4 and showed significantly increased therapeutic effect of the combination. These preclinical studies led to a clinical trial with prostate GVAX and anti-CTLA-4 that, although initially showing some promise, ultimately failed to show substantial clinical activity.[82,83] Subsequently, as the phase III trial of anti-CTLA-4 was in development, an arm that included the gp100 peptide vaccine in incomplete Freund adjuvant (IFA) plus anti-CTLA-4 was included.[84] Although anti-CTLA-4 provided a significant increase in progression-free survival, the group that included vaccine fared worse. These and other studies raised the specter that cancer vaccines were having a negative effect on patients.[85] Recent work from the laboratory of Overwijk confirm the suspicions and show in animal models why short peptide vaccines in IFA is ineffective in combination, how it leads to sequestration of anticancer T cells at the vaccine site, and to their exhaustion.[86] These preclinical data also raise concern for the large number of combination immunotherapy clinical trials using short peptide vaccines in IFA. In contrast to results of peptide vaccines in IFA, and consistent with the early work of Allison, other vaccine strategies in preclinical models were augmented with anti-CTLA-4 or checkpoint blockade.[87]

Additional studies have shown that vaccines combined with T-cell agonists can significantly augment therapeutic efficacy. This work is based on the hypothesis that priming with antigen results in upregulation of the agonist receptor, which is then susceptible to targeting via therapy. Examples of this have been vaccines combined with anti-CD27, anti-OX40, anti-4-1BB, or anti-GITR.[88–91] Because these preclinical studies have reported substantially improved antitumor efficacy, clinical trials exploring these combinations need to be explored and represent an important future research goal.

SUMMARY

The authors recognize that there are many additional therapeutic strategies to modify existing anticancer immunity. Some of the most promising include modifying the microbiome; oncolytic viruses; epigenetic modifiers of DNA methyltransferase and histone deacetylase; drugs targeting the immunosuppressive metabolic enzymes indoleamine 2,3-dioxygenase, arginase, and inducible nitric oxide synthase; and intracellular signaling molecules or transcription factors, such as stimulator of interferon genes. Perhaps one of the most exciting approaches is the development of synthetic immune agents designed to direct effector T cells to tumor cells (ie, DARTs, BiTEs), stimulate two or more receptors immune receptors, combine T-cell agonists with checkpoint blockade, or with strategies to neutralize immune suppressive mediators.

Additionally, we expect to see substantial growth for adoptive immunotherapy treatments using TIL, chimeric antigen receptor, and TCR constructs. Although substantial barriers exist, we also expect the search for off-the-shelf cell therapy products, either T cell or natural killer cell, will be explored. In the autologous setting, improved sterile sorting technologies coupled with recent identification of membrane markers identifying tumor-reactive T cells provide opportunities to sort and expand T cells enriched for anticancer function.[92]

Another future research goal is to understand and develop strategies to offset the negative impact that surgery can have on immunity.[93] Given the current understanding and spectrum of pharmaceutical agents under development, we believe there are at least two areas of surgical/immunotherapy research that are ripe for exploration. First, what can be done to further characterize the mechanisms of action for the apparent postsurgical immune defects and develop strategies to counteract said mechanisms. Second, development of neoadjuvant and surgical interventions that will result in augmented anticancer immunity.

REFERENCES

1. Dudley ME, Wunderlich JR, Yang JC, et al. Adoptive cell transfer therapy following non-myeloablative but lymphodepleting chemotherapy for the treatment

of patients with refractory metastatic melanoma. J Clin Oncol 2005;23(10): 2346–57.

2. Rosenberg SA. IL-2: the first effective immunotherapy for human cancer. J Immunol 2014;192(12):5451–8.

3. Brahmer JR, Tykodi SS, Chow LQ, et al. Safety and activity of anti-PD-L1 antibody in patients with advanced cancer. N Engl J Med 2012;366(26):2455–65.

4. Grupp SA, Kalos M, Barrett D, et al. Chimeric antigen receptor-modified T cells for acute lymphoid leukemia. N Engl J Med 2013;368(16):1509–18.

5. Kochenderfer JN, Rosenberg SA. Treating B-cell cancer with T cells expressing anti-CD19 chimeric antigen receptors. Nat Rev Clin Oncol 2013;10(5):267–76.

6. Herbst RS, Soria J-C, Kowanetz M, et al. Predictive correlates of response to the anti-PD-L1 antibody MPDL3280A in cancer patients. Nature 2014;515(7528): 563–7.

7. Ulloa-Montoya F, Louahed J, Dizier B, et al. Predictive gene signature in MAGE-A3 antigen-specific cancer immunotherapy. J Clin Oncol 2013;31(19):2388–95.

8. Pages F, Mlecnik B, Marliot F, et al. International validation of the consensus Immunoscore for the classification of colon cancer: a prognostic and accuracy study. Lancet 2018;391(10135):2128–39.

9. Galon J, Costes A, Sanchez-Cabo F, et al. Type, density, and location of immune cells within human colorectal tumors predict clinical outcome. Science 2006; 313(5795):1960–4.

10. Sharma P, Hu-Lieskovan S, Wargo JA, et al. Primary, adaptive, and acquired resistance to cancer immunotherapy. Cell 2017;168(4):707–23.

11. Bethmann D, Feng Z, Fox BA. Immunoprofiling as a predictor of patient's response to cancer therapy-promises and challenges. Curr Opin Immunol 2017;45:60–72.

12. Chae YK, Pan A, Davis AA, et al. Biomarkers for PD-1/PD-L1 blockade therapy in non-small-cell lung cancer: is PD-L1 expression a good marker for patient selection? Clin Lung Cancer 2016;17(5):350–61.

13. Kim H, Kwon HJ, Park SY, et al. PD-L1 immunohistochemical assays for assessment of therapeutic strategies involving immune checkpoint inhibitors in non-small cell lung cancer: a comparative study. Oncotarget 2017;8(58):98524–32.

14. Stack EC, Wang C, Roman KA, et al. Multiplexed immunohistochemistry, imaging, and quantitation: a review, with an assessment of Tyramide signal amplification, multispectral imaging and multiplex analysis. Methods 2014;70(1):46–58.

15. Feng Z, Puri S, Moudgil T, et al. Multispectral imaging of formalin-fixed tissue predicts ability to generate tumor-infiltrating lymphocytes from melanoma. J Immunother Cancer 2015;3:47.

16. Feng Z, Bethmann D, Kappler M, et al. Multiparametric immune profiling in HPV-oral squamous cell cancer. JCI Insight 2017;2(14). https://doi.org/10.1172/jci.insight.93652.

17. Corredor G, Wang X, Zhou Y, et al. Spatial architecture and arrangement of tumor-infiltrating lymphocytes for predicting likelihood of recurrence in early-stage non-small cell lung cancer. Clin Cancer Res 2018. https://doi.org/10.1158/1078-0432.CCR-18-2013.

18. Ascierto PA, Brugarolas J, Buonaguro L, et al. Perspectives in immunotherapy: meeting report from the Immunotherapy Bridge (29-30 November, 2017, Naples, Italy). J Immunother Cancer 2018;6(1):69.

19. Ayers M, Lunceford J, Nebozhyn M, et al. IFN-gamma-related mRNA profile predicts clinical response to PD-1 blockade. J Clin Invest 2017;127(8):2930–40.

20. Thorsson V, Gibbs DL, Brown SD, et al. The immune landscape of cancer. Immunity 2018;48(4):812–30.e14.
21. Stahl PL, Salmen F, Vickovic S, et al. Visualization and analysis of gene expression in tissue sections by spatial transcriptomics. Science 2016;353(6294):78–82.
22. Rizvi NA, Hellmann MD, Snyder A, et al. Cancer immunology. Mutational landscape determines sensitivity to PD-1 blockade in non-small cell lung cancer. Science 2015;348(6230):124–8.
23. Nowicki TS, Hu-Lieskovan S, Ribas A. Mechanisms of resistance to PD-1 and PD-L1 blockade. Cancer J 2018;24(1):47–53.
24. Riaz N, Havel JJ, Makarov V, et al. Tumor and microenvironment evolution during immunotherapy with nivolumab. Cell 2017;171(4):934–49.e15.
25. Spranger S, Luke JJ, Bao R, et al. Density of immunogenic antigens does not explain the presence or absence of the T-cell-inflamed tumor microenvironment in melanoma. Proc Natl Acad Sci U S A 2016;113(48):E7759–68.
26. Mlecnik B, Bindea G, Angell HK, et al. Integrative analyses of colorectal cancer show immunoscore is a stronger predictor of patient survival than microsatellite instability. Immunity 2016;44(3):698–711.
27. Weber JS, Sznol M, Sullivan RJ, et al. A serum protein signature associated with outcome after anti-PD-1 therapy in metastatic melanoma. Cancer Immunol Res 2018;6(1):79–86.
28. Weiss GJ, Beck J, Braun DP, et al. Tumor cell-free DNA copy number instability predicts therapeutic response to immunotherapy. Clin Cancer Res 2017;23(17):5074–81.
29. Adalsteinsson VA, Ha G, Freeman SS, et al. Scalable whole-exome sequencing of cell-free DNA reveals high concordance with metastatic tumors. Nat Commun 2017;8(1):1324.
30. Whiteside TL. The emerging role of plasma exosomes in diagnosis, prognosis and therapies of patients with cancer. Contemp Oncol (Pozn) 2018;22(1A):38–40.
31. Goronzy JJ, Qi Q, Olshen RA, et al. High-throughput sequencing insights into T-cell receptor repertoire diversity in aging. Genome Med 2015;7(1):117.
32. Glanville J, Huang H, Nau A, et al. Identifying specificity groups in the T cell receptor repertoire. Nature 2017;547(7661):94–8.
33. Kanderova V, Kuzilkova D, Stuchly J, et al. High-resolution antibody array analysis of childhood acute leukemia cells. Mol Cell Proteomics 2016;15(4):1246–61.
34. Xu GJ, Kula T, Xu Q, et al. Comprehensive serological profiling of human populations using a synthetic human virome. Science 2015;348(6239):aaa0698.
35. Larman HB, Zhao Z, Laserson U, et al. Autoantigen discovery with a synthetic human peptidome. Nat Biotechnol 2011;29(6):535–41.
36. Kwek SS, Dao V, Roy R, et al. Diversity of antigen-specific responses induced in vivo with CTLA-4 blockade in prostate cancer patients. J Immunol 2012;189(7):3759–66.
37. Nagele EP, Han M, Acharya NK, et al. Natural IgG autoantibodies are abundant and ubiquitous in human sera, and their number is influenced by age, gender, and disease. PLoS One 2013;8(4):e60726.
38. Tripathi SC, Peters HL, Taguchi A, et al. Immunoproteasome deficiency is a feature of non-small cell lung cancer with a mesenchymal phenotype and is associated with a poor outcome. Proc Natl Acad Sci U S A 2016;113(11):E1555–64.
39. Yuan J, Adamow M, Ginsberg BA, et al. Integrated NY-ESO-1 antibody and CD8+ T-cell responses correlate with clinical benefit in advanced melanoma patients treated with ipilimumab. Proc Natl Acad Sci U S A 2011;108(40):16723–8.

40. Hulett TW, Jensen SM, Wilmarth PA, et al. Coordinated responses to individual tumor antigens by IgG antibody and CD8+ T cells following cancer vaccination. J Immunother Cancer 2018;6(1):27.

41. Marin-Acevedo JA, Dholaria B, Soyano AE, et al. Next generation of immune checkpoint therapy in cancer: new developments and challenges. J Hematol Oncol 2018;11(1):39.

42. Tran B, Carvajal RD, Marabelle A, et al. Dose escalation results from a first-in-human, phase 1 study of the glucocorticoid-induced TNF receptor-related protein (GITR) agonist AMG 228 in patients (Pts) with advanced solid tumors. J Clin Oncol 2017;35:2521.

43. Burris HA, Infante JR, Ansell SM, et al. Safety and activity of varlilumab, a novel and first-in-class agonist anti-CD27 antibody, in patients with advanced solid tumors. J Clin Oncol 2017;35(18):2028–36.

44. Cabo M, Offringa R, Zitvogel L, et al. Trial watch: immunostimulatory monoclonal antibodies for oncological indications. Oncoimmunology 2017;6(12):e1371896.

45. Curti BD, Kovacsovics-Bankowski M, Morris N, et al. OX40 is a potent immune-stimulating target in late-stage cancer patients. Cancer Res 2013;73(24):7189–98.

46. Bell RB, Duhen R, Leidner RS, et al. Neoadjuvant anti-OX40 (MEDI6469) prior to surgery in head and neck squamous cell carcinoma. J Clin Oncol 2018;36(suppl) [abstract: 6011].

47. Infante JR, Hansen AR, Pishvaian MJ, et al. A phase Ib dose escalation study of the OX40 agonist MOXR0916 and the PD-L1 inhibitor atezolizumab in patients with advanced solid tumors. J Clin Oncol 2016;34(15):101.

48. Messenheimer DJ, Jensen SM, Afentoulis ME, et al. Timing of PD-1 blockade is critical to effective combination immunotherapy with anti-OX40. Clin Cancer Res 2017;23(20):6165–77.

49. Messenheimer DJ, Feng Z, Wegmann KW, et al. Timing of PD-1 blockade is critical to successful synergy with OX40 costimulation in preclinical mammary tumor models. Cancer Res 2016;76(14 Suppl) [abstract number: 4361].

50. Shrimali RK, Ahmad S, Verma V, et al. Concurrent PD-1 blockade negates the effects of OX40 agonist antibody in combination immunotherapy through inducing T-cell apoptosis. Cancer Immunol Res 2017;5(9):755–66.

51. Pulliam SR, Uzhachenko RV, Adunyah SE, et al. Common gamma chain cytokines in combinatorial immune strategies against cancer. Immunol Lett 2016;169: 61–72.

52. Spolski R, Gromer D, Leonard WJ. The gamma c family of cytokines: fine-tuning signals from IL-2 and IL-21 in the regulation of the immune response. F1000Res 2017;6:1872.

53. Payne R, Glenn L, Hoen H, et al. Durable responses and reversible toxicity of high-dose interleukin-2 treatment of melanoma and renal cancer in a Community Hospital Biotherapy Program. J Immunother Cancer 2014;2:13.

54. Spangler JB, Moraga I, Mendoza JL, et al. Insights into cytokine-receptor interactions from cytokine engineering. Annu Rev Immunol 2015;33:139–67.

55. Charych D, Khalili S, Dixit V, et al. Modeling the receptor pharmacology, pharmacokinetics, and pharmacodynamics of NKTR-214, a kinetically-controlled interleukin-2 (IL2) receptor agonist for cancer immunotherapy. PLoS One 2017; 12(7):e0179431.

56. Garber K. Cytokine resurrection: engineered IL-2 ramps up immuno-oncology responses. Nat Biotechnol 2018;36(5):378–9.

57. Conlon KC, Lugli E, Welles HC, et al. Redistribution, hyperproliferation, activation of natural killer cells and CD8 T cells, and cytokine production during first-in-

human clinical trial of recombinant human interleukin-15 in patients with cancer. J Clin Oncol 2015;33(1):74–82.

58. Burkett PR, Koka R, Chien M, et al. Coordinate expression and trans presentation of interleukin (IL)-15Ralpha and IL-15 supports natural killer cell and memory CD8+ T cell homeostasis. J Exp Med 2004;200(7):825–34.

59. Ng SSM, Nagy BA, Jensen SM, et al. Heterodimeric IL15 treatment enhances tumor infiltration, persistence, and effector functions of adoptively transferred tumor-specific T cells in the absence of lymphodepletion. Clin Cancer Res 2017;23(11):2817–30.

60. Van der Jeught K, Bialkowski L, Daszkiewicz L, et al. Targeting the tumor microenvironment to enhance antitumor immune responses. Oncotarget 2015;6(3): 1359–81.

61. Heller L, Merkler K, Westover J, et al. Evaluation of toxicity following electrically mediated interleukin-12 gene delivery in a B16 mouse melanoma model. Clin Cancer Res 2006;12(10):3177–83.

62. Lucas ML, Heller L, Coppola D, et al. IL-12 plasmid delivery by in vivo electroporation for the successful treatment of established subcutaneous B16.F10 melanoma. Mol Ther 2002;5(6):668–75.

63. Cutrera J, King G, Jones P, et al. Safe and effective treatment of spontaneous neoplasms with interleukin 12 electro-chemo-gene therapy. J Cell Mol Med 2015;19(3):664–75.

64. Daud AI, DeConti RC, Andrews S, et al. Phase I trial of interleukin-12 plasmid electroporation in patients with metastatic melanoma. J Clin Oncol 2008;26(36): 5896–903.

65. Li MO, Wan YY, Sanjabi S, et al. Transforming growth factor-beta regulation of immune responses. Annu Rev Immunol 2006;24:99–146.

66. Massague J. TGFbeta in cancer. Cell 2008;134(2):215–30.

67. Marwitz S, Depner S, Dvornikov D, et al. Downregulation of the TGFbeta Pseudoreceptor BAMBI in non-small cell lung cancer enhances TGFbeta signaling and invasion. Cancer Res 2016;76(13):3785–801.

68. Mariathasan S, Turley SJ, Nickles D, et al. TGFbeta attenuates tumour response to PD-L1 blockade by contributing to exclusion of T cells. Nature 2018;554(7693): 544–8.

69. Lan Y, Zhang D, Xu C, et al. Enhanced preclinical antitumor activity of M7824, a bifunctional fusion protein simultaneously targeting PD-L1 and TGF-beta. Sci Transl Med 2018;10(424). https://doi.org/10.1126/scitranslmed.aan5488.

70. Ward JP, Gubin MM, Schreiber RD. The role of neoantigens in naturally occurring and therapeutically induced immune responses to cancer. Adv Immunol 2016; 130:25–74.

71. Poehlein CH, Ruttinger D, Ma J, et al. Immunotherapy for melanoma: the good, the bad, and the future. Curr Oncol Rep 2005;7(5):383–92.

72. Smith JW 2nd, Walker EB, Fox BA, et al. Adjuvant immunization of HLA-A2-positive melanoma patients with a modified gp100 peptide induces peptide-specific CD8+ T-cell responses. J Clin Oncol 2003;21(8):1562–73.

73. Dols A, Meijer SL, Hu HM, et al. Identification of tumor-specific antibodies in patients with breast cancer vaccinated with gene-modified allogeneic tumor cells. J Immunother 2003;26(2):163–70.

74. Dranoff G, Jaffee E, Lazenby A, et al. Vaccination with irradiated tumor cells engineered to secrete murine granulocyte-macrophage colony-stimulating factor stimulates potent, specific, and long-lasting anti-tumor immunity. Proc Natl Acad Sci U S A 1993;90(8):3539–43.

75. Disis ML, Gooley TA, Rinn K, et al. Generation of T-cell immunity to the HER-2/neu protein after active immunization with HER-2/neu peptide-based vaccines. J Clin Oncol 2002;20(11):2624–32.

76. Chang AE, Aruga A, Cameron MJ, et al. Adoptive immunotherapy with vaccine-primed lymph node cells secondarily activated with anti-CD3 and interleukin-2. J Clin Oncol 1997;15(2):796–807.

77. Gros A, Parkhurst MR, Tran E, et al. Prospective identification of neoantigen-specific lymphocytes in the peripheral blood of melanoma patients. Nat Med 2016;22(4):433–8.

78. Twitty CG, Hu H-M, Fox BA. Tumor Autophagosome-based Cancer Vaccine Combined Immunotherapy With Anti-OX40 Provides Therapeutic Immunity Against Established Breast Cancer. J Immunother 2012;35(9):746.

79. Twitty CG, Jensen SM, Hu HM, et al. Tumor-derived autophagosome vaccine: induction of cross-protective immune responses against short-lived proteins through a p62-dependent mechanism. Clin Cancer Res 2011;17(20):6467–81.

80. Yu G, Li Y, Cui Z, et al. Combinational immunotherapy with Allo-DRibble vaccines and Anti-OX40 co-stimulation leads to generation of cross-reactive effector T cells and tumor regression. Sci Rep 2016;6:37558.

81. van Elsas A, Hurwitz AA, Allison JP. Combination immunotherapy of B16 melanoma using anti-cytotoxic T lymphocyte-associated antigen 4 (CTLA-4) and granulocyte/macrophage colony-stimulating factor (GM-CSF)-producing vaccines induces rejection of subcutaneous and metastatic tumors accompanied by auto-immune depigmentation. J Exp Med 1999;190(3):355–66.

82. Small EJ, Sacks N, Nemunaitis J, et al. Granulocyte macrophage colony-stimulating factor–secreting allogeneic cellular immunotherapy for hormone-refractory prostate cancer. Clin Cancer Res 2007;13(13):3883–91.

83. van den Eertwegh AJM, Versluis J, van den Berg HP, et al. Combined immuno-therapy with granulocyte-macrophage colony-stimulating factor-transduced allogeneic prostate cancer cells and ipilimumab in patients with metastatic castration-resistant prostate cancer: a phase 1 dose-escalation trial. Lancet Oncol 2012;13(5):509–17.

84. Hodi FS, O'Day SJ, McDermott DF, et al. Improved survival with ipilimumab in patients with metastatic melanoma. N Engl J Med 2010;363(8):711–23.

85. Eggermont AMM. Therapeutic vaccines in solid tumours: can they be harmful? Eur J Cancer 2009;45(12):2087–90.

86. Hailemichael Y, Dai Z, Jaffarzad N, et al. Persistent antigen at vaccination sites induces tumor-specific CD8+ T cell sequestration, dysfunction and deletion. Nat Med 2013;19(4):465–72.

87. Hurwitz AA, Yu TFY, Leach DR, et al. CTLA-4 blockade synergizes with tumor-derived granulocyte–macrophage colony-stimulating factor for treatment of an experimental mammary carcinoma. Proc Natl Acad Sci U S A 1998;95(17):10067–71.

88. Yu G, Li Y, Cui Z, et al. Combinational immunotherapy with Allo-DRibble vaccines and anti-OX40 co-stimulation leads to generation of cross-reactive effector T cells and tumor regression. Sci Rep 2016;6(1). https://doi.org/10.1038/srep37558.

89. Munks MW, Mourich DV, Mittler RS, et al. 4-1BB and OX40 stimulation enhance CD8 and CD4 T-cell responses to a DNA prime, poxvirus boost vaccine. Immunology 2004;112(4):559–66.

90. Liu Z, Hao X, Zhang Y, et al. Intratumoral delivery of tumor antigen-loaded DC and tumor-primed CD4(+) T cells combined with agonist alpha-GITR mAb promotes

durable CD8(+) T-cell-dependent antitumor immunity. Oncoimmunology 2017; 6(6):e1315487. https://doi.org/10.1080/2162402X.2017.1315487.

91. Wei SM, Fei JX, Tao F, et al. Anti-CD27 antibody potentiates antitumor effect of dendritic cell-based vaccine in prostate cancer-bearing mice. Int Surg 2015; 100(1):155–63.

92. Duhen T, Duhen R, Montler R, et al. Co-expression of CD39 and CD103 identifies tumor-reactive CD8 T cells in human solid tumors. Nat Commun 2018;9(1):2724.

93. Bakos O, Lawson C, Rouleau S, et al. Combining surgery and immunotherapy: turning an immunosuppressive effect into a therapeutic opportunity. J Immunother Cancer 2018;6(1):86.

Moving?

Make sure your subscription moves with you!

To notify us of your new address, find your **Clinics Account Number** (located on your mailing label above your name), and contact customer service at:

Email: journalscustomerservice-usa@elsevier.com

800-654-2452 (subscribers in the U.S. & Canada)
314-447-8871 (subscribers outside of the U.S. & Canada)

Fax number: 314-447-8029

Elsevier Health Sciences Division
Subscription Customer Service
3251 Riverport Lane
Maryland Heights, MO 63043

*To ensure uninterrupted delivery of your subscription, please notify us at least 4 weeks in advance of move.

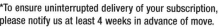

Printed and bound by CPI Group (UK) Ltd, Croydon, CR0 4YY

03/10/2024

01040481-0016